PARAPROFESSIONALS IN MENTAL HEALTH

Theory and Practice

Edited by

Sam R. Alley, Ph.D.
Judith Blanton, Ph.D.
Ronald E. Feldman, Ph.D.

Social Action Research Center
San Rafael, California

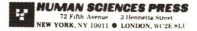

HUMAN SCIENCES PRESS
72 Fifth Avenue   3 Henrietta Street
NEW YORK, NY 10011 ● LONDON, WC2E 8LU

Library of Congress Catalog Number 79-11115

ISBN: 0-87705-420-7

Printed in the United States of America
9 987654321

Credits
Table 1–3 (p. 26) and Table 1–5 (p. 28) reprinted with permission from Francine Sobel, *The nonprofessional revolution in mental health*, Columbia University Press, New York, 1970, pp. 104 and 159, respectively.
Table 1–4 (p. 27) reprinted with permission from C. E. Young, J. E. True, and M. E. Packard, A national survey of associate degree mental health and human services workers, *Journal of Community Psychology*, 1976, *4*, 92–93.
Table 1–6 (p. 33) reprinted with permission from B. D. Bartels and J. D. Tyler, Paraprofessionals in the community mental health center, *Professional Psychology*, 1975, *6*, p. 446.

Library of Congress Cataloging in Publication Data

Main entry under title:

Paraprofessionals in mental health.

 Bibliography
 Includes index.
 1. Allied mental health personnel. 2. Mental health services. I. Alley, Sam. II. Blanton, Judith. III. Feldman, Ronald A. IV. Social Action Research Center. [DNLM: 1. Allied health personnel. 2. Community mental health services—Manpower—United States. WM21 P223]
RC440.2.P38   610.69'53   79-11115
ISBN 0-87705-420-7

CONTENTS

FOREWORD

The National Institute of Mental Health is committed to improving the access, quality, and quantity of mental health services to individuals in need. The challenge of meeting these goals is becoming increasingly difficult, however, because of the diversity and complexity of the new and different mental health service configurations and requirements that are emerging. Among the areas of immediate and special consequence are: the acceleration of the process of deinstitutionalization; development and refinement of community service networks; adoption of service strategies which give key roles to community support systems, including expanded self-help mutual aid groups; increased concern and attention for underserved groups (viz., minorities, youth, older persons, those in rural areas, chronically disabled, etc.); greater attention to prevention; and the implementation of the 1975 amendments to P.L. 94-63. These amendments alone add seven service areas to the five required in the original legislation.

The successful implementation of these new, but nevertheless very important and needed services lies, in part, in the preparation and effective utilization of competent, cost-effective personnel to provide the new services in new ways and in different settings. A very promising manpower resource that meets this requirement is the paraprofessional. As Francine Sobey, among others, clearly documents, paraprofessionals can and do contribute to the development and delivery of new services relevant to community needs. Furthermore, paraprofessionals are a cost-effective means for reaching the traditionally neglected minority, economically disadvantaged, and geographically isolated populations which have the greatest need for outreach and follow-up services. The cost benefit arising from the use of paraprofessionals is extremely important given the present and future budget constraints.

Although paraprofessional personnel have been involved in providing mental health services for as long as we have had organized systems of care, it was not until the decade of the 60s that their real and potential contributions became formally recognized. The Division of Manpower and Training, recognizing the significance of this new manpower resource, initiated two types of paraprofessional training programs.

In 1971, the Division initiated systematic support for a nationwide network of associate of arts degree (AA) training programs in community colleges. These training programs represent a planned strategy for producing generalists who can provide needed mental health functions in a wide variety of service agencies and settings. Shortly thereafter, in 1972, the Division also initiated support for a nationwide network of New Careers training programs that were designed to simultaneously prepare paraprofessionals to offer needed services and to provide opportunities for upward mobility to persons from economically disadvantaged backgrounds. These New Careers programs provided an opportunity needed for career advancement, while retaining high educational and service standards. The basing of decisions regarding promotion on the individuals' experience and demonstrated capability, as well as on the completion of formal educational requirements, was a principle supported by these programs.

The last seven years of experience with the paraprofessional initiatives has also suggested that a number of other important principles can be promoted by the use of paraprofessionals. For example, the development, employment, and appropriate utilization of paraprofessionals can be an effective strategy to aid in: (a) increasing and maintaining an adequate supply of mental health specialists, both professional and paraprofessional, to provide mental health services to this and future generations; (b) the development of a manpower service strategy that is based on a clearly articulated and anticipatory national mental health service strategy; (c) the promotion of a one-class system of mental health care in which every citizen is entitled to quality services delivered by appropriately trained specialists; (d) meeting the mental health service needs of underserved populations; and (e) the placement of a high priority on appropriate manpower development programs for minority groups. These principles are consistent with and responsive to the recommendations made by the President's Commission on Mental Health.

The need and importance of the paraprofessional mental health worker should be beyond debate. At the present time, paraprofessional personnel comprise the largest single category of direct service personnel working in the nation's mental health facilities. They are there every working day, providing a wide range of important and absolutely necessary direct mental health services. Moreover, the paraprofessional workers are effective in performing their functions.

In the face of the history and proven validity of the paraprofessional workers, their level acceptance and legitimation has not been commensurate with their importance. For this reason, the Paraprofessional Manpower Development Branch of our Division provided support for the completion of this volume as part of a larger effort. The goal of this book is to make available up-to-date information on paraprofessionalism. The authors represent many of the most qualified authorities in the nation. Collectively, they have provided the public with the most current and the most comprehensive book on paraprofessionals. It is our hope that this book will be useful for paraprofessionals, professionals, scholars, and consumer representatives who share a desire to make available to the public highly effective and relevant mental health services.

William H. Denham, Ph.D.
Director
Division of Manpower and Training Programs

Vernon R. James, M.Ed.
Chief
Paraprofessional Manpower Development Branch
Division of Manpower and Training Programs

ACKNOWLEDGMENTS

Many persons, in addition to the authors themselves, made the conception and production of this anthology possible. We wish to thank each of these individuals for their contributions.

Vernon James, Chief of the Paraprofessional Development Division of National Institute of Mental Health, recognized the potential value of this volume and supplied the funds necessary for its completion. These funds were provided by contract number 5 T41 MH14487. We also wish to express appreciation to George White and Donald Fisher who provided support and guidance in compiling this anthology, and to Mary Bilstad, Vieva Monteau, and Carolyn Snowden who helped us through many basic activities without which this volume could not have been produced.

The editors, Andree Abecassis, Sandy Boucher, Mary Lou Fitzgerald, and Susan McElroy, worked diligently to refine the chapters. Herbert Highstone, Karen Mann, and Marge Mysyk gave additional editorial assistance, carefully proofread the chapters and scrutinized each manuscript for conformance with the stylistic requirements codified by the American Psychological Association. And Duane Welsch, the Administrative Assistant for our project, masterfully carried out the responsibilities for keeping track of each draft of each manuscript and for coordinating the editing efforts.

In addition to writing the chapters and carrying out the relevant background research, the authors were each very responsive to our suggestions for relevant topics as well as to our ideas for revision of early drafts. We enjoyed working with and learning from each author.

INTRODUCTION

This anthology presents in one accessible location original and up-to-date papers written both by theoreticians and practitioners knowledgeable about the use of paraprofessionals in mental health. The book is broad in its coverage, containing chapters on topics ranging from the roles played by paraprofessionals in two specific community mental health centers (chapters 10 and 11) to the literature documenting the effectiveness (chapter 4) and the economic efficiency (chapter 3) of this growing work force. Overall, the volume focuses on the use of paraprofessionals as an important strategy for improving the quality of services, not as an end in itself. The chapters on paraprofessionals are supplemented by papers (chapters 13 and 14) on the related topics of volunteers and self-help groups.

The book should prove to be useful to a variety of readers, including persons responsible for: college-based training programs for mental health paraprofessionals or professionals; agency-based, in-service training programs for paraprofessional and professional staff members; policy decisions at agency, city, county, state or federal levels; and scholarly and research activities. Most of the chapters are written in a relatively non–technical style; however, chapters 3 and 4 are more scholarly in thrust and are oriented toward academicians and state or federal policy makers.

For purposes of this anthology a mental health "paraprofessional" is defined as a regularly employed and fully salaried staff member whose formal degree in mental health does not exceed the baccalaureate (BA or BS level).

Thus, a person with a master's degree in psychology would not be classified as a paraprofessional, while an individual with a PhD in philosophy would be categorized as a paraprofessional in mental health. Also, a volunteer with a BA would not be a paraprofessional, while a salaried staff member who has not completed high school would be classified as a paraprofessional.

Categorical generalizations about paraprofessionals are limited in validity, for individual paraprofessionals differ in both their backgrounds and their reasons for having sought their employment positions. For purposes of clarification, however, three major categories of paraprofessionals can be distinguished.

The first type consists of persons who are natives of the community and/or the subculture being served by the mental health agency. These paraprofessionals may be especially well equipped with knowledge about the local community and with skills useful in communicating with local clients and organizations. Frequently described as "indigenous," these paraprofessionals often, but not necessarily, are members of minority groups or economically disadvantaged populations.

Some paraprofessionals are graduates of New Careers training programs. Designed as a strategy to train and to employ economically disadvantaged persons to serve their local communities, these programs ideally provide academic credit both for relevant life and work experience and for the completion of formal course work. A comprehensive New Careers strategy combines a training program with (a) paid time off from work for training, and (b) a career ladder that opens up the opportunity structure to qualified persons regardless of their economic backgrounds. Based on ideas articulated by Pearl and Riessman (1965), and others, the New Careers strategy has been analyzed and evaluated in a recent book (Cohen, 1976). Chapters 5, 10, 11, and 12 should be of greatest interest to readers whose interests focus on issues related to the New Careers strategy.

A second category is comprised of paraprofessionals who have successfully overcome specific psychological difficulties and who, consequently, may be able to provide special insights and skills in serving particular clients. For example, a former drug addict may be better able than other staff members to enhance the credibility of an agency's services, demonstrate by example that drug abuse can be overcome, and offer advice useful to a client who is coping with the day-to-day difficulties involved in "kicking the habit."

The third type of paraprofessional consists of persons with some college education. Many of these persons possess AA or BA degrees from paraprofessional training programs or BA degrees in one of the behavioral sciences. These college-trained persons, at the time of employment, may be equipped with considerable academic knowledge about mental health as well as with practical skills acquired through supervised fieldwork experiences. Furthermore, they may be especially adept at the performance of tasks such as writing diagnostic reports or compiling public education materials. Paraprofessionals from any of the three categories may be highly upwardly mobile, wishing eventually to achieve a graduate degree or otherwise to become eligible for a position offering greater responsibility and higher pay.

Paraprofessionals, thus, can both complement professionals by providing new services and perspectives, and supplement professionals by giving assistance on tasks. The fact that paraprofessionals complement professionals has been documented in many reports, including three nationwide interview studies in which information was gathered from professionals (Bartels & Tyler, 1975; Sobey, 1970; Young, True, & Packard, 1976).

The reader interested in additional items on paraprofessionals is referred to a recently completed bibliography (Social Action Research Center, 1978). Covering the literature published from 1966 through the first six months of 1977, this bibliography contains entries on both general issues (e.g., the training of paraprofessionals) and on specific functions performed by paraprofessionals (e.g., services for the elderly).

Another publication (Alley, Blanton, Feldman, Hunter, & Rolfson, 1979) contains descriptions of 12 effective programs in which paraprofessionals play major roles and perform innovative functions. Representing the twelve services required by the Community Mental Health Amendments of 1975 (Public Law 94-63), the programs are all located within community mental health centers or similar settings. The case studies describe broader issues (e.g., selection, training, supervision, morale, and career mobility) as well as the specific functions performed by the paraprofessional staff members.

This anthology is organized into five sections, progressing from general to specialized issues. Part I, "Philosophy and History of the Use of Paraprofessionals," contains chapters designed to provide the reader with a framework for assimilating the more specialized topics covered in the remaining sections. Pertinent to all readers, these chapters would ideally be read prior to the other chapters.

Part II, "General Issues in Service Programs Involving Paraprofessionals," focuses on issues relevant to all mental health service areas, regardless of whether the services are offered by community mental health centers or by other agencies. Pertinent to all readers, these chapters should be of special interest to government policymakers.

Part III, "Specialized Roles for Paraprofessionals," contains chapters describing nontraditional functions that can be performed by paraprofessionals. The roles in psychosocial rehabilitation programs are especially relevant to community mental health centers, while that of the indigenous change agent is relevant to a wide variety of organizational settings.

Part IV, "The Involvement of Paraprofessionals in Community Mental Health Centers," contains chapters that focus explicitly on the role of paraprofessionals in community mental health programs. The first three chapters are explicitly relevant to all service areas, while the fourth (chapter 12) describes how paraprofessionals in a consultation and education program helped to create a collaborative relationship between a mental health center and the surrounding community.

Part V, "Volunteers and Self-Help," contains two chapters describing the functions of two groups of nonprofessionals in mental health. The chapters also contain discussions of the relationship between paraprofessionals and these nonprofessional resources.

Brief summaries, written by the editors, precede each chapter. These summaries are designed both to assist readers in selecting those chapters that are most pertinent to their interests and to highlight major themes contained in the entries.

REFERENCES

Alley, S. R., Blanton, J., Feldman, R. E., Hunter, G. D., & Rolfson, M. *Case studies of mental health paraprofessionals: Twelve effective programs.* New York: Human Sciences Press, 1979.

Bartels, B. D., & Tyler, J. D. Paraprofessionals in the community mental health center. *Professional Psychology,* 1975, *6,* 442–453.

Cohen, R. *"New Careers" grows older: A perspective on the paraprofessional experience, 1965–1975.* Baltimore, Md.: Johns Hopkins University Press, Policy Studies in Employment and Welfare, No. 26, 1976.

Pearl, A., & Riessman, F. *New careers for the poor.* New York: Free Press, 1965.

Sobey, F. *The nonprofessional revolution in mental health.* New York: Columbia University Press, 1970.

Social Action Research Center. *Paraprofessionals in mental health: An Annotated bibliography—1966 to 1977.* San Rafael, Calif. Author, 1978.

Young, C. E., True, J. E., & Packard, M. E. A national study of associate degree mental health and human services workers. *Journal of Community Psychology,* 1976, *4,* 89–95.

PHILOSOPHY AND HISTORY OF THE USE OF PARAPROFESSIONALS

Chapter 1

PARAPROFESSIONALS IN MENTAL HEALTH: A FRAMEWORK FOR THE FACTS

Vernon James*

Who are paraprofessionals? Why are they needed? How effective are they? How can their performance be improved? This chapter provides answers to these questions through descriptions of effective programs, analysis of existing information, and policy recommendations. It appears at the beginning of the anthology to introduce the other, more specialized chapters.

In addition to supplementing professionals as aides or assistants, paraprofessionals also complement professionals. They help agencies to engage in new functions and to reach traditionally underserved populations (e.g., chronic patients, the elderly, minorities, the homebound, and the poor). The author illustrates this theme by survey research findings and descriptions of effective programs in which paraprofessionals play key roles. This chapter also highlights the most common problems in programs that use paraprofessionals and offers recommendations for the amelioration of these problems.

The most persuasive reason for acknowledging and understanding the role of paraprofessionals in mental health is that they are physically *there*, every working day, delivering a significantly large portion of the actual direct services in our national mental health system. Planners, legislators, policy makers, and administrators must take this fact into account, for the contribution

*Chief, Paraprofessional Manpower Development Branch, Division of Manpower and Training Programs, National Institute of Mental Health, Rockville, Maryland 20852.

of paraprofessionals is now irreplaceable. They do far more than merely deliver, at a lower cost, many services formerly provided by professionals. The
variety of their service contributions and the versatility of their response to
community needs have overflowed the traditional boundaries of professional
practice. As a consequence, much of the action is now with paraprofessionals;
to underestimate their contribution is to be ignorant of large parts of the
mental health system; to underutilize them is to reduce the effectiveness and
efficiency of the national mental health systems in providing services to those
in need.

This chapter presents a pragmatic framework for comprehending the
significance and the use of paraprofessionals in various mental service programs, citing empirical evidence, describing some exemplary programs, and
offering policy recommendations. The following questions are answered: Who
are paraprofessionals? How many paraprofessionals are there? Why are they
needed? How effective are they? How can paraprofessional performance be
improved?

WHO ARE PARAPROFESSIONALS?

Paraprofessionals are paid workers who are presently functioning, or who are
being trained to function, in mental health service delivery positions which
require a baccalaureate degree, an associate degree, a certificate in specialized
competencies, a high school diploma, or their equivalent in experience. Formerly these workers were called subprofessionals, nonprofessionals, or aides.
The change in title reflects a positive shift in attitudes toward paraprofessionals
due to a recognition of the significance of the services they provide, and the
well-documented evidence of their competence. The *work* of paraprofessionals
can now be a *career* in which the development of competence and job performance is matched with increasing responsibility and salary.

The term paraprofessional is currently being used broadly to describe an
entire class or category of personnel encompassing all occupational groups
below the master's degree level. While this concept is not unanimously agreed
upon, it does provide a framework for understanding the paraprofessional
occupational field while simultaneously allowing the individual workers to
have titles descriptive of their work. Also significant to note is that the term
paraprofessional is not, by definition, a negative or second-class term. Webster's Dictionary[1] defines "para" as "alongside of; beside" rather than as
"below" or "sub." By implication, paraprofessionals are potentially equal to,
but different from, professionals.

McPheeters (Note 1), in his paper entitled "Roles and Functions of
Mental Health Personnel," provides a useful scheme for understanding this
broad category of personnel. He describes four levels of workers around which
the many different paraprofessional and professional occupational classes can

be organized. The first three levels, corresponding to the broader concept of the term paraprofessional, are (a) the *entry level*—persons with no job-specific training prior to entering employment, (b) the *technical level*—persons with one or two years of specific training for their work, who may have a certificate or an associate degree, and (c) the *associate level*—persons with a baccalaureate degree or approximate equivalent with specific training in the field.

Within this same broad context, the Paraprofessional Manpower Development Branch, NIMH, describes paraprofessionals in the following manner:

> These workers perform a wide variety of direct and indirect mental health related functions on behalf of clients and their families in hospitals, community mental health centers and other organized mental health/human service systems. These workers perform these functions independently, but usually under the general supervision of other mental health professionals. The degree of autonomy relates primarily to the functional level and employment status of the workers. The paraprofessional is usually categorized into three levels: *entry level* (aide or beginning New Careers enrollee); *technical level* (or apprentice or assistant level), usually requiring an AA degree; and *associate level*, usually demanding the BA degree.

McPheeters (Note 1) has developed a scheme which illuminates the organization of service functions of paraprofessionals and the emergence of their occupational class. He describes five different arrangements for structuring paraprofessionals' roles and functions: (a) as *aides to single professions*, e.g., social work aides, psychology aides, (b) around *specific tasks*, e.g., intake interviews, administration of tests, (c) around *major functions*, e.g., intake workers, rehabilitation workers, (d) around *administrative arrangements*, e.g., day ward aides, night supervisors, and (e) around *total needs of a small group of clients*, e.g., the developing generalist model.

As suggested by this scheme, paraprofessionals can *supplement* the work of professionals. By performing tasks that require less formal education, they can enable professionals to devote more of their time to those specialized tasks requiring graduate level training. This role of aide to single professionals is the oldest of the five arrangements. These aides may themselves become professionals, over time, adding training to the important dimension of life experience which they bring to their work.

Paraprofessionals can also *complement* professionals. They have provided many services in areas that are generally outside the specialized training of professionals. They have served as ombudspersons, expeditors, referral agents; they have assisted clients in solving problems of daily living and in coping with service agencies. Indigenous paraprofessionals have helped to communicate the needs of the community to the mental health center and to increase trust in and use of mental health services by the community. These complementary service functions and utilization models are used in a wide variety of service settings. Paraprofessionals can perform complementary functions in the four roles other than that of aide, and are particularly effective in complementing professionals when they serve as generalists. As generalists, paraprofessionals are trained in skills based on the needs of clients rather than on the traditions of professional disciplines.

How Many Paraprofessionals Are There?

Paraprofessionals are the single largest category of personnel providing direct services in the 3,300 mental health facilities in the nation. The relative numbers and percentages of paraprofessionals as compared to other direct service personnel in mental health facilities are made graphically clear in Tables 1-1 and 1-2. These tables portray some startling facts. In 1976, for instance, mental health workers with less than a BA degree made up 45.1% (N = 130,021) of all the mental health service personnel in mental health facilities surveyed. The other categories of paraprofessionals, LPN and LVN, made up 5.3% (N = 15,337) of mental health services personnel. Together these two groups represented 50.4% (N = 145,358) of all the mental health service personnel in the facilities surveyed in 1976. These figures do not include BA-level workers in the "Other Mental Health Professionals" category (11.9%, N = 34,249) or the BA workers included under the "Social Work" and "Psychologist" categories. Data on the number of paraprofessionals in these latter two categories do not exist, but indications are that the number is high.

When community mental health centers are considered alone (Table 1-2), the number of paraprofessionals is somewhat reduced. However, their numbers are still higher than any other single category of personnel. In CMHCs, paraprofessional mental health workers, LPNs, and LVNs constitute 29.6% (N = 10,561) of the personnel in 1976 and higher percentages in other years reported. Other data suggest that the paraprofessionals' contribution is proportionate to their numbers. Steinberg, Freeman, Steele, Balodis, and Batista (1976) estimate that at least 30% of all *direct* mental health services provided in federally funded community mental health centers are delivered by paraprofessionals.

Why Are Paraprofessionals Needed?

Manpower Needs in Mental Health

Community mental health centers are mandated to provide mental health services to all persons in need, regardless of income. Expanding services and numbers of centers within community mental health and other domains have

Table 1–1   Distribution of Personnel by Discipline in
All Mental Health Facilities, United States, 1970–1976

| | Year | | | |
Discipline	1968	1972	1974	1976
Full-time equivalent positions, by discipline				
Psychiatrists	9,891	12,938	14,947	15,339
Other physicians	2,736	3,991	3,548	3,356
Psychologists	5,212	9,443	12,597	15,251
Social workers	9,755	17,687	22,147	25,887
Registered nurses	24,256	31,110	34,089	39,392
Other MH professionals (BA+ or =)	12,136	17,514	29,325	34,249
Physical health	—	8,203	10,507	9,631
Total professional patient care staff	63,986	100,886	127,160	143,105
LPN, LVN		19,616	17,193	15,337
MH worker (BA–)		120,753	128,529	130,021
Total patient care staff		241,255	272,882	288,463
Administration, clerical, maintenance		134,719	130,142	134,795
TOTAL POSITIONS		375,974	403,024	423,258
Disciplines as a percentage of total patient care staff				
Psychiatrists		5.4	5.5	5.3
Other physicians		1.7	1.3	1.2
Psychologists		3.9	4.6	5.3
Social workers		7.3	8.1	9.0
Registered nurses		12.9	12.5	13.7
Other MH professionals (BA+ or =)		7.3	10.7	11.9
Physical health		3.4	3.9	3.3
Total professional patient care staff		41.9	46.6	49.6
LPN, LVN		8.1	6.3	5.3
MH worker (BA–)		50.1	47.1	45.1
TOTAL PATIENT CARE STAFF		100.0	100.0	100.0

Note. Data in this table from Preliminary Working Draft of the Final Report of the Task Panel on Personnel to the President's Commission on Mental Health, December, 1977, based on a compilation of NIMH Division of Biometry and Epidemiology data.

created a shortage of professional staff members trained in a combination of community and clinical skills. While enormous numbers of professional clinicians have been trained since that time, the conclusions about professional manpower reached by the Joint Commission on Mental Illness and Health in 1959 (Albee, 1959) still seem to hold (e.g., Arnhoff, Jenkins, & Speisman, 1969; Matarazzo, 1971), particularly for the community service area. As expressed in the 1959 Albee volume:

Table 1-2 Distribution of Personnel by Discipline in
Community Mental Health Centers, United States, 1970–1976

Discipline	Year			
	1970	1972	1974	1976
Full-time equivalent positions, by discipline				
Psychiatrists	1,394	1,583	1,848	2,292
Other physicians	103	241	270	274
Psychologists	1,005	1,807	2,994	4,543
Social workers	1,989	3,044	4,418	6,752
Registered nurses	1,989	2,722	3,459	4,588
Other MH professionals (BA+ or =)		2,441	4,306	6,336
Physical health		158	252	305
Total professional patient care staff		11,996	17,546	25,090
LPN, LVN		1,244	1,367	1,288
MH worker (BA−)		5,574	7,605	9,273
Total patient care staff	13,123	18,814	26,518	35,651
Administration, clerical, maintenance		5,841	8,791	12,816
TOTAL POSITIONS		24,655	35,309	48,467
Disciplines as a percentage of total patient care staff				
Psychiatrists	10.6	8.4	7.0	6.4
Other physicians	0.8	1.3	1.0	0.8
Psychologists	7.7	9.6	11.3	12.7
Social workers	15.2	16.2	16.7	18.9
Registered nurses	15.2	14.5	13.0	12.9
Other MH professionals (BA+ or =)		13.0	16.2	17.8
Physical health		0.8	0.9	0.9
Total professional patient care staff		63.8	66.1	70.4
LPN, LVN		6.6	5.2	3.6
MH worker (BA−)		29.6	28.7	26.0
TOTAL PATIENT CARE STAFF		100.0	100.0	100.0

Note. Data in this table from Preliminary Working Draft of the Final Report of the Task Panel on Personnel to the President's Commission on Mental Health, December, 1977, based on a compilation of NIMH Division of Biometry and Epidemiology data.

The long-standing shortage of professionals . . . has been aggravated rather than relieved by a tremendously increased demand for mental health services in other agencies—for example schools, courts, and prisons as well as in private practice (p. xi, Staff Review Introduction).

The lengthy educational preparation of professional personnel in the field of mental illness and mental health makes pessimistic the prospect that their number can be increased sufficiently to meet social needs (p. 256).

What we need are techniques and methods enabling far more people to be reached per professional person. If we do not at present have such techniques, then we should spend time looking for them. The logic of the manpower situation in which we find ourselves makes other solutions unrealistic (p. 254).

Maintaining Quality Services at Lowered Cost

Appropriately trained and supervised paraprofessionals can deliver quality services at a cost considerably less than required for compensation of professionals.[2] Various studies support the contention that paraprofessionals are effective. Following are descriptions of three such studies: Durlak's (1973) review of research studies, Sobey's (1970) survey of key personnel in 185 NIMH-funded projects, and Young, True, and Packard's (1976) survey of supervisors of AA-level paraprofessionals concerning the performance of their supervisees.

Durlak (1973) summarizes his findings succinctly, distinguishing studies in which experimental procedures have been employed from the more general research:

> The present author undertook a systematic but not necessarily exhaustive search of the professional literature of the last ten years. Over 300 references were obtained relevant to the selection, training and therapeutic functioning of nonprofessionals.
>
> There are 14 studies that have used various experimental procedures to compare directly the therapeutic effectiveness of non-professional and professional personnel. In 7 of the 14 studies, lay therapists had achieved significantly better therapeutic results than professionals; in the other 7 studies, results for the two groups were similar. *In no study have lay persons been found to be significantly inferior to professional workers* (pp. 301–302).

In her survey of contributions to service improvement by nonprofessionals (both paid paraprofessionals and unpaid volunteers), Sobey (1970) discovered that most agencies rated the contributions by nonprofessionals as "substantial." Categorized by area of service improvement, these findings are presented in Table 1-3 (adapted from Sobey, p. 159). Especially noteworthy is the fact that paraprofessionals help other staff members gain new viewpoints on the population served.

Young et al. (1976) conducted on-site interviews of more than 100 employed graduates of AA-degree programs in the mental health human services. Both paraprofessionals and their supervisors were interviewed. Table 1-4 is adapted from the more extensive table contained in the authors' 1976 report (pp. 92–93). It includes only the tasks from the original table that 45% or more of the paraprofessionals reported performing "much or most of the time." As

Table 1–3   Contributions by Nonprofessionals to
Improvements in Service

Specific service improvement	Impact of nonprofessional contribution on specific service improvement (given in percentage of total responses)			
	Substantial	Moderate	Slightly or not at all	Total number of project responses
Service initiated and completed faster	54	31	15	80
Able to serve more people	59	32	9	127
New services provided	57	27	16	141
More professional time made available for treatment	45	31	24	106
New viewpoints gained by project staff re population served	53	31	16	135

is indicated in the table, usually two-thirds or more of the supervisors gave "excellent" or "good" ratings to the paraprofessionals performing these tasks. Also noteworthy is the wide range of roles performed by paraprofessionals on the job.

Performance of New Roles in Mental Health

A more complete understanding of mental health is constantly evolving, and new ways of contributing to the health of communities are periodically tried. Priorities of service delivery undergo repeated change and elaboration. Because of their broad range of skills and interests, paraprofessionals have been in the forefront of innovation, well placed to meet new demands and challenging mandates.[3] The shorter duration of their training can render them more adaptable than professionals to changing circumstances and more willing to switch tactics.

These new roles are documented by the previously reported findings of Young et al. (1976) contained in Table 1-4. The nontraditional functions performed by paraprofessionals "much or some of the time" include: motivating patients to improve personal hygiene (62%); milieu therapy (62%); serving as a spokesman (woman) for patients in dealing with treatment staff (92%); helping patients obtain legal, financial or other treatment/educational assistance (84%); aiding patients and families upon discharge (46%); reporting back to treatment team on patient's progress (59%).

Table 1–4   Graduates' Work Activities and Supervisors' Ratings

Task	Frequency with which the paraprofessionals report performing the task much or some of the time	Frequency with which supervisors rate the para-professionals' performance as good or excellent
Screening and evaluation		
Conduct intake interviews	54%	75%
Assist in gathering information on the patients' immediate life situation	78%	75%
Record history/background information on patient	60%	69%
Make recommendations for treatment discharge, follow-up	76%	74%
Direct client-contact activities		
Individual therapy	74%	73%
Group therapy	68%	64%
Work with families of patients	46%	76%
Motivate patients to improve personal hygiene such as PET	62%	73%
Milieu therapy	62%	73%
Procedures and records		
Record keeping	97%	71%
Scheduling appointments or meetings	57%	66%
Participation in staff meetings, treatment team meetings, etc.	99%	75%
Read patients' files, records	92%	80%
Advocacy		
Serve as spokesperson for patient in dealing with treatment staff	92%	79%
Help patients obtain legal, financial, or other treatment/educational assistance	84%	77%
Community adjustment/liaison		
Aid patients and families upon discharge	46%	82%
Report back to treatment team on patients' progress	59%	77%

Further documentation comes from Sobey's (1970) nationwide study of paraprofessionals and volunteers employed in NIMH-funded programs. Sobey states:

> Quite disparate opinions have been confidently expressed about the impact of nonprofessionals in mental health work. These have ranged from the claim that nonprofessionals are taking over most of the professionals' tasks to the other extreme that nonprofessionals are only being given the most routine, menial tasks which professionals wish to be rid of anyhow. There is no evidence to support either extreme contention. Rather . . . nonprofessionals, to a highly significant degree, are engaged in new roles and functions not previously performed by either professionals or nonprofessionals. And, many of these roles are therapeutic in nature (p. 97).

Sobey substantiates her generalization with data. Presented in Table 1-5 (adapted from p. 104 of Sobey), these data indicate that paraprofessionals (a) perform a wide variety of roles and (b) are more likely than professionals to perform various newer roles. These latter roles include: caretaking; social relationship, activity group, and milieu therapy; retraining in special skills; and

**Table 1–5   Project Distribution
Showing Differential Performance of Functions**

Functions	Functions performed (in 185 projects)		
	Mainly by non-professionals	Mainly by professionals	Equally by both
Caretaking (e.g., ward care, day care)	37	5	12
Socializing relationships (individual or group)	36	17	32
Activity group therapy	27	14	21
Tutoring	25	10	6
Milieu therapy	22	17	20
Facilitate access to community services	22	22	13
Individual counseling	19	35	25
Reception orientation to service	18	13	25
Retraining (special skill functions)	18	5	4
Resource finding (home, job)	17	22	11
Group counseling	15	27	24
Other special skills	14	3	5
Other therapeutic functions	12	2	6
Case finding and facilitation of access to project service	11	17	22
Screening (nonclerical)	11	32	17
Community improvement	10	11	3

tutoring. Professionals are more likely to provide the following somewhat more traditional services: individual counseling, group counseling, case finding and facilitation, and nonclerical screening.

Poorer and Marginal Populations

Mental health professionals are not necessarily well prepared to meet the needs of persons from the lower socioeconomic groups or of persons who are barely able to cope with the demands of society. Yet one of the primary motivating factors in creating a nationwide network of community mental health centers is to make quality services available to these underserved populations.

It has been well documented that middle-class professionals find lower-class patients more difficult to treat, while paraprofessionals have willingly accepted such challenges (Arnhoff et al., 1969; Lorion, 1973; Alley, Blanton, Feldman, Hunter & Rolfson, 1979). Paraprofessionals have also performed most creditably in areas of high drug use, alcoholism and delinquency, which in many cases become "afflictions of a neighborhood."

SOME EXAMPLES OF PARAPROFESSIONAL WORK IN SPECIFIC PROGRAMS

Case Studies of Mental Health Paraprofessionals: Twelve Effective Programs (Alley et al., 1979) was designed as a companion volume to this anthology. From its description of effective community mental health center programs, I have drawn examples of key roles filled by paraprofessionals and noted how paraprofessionals contribute to the following ideals, which are particularly characteristic of the community mental health movement.

The Best Available Services for All Citizens Regardless of Income, Ethnicity, or Age

The child and parent program of the Huntsville-Madison County Community Mental Health Center in Huntsville, Alabama, places paraprofessional consultants (BA level) within county schools to assist teachers and make referrals to the service's day treatment program. This program is itself staffed by paraprofessionals who keep careful records of the treatment and the progress of each child referred. These records are closely scrutinized, and the overall work is supervised and evaluated by a professional who directs the program.

Care Provided in Accessible Community Locations

The transitional care service of the Weber Mental Health Center in Ogden, Utah, employs paraprofessionals to deliver services within a "hotel" in a run-down central city location. Neighborhood residents can drop in for social events and/or for day treatment. There are rooms for those who need to stay. Trained and supervised paraprofessionals act as hosts and helpers.

Engaging in Outreach Efforts to Serve Consumers in Locations Appropriate to Their Needs

The aging program of the Hillsborough Community Mental Health Center in Tampa, Florida, employs paraprofessionals who seek new clients and provide direct clinical services to aging clients in less accessible sites. Nonambulatory clients are served in their homes and can be transported to such places as welfare agencies, medical and psychiatric clinics, grocery stores, and to recreational events. The paraprofessionals also consult with and advise nursing home personnel.

Provision of a Wide Variety of Service Options Appropriate to Differing Populations Within the Catchment Area

The screening service of the Roxbury Court Clinic in Roxbury, Massachusetts, employs paraprofessionals and professionals to determine whether clients incarcerated for crimes related to drugs or alcohol can benefit from mental health services offered as an alternative to imprisonment. These agency-based staff members collaborate with paraprofessionals in community-based treatment programs. Options for this set of clients include: inpatient, halfway house, day treatment, outpatient, and self-help settings. Two types of specialized treatment programs are an inpatient program for drug-abusing women with children, and services provided by Spanish-speaking staff members for Spanish-speaking clients.

Provision of Emergency Care in Appropriate Settings with Minimal Restrictions on Clients

The emergency service of the Southwest Denver Community Mental Health Services in Denver, Colorado, employs supervised and trained paraprofessionals to provide services to citizens in crises. The clients are rarely referred to inpatient wards. Usually clients receive services that enable them to stay at home. Alternatively, they may be transferred for short stays with healthy families living in single-family homes. The paraprofessionals provide backup services to the healthy family members so that they can maintain normal living patterns without involvement in therapy. This procedure both saves on the use of inpatient facilities and avoids the stigma of being institutionalized.

Creation of Normal Growth-Enhancing Environments as an Alternative to Medical Treatment

The partial hospitalization service of the Rutgers Community Mental Health Center-Rutgers Medical School in Rutgers, New Jersey, employs paraprofessionals who work with discharged mental patients within a "club" (rather than a "clinic" or "hospital") setting. The work and help of club "members" (the discharged patients) is vital to the functioning of the program; for example, they perform the functions of workers such as clerks, janitors, and cooks, thus strengthening their vocational and living skills. Eventually the members assume paid positions throughout the entire mental health center and in businesses in the community. Paraprofessionals from the club assist in skill training and "understudy" the work roles so that they can substitute at short notice for an absentee.

Provision of Continuity of Care by Mental Health Generalists

The aftercare service of the Cambridge-Somerville Mental Health and Retardation Center in Cambridge, Massachusetts, employs multiskilled paraprofessionals to work on a one-to-one basis with clients, from the time the clients are admitted to a nearby state mental hospital to the date they are discharged. This helps clients in post-discharge adjustment in their home communities. Within the state hospital, the paraprofessionals plan with their clients for discharge, helping them to house-hunt, to shop, or to gain assistance from welfare. After discharge, the paraprofessionals counsel on the availability of skill training, recreation, medication, and other services, and also help to mediate disputes—with landlords, for example. If staff members of the center's emergency unit are considering readmitting a discharged client to the state hospital, the appropriate aftercare paraprofessional is available to help the client to resolve personal crises and to provide advice on the decision and complications of readmission.

Prevention of Mental Health Problems Through Enhancing the Competencies of Individuals and Organizations in the Community

The consultation and education service of the Dr. Solomon Carter Fuller Community Mental Health Center in Boston, Massachusetts, employs paraprofessionals to consult, educate, and organize in the community. Working in teams with professionals or with one another, these paraprofessionals provide many services. They have taught seminars on mental health issues to pastors, consulted both with professionals in public agencies and citizens in grass roots

als. Secondly, an important problem is the unexplained lack of acceptance of paraprofessionals by professionals. Also of importance is the absence of concerns, such as those voiced by Gartner and Riessman, about cooptation and the perpetuation of traditional services.

The Perspective of Paraprofessionals

A complementary perspective on problems from the viewpoint of paraprofessionals themselves is provided by the findings of a study (described earlier) by Young et al. (1976). The results of the study indicate that the associate degree program prepares MHAs (mental health associates) for a wide range of mental health activities in multiple settings. However, the authors stressed the need for additional efforts by educational institutions and service agencies to promote further development of programs to meet local manpower needs, establish linkages between the programs and the community agencies, develop MHA roles within service delivery teams in agencies, implement career ladders for MHAs, and improve supervision.

These investigators summarize in detail the descriptions of problems within the mental health service agencies. Noteworthy is the need for more guidance on using paraprofessionals, as well as failure to use paraprofessionals optimally in roles complementary to those performed by professionals. In the authors' words:

> We did note that the MHAs in our sample received less supervision than we had expected. It seems unrealistic for new graduates to be job-ready for the entire range of potential jobs and client populations in the human services. For this reason, specific in-service training and closer supervision of new MHAs seems advisable. Most of the user agencies studied had not adequately developed such programs. More recent graduating classes may well have a greater need for this assistance in order to perform as capably and as quickly as the MHAs in our sample.
>
> One reason for the lack of such in-service programs is the uncertainty on the part of some agencies as to how MHAs could best be used and how much responsibility and authority to give them in working with patients. These factors suggest that MHAs and their college faculty need to inform employers and other MH/HS [mental health/human service] professionals about the training and education components of their associate degree MH/HS programs. One objective of many programs has been to prepare people for roles not currently being carried out by the MH/HS agency (e.g., client advocate, outreach worker). While MHAs were performing these new roles in some cases, the majority were carrying out traditional functions or an expansion of these functions (p. 94).

Young et al. (1976) also found that 30% of the graduates were dissatisfied with their jobs. The major sources of dissatisfaction were related to nonchallenging or menial work, a salary level that was seen as not being commensurate with their responsibilities, and a lack of acceptance by some colleagues. Moreover, 56% planned to change jobs in the next five years; an important contributing factor was the absence of career ladders for those persons who did not obtain higher degrees.

Status Competition

The problem of status competition between professionals and paraprofessionals is especially important. As indicated in Table 1-6, this problem is one of those most frequently reported by professionals. Furthermore, Sobey (1970) notes that 34% of nonprofessionals report status conflicts between themselves and professionals, while Young et al. (1976) report that 42% of mental health paraprofessionals felt accepted "with some reservations" by "some" of their fellow staff members. In a vivid first-person report (Hines, 1970) an agency paraprofessional describes jealousy from professionals, combined with various approaches to discourage her efforts. Status competition, doubtlessly, originates with paraprofessionals as well as with professionals. The fact that professionals can unwittingly contribute to status competition is illustrated clearly by Heller and Monahan (1977):

> Nonprofessionals are sometimes led to believe what can be patronizing rhetoric: the professional employer convinces them they were hired because they have better interactive skills with low-income populations than do professionals. It is quite natural for them to assume that once they are trained in the special skills and knowledge of the professional they will then be "double smart" . . . and will be even more competent than the professional. There is no way either side can win if the work is described in terms that encourage rivalry (p. 318).

HOW CAN PARAPROFESSIONAL PERFORMANCE BE IMPROVED?

The foregoing discussion has revealed many areas where improvements can be initiated and progress made. However, nothing can be achieved until we first "catch up with facts," to acknowledge what paraprofessionals are actually accomplishing. Unless we can reach beyond the idealized models of professional aspiration, we shall miss much of what is happening "in the front lines," where clients in various degrees of desperation are being sustained on a day-to-day basis. The following steps seem to be the most evident and the most urgent:

1. Increase the knowledge of persons in the mental health field, so that they know what paraprofessionals are doing, are capable of doing, and the myriad ways in which they can be deployed.

2. Strengthen the supervisory skills of professionals and the managerial aspects of their education, so that they are better able to delegate, train, and evaluate the work of paraprofessionals in their charge.
3. Work out alternate career ladders and credentialing systems for paraprofessionals, some of which bring them up to the proficiency of professionals in the core disciplines, and some of which build on skills complementary to those of professionals. In this way, we can keep the mental health system open to new styles of delivery and spontaneous ways of coping that arise from the demands of concrete situations.
4. Experiment in ways of fostering cooperation instead of rivalry between professionals and paraprofessionals. Clarify definitions of paraprofessional roles which point out supplementary/complementary relations with professionals. Equal status contact and opportunities for frank exchange of viewpoints between staff at all levels can play a part.
5. Develop a closer liaison between the colleges and universities which educate paraprofessional workers and the mental health systems which employ them. Discover what paraprofessionals must know and what they could bring to mental health centers, and then apply the knowledge in training programs.
6. The most innovative and ingenious ways of helping to solve clients' problems are lost to the system unless paraprofessionals (and professionals) are carefully evaluated. Mental health centers need to go on discovering what services are valuable and to correct mistakes where these occur.

Paraprofessionals have been and will continue to be an important part of health delivery systems. They work in ways which both complement and supplement professional services. Mental health planners must take account of this important resource in design of new services, supervision systems, in-service education programs, career ladders, and evaluation strategies. Effectively used, paraprofessionals can be an important force in improving mental health care.

NOTES

[1] *Webster's New Collegiate Dictionary.* Springfield, Mass.: G. & C. Merriam, 1976.

[2] Chapter 4 in this source book, by Alan Gartner, reviews the extensive evidence documenting the effectiveness of paraprofessionals; Chapter 3, by Thomas Marschak and Curtis Henke, documents the economic efficiency of paraprofessionals.

[3] This topic is explored in detail in four chapters of this source book: Chapter 9 by Robert Cohen and Melissa Devine; Chapter 10 by Mark Tarail; Chapter 11 by Mansell Pattison, Ernest Kuncel, Frank Murillo and Razmig Madenlian; and Chapter 12 by Bernard Bandler, Ruth Batson and Lyda Peters.

Reference Notes

1. H. McPheeters, *Roles and functions of mental health personnel.* Unpublished manuscript, 1978. (Available from Dr. Harold McPheeters, Southern Regional Education Board, 130 6th St. NW, Atlanta, Ga. 30313.)

References

Albee, G. W. *Mental health manpower trends.* New York: Basic Books, 1959.

Alley, S. R., Blanton, J., Feldman, R. E., Hunter, G. D. & Rolfson, M. *Case studies of mental health paraprofessionals: Twelve effective programs.* New York: Human Sciences Press, 1979.

Arnhoff, F. N., Jenkins, J. W., & Speisman, J. C. The new mental health workers. In F. N. Arnhoff, E. A. Rubenstein, & J. C. Speisman (Eds.), *Manpower for mental health.* Chicago: Aldine Publishing Co., 1969.

Bartels, B. D., & Tyler, J. D. Paraprofessionals in the community mental health center. *Professional Psychology,* 1975, *6,* 442–453.

Durlak, J. A. Myths concerning the nonprofessional therapist. *Professional Psychology,* 1973, *4,* 300–304.

Gartner, A., & Riessman, F. Changing the professions. In R. Gross (Ed.), *The new professionals.* New York: Simon and Schuster, 1972.

Heller, K., & Monahan, D. *Psychology and community change.* Homewood, Ill.: Dorsey Press, 1977.

Hines, L. A nonprofessional discusses her role in mental health. *American Journal of Psychiatry,* 1970, *126,* 1467–1472.

Lorion, R. P. Socioeconomic status and traditional treatment approaches reconsidered. *Psychological Bulletin,* 1973, *4,* 263–270.

Matarazzo, J. D. Some national developments in the utilization of nontraditional mental health manpower. *American Psychologist,* 1971, *26,* 363–371.

Sobey, F. *The nonprofessional revolution in mental health.* New York: Columbia University Press, 1970.

Steinberg, S. S., Freeman, K. A., Steele, C. A., Balodis, I., & Batista, A. L. *Information on manpower utilization, functions, and credentialing in community mental health centers* (Contract No. ADM 45-74-158). Washington, D.C.: Department of Health, Education, and Welfare, National Institute of Mental Health, Division of Manpower and Training, 1976.

Young, C. E., True, J. E., & Packard, M. E. A national study of associate degree mental health and human services workers. *Journal of Community Psychology,* 1976, *4,* 89–95.

Chapter 2

THE PARAPROFESSIONAL: A BRIEF SOCIAL HISTORY

Murray Levine
Steve Tulkin
James Intagliata
Jonathan Perry
Ed Whitson*

This chapter provides historical and cultural perspectives on the current practices, successes, and problems of the paraprofessional movement. A major section of the chapter details the development of paraprofessional-delivered services in Western Europe and the U.S.A. Notable is the fact that the human services began when concerned nonprofessionals organized programs to meet unfilled needs. As the chapter points out, these once informal services have become "professionalized," with consequent drawbacks as well as benefits.

The chapter also discusses the role of nonprofessionals in undeveloped and developing countries. Paraprofessionals entered the scene when traditional services were modernized. Problems that occur when Western mental health models are transplanted to developing countries are described, as well as two examples of organizational solutions to these problems. The chapter concludes by drawing lessons for the present.

All of the modern human services that exist today developed in a similar pattern in the 19th and 20th centuries. These institutions include: mental hospitals; welfare services; probation and parole offices; juvenile courts; institutions for unwed mothers, alcoholics, the retarded, the poor, the sick, and the aged; outpatient clinics; child and family service agencies; and neighborhood service centers. Some concerned members of society recognized there were

*All authors are from Department of Psychology, State University of New York at Buffalo, Buffalo, New York.

people with needs that were unserved by the resources of family and friends or by existing institutions. These concerned individuals who were "amateurs," "nonprofessionals," provided the service themselves as best they could and, in one way or another, convinced their communities to allocate a portion of the community's resources to providing for those in need.

Today's paraprofessionals are very much like the concerned individuals who began our modern services.[1] Like the early amateurs, today's paraprofessionals have been recruited to serve an impoverished and dependent population which was not served or was served inadequately by existing helping services.[2] Like the concerned individuals who began to serve others, the earliest paraprofessionals were not selected because of their education or other formal training. They were often selected, or more often self-selected, for personal traits and for knowledge of the culture of those whom they were to serve. Just as the 19th century workers served as bridges between those in need and members of the larger society, modern paraprofessionals are supposed to provide a bridge between middle-class oriented and staffed agencies and clients who were previously unserved or only poorly served by those agencies.

One important difference exists. Most of the 19th century services developed informally or under private auspices. The pioneer antipoverty agencies of the early 1960s started with private funds or with funds contributed by organizations for experimental purposes. These funds were free of many constraints found in large, government funded, formal organizations. When the experimental phase passed, it was necessary to find permanent funding for positions. Jobs for paraprofessionals were developed in large, formal organizations which are in the main professionally dominated. This change in the circumstances of employment has important implications. Paraprofessionals today are often required to act in terms of government and agency policies, rather than their personal motivations and instincts.

The first part of this chapter will discuss amateurs and paraprofessionals in several fields of human service. Although we will concentrate on social work in the United States, as it developed in the 19th and 20th centuries, we will touch briefly on examples from other disciplines. We will show that agencies and services changed dramatically when they became professionalized. Although originally intended to service impoverished populations, the change in services resulted in a failure of service to reach large segments of the population. Paraprofessionals were introduced into the service system to help redress the imbalance. The second part of the paper will trace the development of the paraprofessional movement in the 1960s, when we saw a renewed concern for human services. This movement received great impetus during the Kennedy administration, which was instrumental in the widespread development of community mental health programs. While creating these programs, the political leadership recognized the lack of trained personnel to staff them. Subsequently they began to turn to paraprofessionals for help. The paraprofessional movement continued under President Johnson as he advanced the social and welfare programs which constituted the Great Society. During this period of enormous growth, conflict often developed between the new paraprofessionals and the professionals who had long dominated the field. At about the same time, a need and a desire for training was recognized. Accordingly, both New Careers training programs and associate of arts/bachelor of arts degree programs in the human services were established to provide training for paraprofessionals. These programs will be described along with their implications for paraprofessionals in human services. Finally, in order to provide some perspective on helping roles in our own culture, we will review some paraprofessional helping roles in other cultures.

THE PARAPROFESSIONAL IN HISTORY

At the end of the middle ages, as a result of wars and complex social changes following the breakdown of the feudal system, a large, visible "underclass" emerged. This class, consisting of the poor, the unemployed, the disabled, widows, unwed mothers, the dependent young, the aged, the insane, and the retarded, had previously been absorbed on the feudal estates. When those estates broke up, masses of poor began wandering, frequently settling in the cities. The attendant social problems were serious and distressing. In France during the middle 1600s, large institutions were built to contain the unemployed people. The staff members of these institutions had no training for their vocations. They had only the mission of trying to get work out of those who were otherwise dependent. Those persons who could not work, such as the violent insane, were kept in chains (Foucalt, 1965).

In England, the Elizabethan Poor Laws of 1601 established a tradition of local responsibility for persons in need. A citizen, with no further specification of qualifications, was appointed overseer of the poor in each community, and each community made provisions for those in need. The poor and the dependent presented a moral dilemma to the English. On the one hand their Judeo-Christian heritage obliged them to help those in need; on the other hand, if this underclass was deemed responsible for its own troubles because of its perceived immorality, sinfulness, or laziness, then society's responsibility was diminished. The community's efforts to assist reflected this ambivalence, and its solutions were often unkind. For example, in the early 19th century it became apparent that welfare costs were heavy. A system of district workhouses was developed. The workhouses were designed to be considerably less attractive than the living conditions of ordinary working people. If sufficiently unattractive, they would repel ablebodied workers, and people would be encouraged to save for their old ages so that they would not have to enter the workhouse. The workhouses were governed by local citizens but often staffed with ex-army men or others not much better off than those they served. Needless to say, the aim of making these workhouses uncomfortable places was quickly realized. Some exceeded the bounds of decency and could aptly be described as concentration camps (Longmate, 1974).

English tradition influenced the care of the same class of people in colonial America (Deutsch, 1949). Some change from the pattern of begrudging, harsh care for members of the underclass emerged late in the 18th century. The period known as the Enlightenment was marked by a rise in scientific ideals. The humanistic and democratic ideals of the French Revolution also influenced the thinking of educated people. Some persons came to view the underclass in a more humane fashion, accepting its members as people deserving consideration, with faith that a scientific approach could ameliorate some of the problems. By the early 19th century, however, problems of welfare forced themselves on public attention. With America's increasing urbanization, the underclass was concentrated in the cities. In the middle 19th century and later, massive immigration compounded the problems. Other social changes due to developing industrialism also aroused concern about human problems (Levine & Levine, 1970).

Wealthy individuals, seeking ways to solve social problems, express personal ideals, or (in some instances) justify the concept that the private concentration of wealth was for the public good, became involved in organizing, systematizing, and reforming institutions. Thus, in the early 19th century, many public and private institutions were developed: mental hospitals, almshouses, workhouses, penitentiaries, and institutions for unwed mothers, orphans, and delinquent youths (Grob, 1973; Rothman, 1971).

Private citizens within cities organized societies to standardized methods of providing charity, overseeing institutions, and trying to coordinate services, which even at that early date threatened to become fractionated. Eventually these local organizations grew into influential national societies. The laymen and volunteers who were involved in them seemed to feel a mixture of fear, contempt, and sympathy for those persons whose care they undertook (Cohen, 1958).

As service organizations developed, and as charity became formalized and expressed through privately-supported local charity organizations, a need developed for full-time salaried workers. The leaders of the social welfare field believed that these workers could be trained to avoid their own past errors, to take advantage of accumulated wisdom, and to apply scientific approaches to make charitable work more efficient and more effective. In the case of relief, they sought to distinguish between the deserving and undeserving poor, so that charitable funds would not be used to support individuals viewed as being idlers, loafers, or other inferior beings. The first workers had been fairly well-to-do volunteers and amateurs who created their own private organizations or served on government commissions. These workers developed into a group which had no precise professional identity. However, as they grew in expertise an identified quasi-professional field developed. The members increasingly sought control over the field, and some had ambitions for professional status. By the early 1900s the first professional schools of social work had been established (Levine & Levine, 1970; Lubove, 1965). There was still room for volunteers in service organizations, and agencies and institutions continued to hire untrained people for most service positions; however, a new pattern of hiring trained persons had been established.

Public and private charities and services continued to exist side by side for some time. By the middle of the 19th century, however, private agencies were unable to manage the myriad of welfare problems, and demands on public agencies grew. Public welfare costs grew simultaneously with a desire on the part of citizens and politicians to centralize control over services with a goal of improving their effectiveness and efficiency. Following a struggle between local and state level authorities, controls emerged in the form of state and local bureaucracies which operated by rules and had a primary concern for limiting costs (Grob, 1973). For workers in the field, these controls meant that their own interests in helping others could be expressed only within the constraints of a formal bureaucratic organization and its supervisory structure.

As the field of social work developed a formal occupational structure with specific salary and benefit levels and with definite training requirements, the people who were attracted were no longer the well-to-do, well-educated reform- and service-minded people. More and more people entered the field who viewed social work as a way to attain social and economic security and personal advancement, as well as a way of expressing a desire to serve. The field was becoming professionalized, and it attracted people with different motivations, and from different backgrounds.

As Wilensky (1964) points out, the process of professionalization leads to an attempt to define training, to define the core functions of a field, and to protect professional turf against the encroachment of other fields. Moreover, the bureaucratic structure of agencies tends to lead each agency to concentrate on certain areas of service. Within those areas workers tend to concentrate their efforts on those people whom they believe they can help with the methods learned in professional schools. Theory, research, and ideology support the idea that to try to help "poor risks" is a waste of scarce resources. While training and the standardization of services was undoubtedly salutory for the field and for the public it served, many problem areas were overlooked. Equally important, some aspects of professionalization and bureaucratization resulted in a loss of vitality and self-renewal in the helping fields.

Personal Experience and Traits as Qualifications

Early leaders recognized that not everyone was equally able to render sympathetic and effective service. Many volunteers provided services in a manner which irritated and put off the recipients of their well-intended offerings. Some individuals, however, seemed to have a natural aptitude for service and could relate well to others, particularly to people who were shunned and rejected by the larger society. Pinel (1806), who removed the chains from mental patients in Parisian institutions after the French Revolution, noted that some individuals worked very well with mental patients, while others had no understanding at all. He preferred ex-patients as attendants.

William Booth, who created the Salvation Army in England in the late 19th century, also understood that personal experience with the problems and circumstances of people who were in need made for a more sympathetic approach. The Salvation Army had a Prison Gate Brigade which met prisoners at the gate as soon as they were released and attempted to provide them with help in reentering the community. He noted that many of his best officers had themselves experienced terms of penal servitude and therefore knew the prison at both ends. He attributed the greatest importance for their effectiveness to the attitudes of the Brigade members toward the ex-convicts (Booth, 1890).

A different, but related, history occurred in the settlement house movement during the late 19th and early 20th centuries in the United States. The first settlement house workers tried to help in the immigrant ghettos and were not indigenous to the communities in which they worked. In fact, many were well-educated, upper-class women, members of the first generation of women to have college and professional educations. These workers moved to the neighborhoods in which they served in order to share as much as they could of the lives of their constituents. They were not trained for their occupation, but they made an enduring commitment; some workers, for example Jane Addams, eventually served as sympathetic communicators of the life-style and problems of the poor to the larger middle class. These were risk-taking individuals who opened themselves to new experiences (Levine & Levine, 1970). What they lacked in early life experience they tried to make up by understanding the culture of those with whom they worked.

An early example of an indigenous nonprofessional who became a salaried paraprofessional was Mrs. Alzina Stevens, a resident in Hull House, the famous settlement in Chicago. Mrs. Stevens had lost the finger of one hand while working as a laborer in a mill as a child. She worked in printing and was active in her union. At Hull House she started working with wayward youth on an informal basis because she related so well to children in difficulty. When, with the assistance of the Hull House group, the first Juvenile Court was established in Chicago in 1899, Mrs. Stevens was a natural choice for the position of Chief Probation Officer (Levine & Levine, 1970).

Thus, personal knowledge, familiarity with the life-style and culture of the people to be served, and traits of sympathy and empathy were recognized as critical for effective services. Yet when human services became a part of a care-giving bureaucracy, these personal qualities were not the major criteria for selecting people for jobs.

The Effects of Bureaucratization and Professionalization

As the provision of help became a full-time occupation, the services which were delivered through formal organizations were frequently affected by their funding sources. As in so many matters, he who pays the piper calls the tune, and changes in services reflected that fact. The early settlement workers, at least those who were in the major centers in New York, Chicago, and Boston, were very much concerned with social reform and community organization. They were activists who fought City Hall for many years. The first workers were also well-to-do individuals who supported themselves. Later, in the 1920s, when the settlement houses were established as voluntary agencies, they developed large budgets requiring stable sources of income; as a result they abandoned controversial work, because in the social climate of the 1920s radical work threatened financial stability. Also, the professionally trained workers who came to take jobs in the settlements in the 1920s were less concerned with social reform. They had been taught methods of casework and group work. Most no longer lived in the neighborhoods they served. While many were sincerely dedicated to their professions, they were no longer part of an exciting, innovative movement. They became more like employees doing a job (Levine & Levine, 1970).

The professionalization of probation workers illustrates recurring themes in the history of paraprofessionals. The earliest practice in the United States comparable to the modern conception of probation was begun by Judge Peter O. Thatcher of Boston, who in 1831 was placing youthful offenders under the supervision of sheriffs, constables, and others (Barnes & Teeters, 1951). Ten years later, John Augustus, a shoemaker, introduced the concept of "friendly supervision" to the Boston courts. Augustus spent much time visiting the courts. He became interested in helping common drunks and other local unfortunates. His technique involved bailing out the offender and/or paying his fine, then using this action as an opening to become involved in the offender's personal life. He would help the offender obtain a job and aid the family in various ways. Apparently a great deal of the expense incurred in this process was covered by Augustus himself from the earnings he made as a shoemaker. Augustus was the first person to use the term "probation." Similar work was carried on by the Massachusetts Children's Aid Society under the direction of Father Rufus R. Cook and Miss L. P. Burnham (Barnes & Teeters, 1951).

Eventually probation became an official legal process, falling under the jurisdiction of the legal bureaucracy. When it did, sheriffs and other law enforcement officers were appointed to the task of supervision. The role of parole officer, with concomitant special training, developed. With its development the process of self-selection based on interest and talent ended.

This trend is illustrated by the history of Mrs. Stevens of Hull House, mentioned previously. She was a model indigenous worker, recognized by her contemporaries for her personal skill in working with children. When a Juvenile Court was established in Chicago in 1899, Mrs. Stevens became its chief probation officer. Even though she was selected for the position because of her personal qualifications and not because of her education or formal training, Mrs. Stevens could not guarantee that persons resembling her would continue to be selected as probation workers. At first probation workers had been paid from private funds and could be selected for personal qualities. A few years later, when the positions had become funded by the State of Illinois, workers were selected by civil service examination. Although the settlement workers had supported civil service as a way of breaking the hold of corrupt municipal political machines, the civil service examination made it difficult to select people for intangible personal qualities. People who could pass civil service examinations were not necessarily those who would do the best job, nor were they the most adventurous and risk-taking. Moreover, because public support for probation was never generous, case loads were very large, and services became relatively ineffective. Civil service probation workers were barred from engaging in preventive work in the community. Even worse, the limitations of the services or of the people offering them were not recognized by the probation workers of that day (Levine & Levine, 1970; Platt, 1969).

Another brief example serves to show how changes in the organizational auspices of services led to change in the service itself. Settlement workers, some of whom were originally trained as teachers, began to do social work within the school in the early 1900s. They worked cooperatively with the schools but had as their organizational base a settlement house. As residents of the neighborhoods, they could easily visit homes during evenings and weekends. Because the program had been successful, the New York Board of Education agreed in 1913 to fund a few positions for social workers. The subsequent social work literature became filled with discussions of qualifications, functions, responsibilities, hours of work, and other organizational issues that never concerned the early settlement workers. When the work was integrated into the organizational setting of the schools, thereby changing its organizational base, the job description also changed. Much of the effort of the early workers to work with the larger community dissipated (Levine & Levine, 1970).

The Culture of the Helper and the Culture of the Client

Not only did the organizational base of services make a difference in the determination of the type of services to be provided, but the organization also limited the selection of people to be trained. The provision of human services is facilitated when helping people relate to clients who are similar to them in culture and life-style. The following examples will show that when greater distance was introduced between the helper and those receiving help, services changed in unanticipated ways.

Worcester State Hospital in Massachusetts opened its doors in 1833 as a model state institution. Its treatment program was called moral therapy and consisted of a regime of regular living, a simple but substantial diet, an emphasis on personal cleanliness, occupational therapy, religious exercises, reading, amusements, and sports. Its chief psychiatrist, Samuel Woodward, emphasized the importance of a mutually respectful relationship between staff and patients. He trained his attendants carefully, gave them important treatment responsibilities, and had these paraprofessionals report directly to him.

The attendants, coming from Worcester, were native American Protestants of English stock, from small towns, as were the bulk of the patients. Although the patients were often indigent, they were still considered to be people very much like the staff. After 1847, Irish Catholic immigrants entered the country in large numbers. Because of the difficult conditions of their lives, they became patients in the mental hospital out of proportion to their numbers. Americans had an unfavorable view of the Irish who had a different language and culture, as well as a history of conflict with the English. Native Americans described the Irish as dirty, ignorant, jealous, drunken debauchers, victims of their own bad habits, rather than as fellow human beings in difficulty because of the onerous conditions of their lives. The staff felt that the Irish did not trust them and that they could not communicate with the Irish. Because the staff found the Irish to be unresponsive, they believed that moral therapy was inapplicable. Eventually moral therapy declined. Hospitals began to emphasize custodial care, and the status of the attendant declined to that of a custodian rather than a paraprofessional actively involved in giving care. There were many reasons for the decline of moral therapy, including overcrowding, a chronic patient population, and reduced resources, but the cultural clash between the native American personnel and the Irish Catholic patients was one of the causes (Grob, 1966).[3]

Another example of the effect of cultural difference between the worker and the client can be seen in the way in which child guidance clinics developed in the 1920s. At first, child guidance clinics were designed to work with low-income families to help prevent delinquency. Within a relatively brief time span, however, child guidance clinics worked less with delinquents and lower-class families and more with middle-class families around less serious problems of adjustment. Two tendencies seem to account for the changes. First, social workers coming into child guidance were being trained in professional schools in casework and in interview methods based on psychoanalytic principles. As the middle-class oriented workers applied the talking therapy they had learned, clients came who were willing and able to use the service that was being offered. In a relatively short time the clientele consisted of middle-class mothers who were able to relate easily to middle-class social workers. As the field of social work upgraded itself, it took some pride in the fact that its clientele came from a better class. The rewards and status accruing to a field are partly determined by the wealth and social status of the clients it serves. Thus, over time social work in the child guidance area changed in emphasis from problems of poverty, delinquency, and school adjustment to more tractable concerns such as those centering on the mother-child relationship (Levine & Levine, 1970). The middle-class social workers were no longer serving as a bridge to link low-income families to the caregiving agencies. Without the bridge, the services which were provided became inappropriate for these families.

The Black Church

The black population in the United States, until relatively recently, was cut off from participation in many professional services. During the period of slavery, blacks for the most part received very little care for mental health or social problems. Following emancipation, they were either not served, or they were segregated in facilities which were typically of lower quality than those available to whites (Grob, 1973). There were undoubtedly blacks who took care of other blacks in need, but little of that effort is recorded in most histories. The black church, however, has always been an important institution for providing services, leadership, mutual support and assistance, and a sense of community among American blacks.

The religion of slaves in the pre-Civil War period was an amalgam of Christian and African beliefs and practices. Scholars (Genovese, 1972; Myrdal, 1964) believe that whites taught blacks Christian religion in order to encourage black submissiveness to authority, but also because some felt genuine concern for their spiritual welfare. In the period after 1750, there was an increased religious revival that extended to blacks, and some black preachers of Christianity appeared on the scene. After Nat Turner, a black preacher, led a slave revolt in 1831, whites continued to teach the Christian religion to blacks, but with greater insistence that instruction and practice be supervised by white preachers. Still some black preachers and religious leaders continued to serve, sometimes surreptitiously.

African cultural beliefs eventually were superceded by Christian beliefs, but characteristics of African culture shaped some practices. Conjurers, root doctors and, in some places, voodoo men and Obeah men (a secret cult of medicine men) provided magic and herbs to help solve problems of the physical body, of the mind, the heart, and of relationships. Some of these practitioners had trained for their roles since childhood, and in that sense were more like professionals than amateurs. Black root and herb doctors sometimes enjoyed a considerable reputation, and occasionally were hired out to treat whites. After emancipation, whites tried to eliminate black medicine altogether, but herb doctors persisted, and some even had a white clientele. In black slave communities the role of preacher was sometimes combined with the role of doctor. These figures (preacher, conjurer, doctor) provided important helping functions within the slave community. They healed the sick, interpreted the unknown, comforted those in pain or sorrow, and were agents for maintaining and transmitting black religious feeling through centuries of oppression. Some scholars believe that the role of preacher attracted the natural leaders in the black community, enabling them to serve their fellows, as well as offering them a route to prestige and power.

In the post-Civil War period, black preachers provided many of the reconstruction era political leaders. With the backlash to reconstruction, black preachers typically became intermediaries between whites and blacks, transmitting white wishes to their congregations, and asking favors of whites for their people. However distasteful this role, it was functional in its time in that it enabled the black preacher to obtain some resources for his community. While not an institution which promoted revolutionary social action, the black church helped to maintain community solidarity, offered a base for some social work, and provided a means for blacks to rise in the world. In more recent days, in the 1950s, the Reverend Adam Clayton Powell of New York City was a leader in sponsoring community welfare in the black community; before his downfall, he exercised considerable political influence in the United States Congress. The role of Martin Luther King, Jr., in the contemporary black civil rights struggle is widely acknowledged, and today a man such as the Reverend Jesse Jackson provides ideas and leadership for black self-help and community organization.

Toward the Present

In the 1930s new problems of public welfare emerged with the deepening depression. Individually-oriented services were of little avail when masses of people were unemployed, when the aged had no source of income, and when state and local resources were strained. During the 1930s public attention was fixed not on individuals in need, but on the development of massive programs of financial assistance such as unemployment insurance, social security, and assistance for dependent women and children. Programs such as the Works Progress Administration (WPA) and the Civilian Conservation Corps (CCC) were designed to make work for people who were unemployed. The emphasis was on employment, not on human services. In any event, by the 1930s patterns of professional employment in welfare, in mental health, in child guidance, and in probation had been well established. Depression era programs did not change the existing pattern of employment in human services.

During the late 1950s and early 1960s human service agencies again discovered that there was a large population of underserved urban poor, and they attempted to deal with the variety of social problems that existed in that population. The discovery of these underserved populations came largely as a result of increased attention to problems of mental health during the years just after World War II. Wartime experience with high rates of neuropsychiatric casualties and high rates of rejection for the draft brought home the importance of mental illness as a national problem. In addition, the state hospitals which had been neglected for many years came under critical scrutiny in the public press as well as in the professional literature. During the war years, the military had experimented successfully with active treatment programs using various methods and drawing personnel from many different fields as therapists. The successful military experience and the increase in resources consequent to public concern led some state hospitals to experiment with similar programs (Brand, 1965; Felix, 1967). Because of the shortage of trained professionals, officials turned to alternative sources for personnel. Specifically in response to the shortage and also in recognition of their demonstrated effectiveness, the Joint Commission on Mental Illness and Health (1961) supported the use of individuals with varied training in treatment roles.

In the late 1950s the nation developed a new awareness of the relationship between social class and mental illness, and of the disparities in the delivery of services to different social classes (Hollingshead & Redlich, 1958). Within the social welfare field, growing costs of public welfare and growing numbers of cases of mothers with illegitimate children, concentrated in black populations in the cities and in white populations in rural areas, led to concern about whether the welfare system itself was sufficient to do the job (Steiner, 1966). In particular, Michael Harrington's book, *The Other America* (1962), influenced President Kennedy's recognition that problems of mental illness and retardation were intimately associated with poverty. Other emergency concerns included the rising rates of juvenile delinquency, adolescent gang wars in our cities, and problems in our schools. Efforts were made to work on these problems through the Ford Foundation programs (Marris & Rein, 1967) and through programs developed consequent to the Juvenile Delinquency Control Act. As attempts were made to redevelop cities through urban renewal programs, many of the human problems of poverty became apparent. The bulldozers that leveled the worst slums also uncovered the deplorable conditions of those who lived in the deteriorated areas. In an effort to ameliorate these conditions, "human renewal" programs were developed, again through the Ford Foundation and later through Community Action Agencies established under the Economic Opportunity Act of 1964. Housing acts, welfare amendments, and efforts to provide training and retraining for people in poverty led to further expansion of human service programs (Levitan, 1969; Sarason, Levine, Goldenberg, Cherlin, & Bennett, 1966). It was natural that this antipoverty effort looked toward a nonprofessional source of personnel to meet the needs of rapidly expanding human service agencies.

The history of paraprofessionals in the community mental health movement followed a course similar to that in the antipoverty program. Albee's (1959) work on the mental health manpower shortage stimulated many mental health professionals to attempt new and creative ways of dealing with this shortage.

INDIGENOUS PARAPROFESSIONALS IN THE 1960s

Both the antipoverty program and the community mental health movement were designed to effect positive change in the lives of underprivileged, poor, and disadvantaged minority persons in America. In the case of the antipoverty program the intention was to aid the poor to gain access to the mainstream economy. In the case of the community mental health movement, the intention was to deliver mental health services to a population which presumably could benefit from these services, but rarely utilized them in their existing forms. Both mental health and antipoverty programs used the indigenous paraprofessional to facilitate these ends because of the belief in the inadequacy of traditional modes of service delivery managed and staffed by traditionally trained professionals.

Several characteristics define the indigenous paraprofessional of the 1960s. First, he or she is a member of the target population and has similar values, language, experience, and family background to those typifying the client population. Second, as a result of this background, he or she possesses an ability to identify, and to deal directly and effectively with clients who might not accept a professional. Third, he or she can communicate effectively with agency professionals. Fourth, he or she does not possess the training or credentials of the professional.

The Antipoverty Program

The antipoverty program, as documented by Moynihan (1969), originated in part from the Kennedy Administration's concern with juvenile delinquency and in part from two older programs, the Ford Foundation's "grey areas" program and the Mobilization for Youth program in New York City. Both of the latter programs emphasized a community organization approach to the problems of poverty and juvenile delinquency that plagued urban areas. This community organization principle was eventually translated into the "maximum feasible participation" clause of the 1964 Economic Opportunity Act and became one of the bases for the utilization of indigenous paraprofessionals by community action agencies.

The emphasis on employment of indigenous paraprofessionals was related to two hypotheses. First, indigenous paraprofessionals were perceived as having special competence in mediating between the agency and the client population; they were members of that population and, therefore, presumably possessed a deeper understanding of its problems and characteristics than did middle-class professionals. Second, by hiring individuals from the target population, the agency was attacking the very heart of poverty itself—unemployment. The paraprofessional thus became a "rescued" segment of the target population who could further augment the escape of others from the poverty cycle.

The latter hypothesis formed the basis of the "New Careers" proposal of the middle 1960s. A simple definition of the New Careers approach is providing human service delivery jobs for the unskilled and uneducated poor which will allow ample opportunity for career advancement (Pearl & Riessman, 1965).

The New Careers concept placed emphasis on employment. As jobs developed in service agencies, job descriptions, training and career advancement became important issues, while emphasis on the personal characteristics of the indigenous worker was reduced considerably. The extent to which this new emphasis may have influenced the selection process of paraprofessionals is not yet clear. Selection conceivably began to favor those persons who could successfully negotiate the career ladder. Yet abilities useful in such negotiation, particularly academic abilities, were not necessarily the abilities most valuable for the paraprofessional worker in the role of mediator between lower-income groups and middle-class care-giving agencies.

Another factor contributing to the growing number of paraprofessionals was the civil rights movement. Black activists argued that only blacks could represent other blacks in a meaningful way, and they insisted that black workers be hired to deal with the black clientele. The community action agencies, often already involved in the political organizing and confrontations with local power structures, became the focus of community political activities. When the ghettos later exploded in rioting, these agencies, rightly or wrongly, were often linked with the violence. A horrified reaction to the riots set in, and combined with local political hostility, caused a backlash of bureaucratization that changed the hiring picture radically. Not as many positions were available. No longer was hiring left entirely to the discretion of the agency directors; antipoverty programs were tied more closely to the local governmental structure and to the local civil service system. The focus in personnel selection changed from an emphasis on personal attributes to something more like a standardized civil service procedure. Whereas the earlier, and less formalized system allowed for selection because of personal characteristics, neighborhood reputations, and other intangibles (including political connections at times), civil service procedures rewarded test taking and other skills related to the attainment of educational credentials. Those skills were only peripherally related to the tasks which paraprofessionals were expected to perform. The parallel between this sequence of events and the previous developments involving amateur and nonprofessional care givers is obvious.

The Community Mental Health Movement

Different groups in the community mental health movement approached the manpower problems documented by Albee (1959), with different premises. In an experiment at Harvard over several years, college students worked as volunteers in mental health settings (Umbarger, Dalsimer, Morrison, & Breggin, 1962). At about the same time, at the Connecticut Valley Hospital in Middletown, Holzberg also began experimenting with college student volunteers. He demonstrated that after their experiences volunteers showed more sympathetic attitudes toward mental illness, made fewer moral judgments about people's behavior, and showed greater self-acceptance (Holzberg, Knapp, & Turner, 1967).

Margaret Rioch (1967) developed an innovative project for the training of mental health counselors at the National Institute of Mental Health. Rioch, a psychiatrist, selected middle-aged, college-educated women as her paraprofessional personnel, and exposed them to an elaborate two-year training program concentrating on psychotherapy and counseling. Follow-up studies over a number of years revealed these women functioned quite ably in several mental health settings. However, their previous educations combined with the special training they had received made them comparable to people who would ordinarily work toward professional degrees in social work or psychology (Magoon, Golann, & Freeman, 1969).

While Rioch's counselors showed there was a large pool of potential trainees for outpatient work in the mental health fields, there still existed a need to develop personnel to undertake inpatient treatment programs in institutions. Sanders (1967), who had had experience with socioenvironmental programs in a Veterans Administration Hospital, decided to establish such a program in a large state hospital which had come under public criticism because of its inadequate conditions. Sanders argued that a major problem facing anyone who wished to develop a treatment program was the calibre of personnel attracted to the custodial duties assigned to most of the attendants in the state hospitals. During the Second World War, personnel shortages had affected the hospitals strongly. In some instances, judges gave vagrants the choice of going to jail or taking positions as attendants in state hospitals. In an effort to upgrade the position and attract better qualified candidates, Sanders developed a program aimed at college graduates. The program provided a stipend for a training period and then a full-time job in the state hospital in situations that allowed therapeutic rather than custodial care. Sanders reported positive evaluations of the program and indicated that it would be necessary to establish career development positions within the state system, if the program were to continue to attract and to hold well-qualified workers.

There are examples in which professionalization tendencies did *not* change the original goals and foci of service delivery systems using paraprofessionals. One such example is Klein's (1967) program to recruit, train, and employ human service aides and assistants in child care centers, schools, neighborhood recreation projects, and social research projects. Klein worked with black youth, referred by youth agencies. His group did not attempt to be selective, but accepted many people as trainees who, because of previous histories of instability in school or in employment, looked as if they might be poor risks. The youth were selected because they shared in the "street culture" of those they would serve. Because of their backgrounds, it was necesary to develop a special approach in training. Training emphasized generic skills of observation and recording of observations; ability to relate to supervisors and to use supervision; understanding of community agencies and services; and instruction in interpersonal relationships. The training program oriented the recruits to the work they were to do and taught them relevant skills experientially rather than through reading. In addition, it simultaneously aimed to provide the trainees with experiences which would broaden their horizons—to help them learn about themselves, their community, and indeed, the wider world. For example, the trainees visited educational, social, and cultural institutions. Most of Klein's trainees responded very well to the challenge and the opportunity. Given encouragement and real prospects of desirable employment, many of his poor risk recruits blossomed.

Another example of a paraprofessional program which consciously avoided professionalization and bureaucratization is described by Goldenberg (1971). Goldenberg recognized that in order for a service to be effective, it had to take into account the needs for growth and development not only of the clients, but especially of the staff. Goldenberg had been working as a consultant to a program sponsored by Community Progress, Inc. (CPI), the pioneer antipoverty agency in New Haven, Connecticut. He noticed that many of the paraprofessionals were dissatisified because of constraints that were placed on their work. The problems were aggravated when CPI added a professional social service unit to its neighborhood centers. Goldenberg and the work crew foremen, the paraprofessionals with whom he was working, visited one of the first Job Corps Centers and were disappointed with it. On their return to New Haven, the group decided to develop within the city an alternative to the Job Corps.

Goldenberg's book, *Build Me a Mountain,* describes the development of the Residential Youth Center. When he undertook to develop the center, he articulated a number of principles aimed at overcoming what he perceived as the stultifying effects of service organizations. Two of these principles are discussed here. First, he felt that many service organizations suffered because the important decision-making responsibility for clients rested with people who had little daily contact with the clients. He, therefore, gave every paraprofessional final responsibility for dispositions of their clients. They had an obligation to consult others on their team, but the final responsibility was theirs. Second, he believed that the center should make provision for the personal and "professional" growth of all of its members. Therefore, all staff members (Goldenberg was the only professional) had several program responsibilities in addition to their primary jobs. Staff members rotated through administrative assignments and shared all duties, including night and weekend assignments at the Residential Center. Staff members also participated in sensitivity and growth programs which focused on issues that were developing at the center and on the relationships among the staff. Goldenberg's staff not only worked exceptionally well with the most difficult client population but it maintained its morale and demonstrated effectiveness.

His primary contribution was his ability to articulate the conditions under which people working in a service setting could truly do their jobs and to translate this understanding into reality. His work is in sharp contrast to tendencies to write job descriptions in great detail or to have people who do not share the tasks given to the paraprofessionals supervise them in their work. In short, the success of Goldenberg's program may be attributable to its non-stratification; in contrast to other situations, where paraprofessionals served merely as a bridge between a low-income population and professional care givers, the power in Goldenberg's agency remained with the paraprofessionals.

Thus, in the late 1950s and the early 1960s there were many fruitful experiments in the use of paraprofessional personnel in a variety of fields. One study (Sobey, 1970) reported there were over 10,000 paraprofessionals working in projects funded by the National Institute of Mental Health. Paraprofessional personnel were used in therapeutic roles in city and suburban settings, clinics, hospitals, schools (e.g., Cowen, Trost, Izzo, Lorion, Dorr, & Isaacson, 1975), and social agencies. Moreover, various projects demonstrated that it was possible to find capable human service workers from among the ranks of the well-educated, and the less well-educated, from among blacks and whites, from among males and females, and from among younger and older groups. Most of these programs initially provided their own recruiting, orientation, training, and supervision. These programs also reported benefits to the paraprofessional human service providers, as well as to the client populations. However, they also pointed to the necessity for developing meaningful career tracks and career ladders if employees in the developing field of human services were not to find themselves in dead-end jobs after a few years.

Since the middle 1960s the emphasis in paraprofessional utilization has turned more and more to the New Careers model. To some extent this model may have enhanced the tendency for paraprofessionals to think in ways typical of most workers—importance of salaries and fringe benefits, advancement, maintenance, and survival of the agency. In doing so, they become increasingly like the professionals whose work they were originally intended to facilitate (Gartner & Riessman, 1974).

Training and employment programs for paraprofessionals were supported by several legislative acts during the 1960s. The most important of these acts consisted of the 1966 Scheuer Amendments to the Economic Opportunity Act. This legislation empowered the Department of Labor to promote the career development of persons in such fields as health, education, and welfare.

Building upon earlier efforts within its own organization, the National Institute of Mental Health, in 1971, began a formalized program of support for New Careers training programs in mental health. The goals of this program were threefold: (a) the improvement of mental health services for neglected population groups; (b) the development and institutionalization of accredited work-based education/training programs; and (c) the development and institutionalization of a manpower development, utilization, and career opportunity system. The training program attempted to link academic skills with the actual learning on the job. Paid time off was given to attend classes, which were sometimes held at local colleges and sometimes at the work site. Credit was also given for on-the-job, in-service training and, in some cases, for previous life experience. A recently published empirical study (Blanton & Alley, 1977) of New Careers programs pinpoints factors that contribute to program success, while a monograph (Cohen, 1976) provides an examination of the longer term evolution of the New Careers movement.

It has become unclear whether the paraprofessionals can or should continue to function in their previous manner, or whether they will adopt the function of the professionals. This ambiguity is reflected by the tremendous growth of associate degree (and some bachelor's-level) training programs during the 1970s. People trained in these programs are truly a new breed of paraprofessionals, less frequently indigenous to low-income communities, and therefore less likely to be expected to play the bridging role which had previously been a major function of most paraprofessional workers. An examination of the development of this new approach, and its impact on the mental health field, is necessary for an understanding of the utilization of paraprofessionals today.

IMPACT OF ASSOCIATE DEGREE PARAPROFESSIONALS

Many nonprofessionals and paraprofessionals have been utilized in mental health work, but only the associate degree workers (and those individuals enrolled in New Careers programs) have had a formal program of academic and clinical training to prepare them for their jobs. Thus, unlike other paraprofessionals whose identity as a group may be limited to a community, a special population, or a specific agency in which they share experience, the associate degree workers have a group identity which cuts across state lines as well as specific agency boundaries. In fact, since they hold academic degrees and hence share a formal group identity, it is reasonable to view the associate degree workers as the most "professional" of the paraprofessionals. Their specific training not only makes them distinct from other paraprofessional groups, but also gives them greater legitimacy with which to bargain in a service delivery system controlled by professionals. Their existence as a group may well have exciting implications for both the delivery of human services and the way in which other human service professionals will be trained for service in the future.

Since 1966 when the first associate degree mental health worker program was initiated at Purdue University, the number of such programs has grown to over 170 (Southern Regional Education Board [SREB], 1976). These programs had graduated an estimated 15,000 persons as of June, 1975, and at least 4,000–5,000 more graduates are currently expected each year (SREB, 1975; Young, True, & Packard, 1976). While the majority of current human service associate degree programs are oriented to mental health, they are also being established in other areas, such as gerontology, corrections, social work, child care, and education (SREB, 1975).

Perhaps the major factor which set the stage for the emergence of the associate degree programs was George Albee's (1959) analysis of the gross shortages of health and mental health personnel, an analysis which called attention to a national human services manpower crisis. The revelation that it would be impossible to train enough workers in traditional professional programs to meet projected service needs helped to create a favorable climate for the development of innovative training approaches.

Encouraged by evidence that persons with relatively little formal training could play valuable roles in delivering human services (Fort Logan Mental Health Center, Note 1; Matarazzo, 1971), planners in various regions of the country established the first associate degree training programs. Their goal was not only to train large numbers of personnel in a relatively short period of time, but also to train a new type of human services worker, the "generalist." The key aspects of the generalist concept are the training of workers in a wide variety of generic helping skills and their preparation to serve the whole client. In order to serve the whole client the generalist training model aims to enable workers to carry through a coordinated treatment plan which integrates the efforts of highly specialized professionals (Felton, Wallach, & Gallo, 1974; McPheeters & King, 1971).

The curriculum in human services associate degree programs differs from traditional professional programs in that it places greater emphasis on the development of self-awareness and practical helping skills, and less emphasis on theory or research skills. To heighten students' self-awareness and interpersonal sensitivity, many programs utilize T-group sessions, sensitivity training, and experiential methods (e.g., role-playing) (Simon, Note 2; SREB, 1975). This approach represents a concerted effort by program planners to develop sensitive workers with humanistic attitudes toward clients (Hadley, True, & Kepes, 1970; McPheeters & King, 1971). To sharpen practical skills, course work is heavily applied in nature (e.g., interviewing, establishing token economies, etc.) and is coordinated with extensive field placement experiences (Danzig, 1970; Lubetkin, Note 3; SREB, 1975; True, Young, & Packard, Note 4).

Thus, like other paraprofessionals the associate degree worker is intended to have certain qualities which distinguish him or her from professionals. First, the associate degree worker is a *doer* rather than a theoretician or researcher. Second, these workers are trained as generalists rather than as highly specialized professionals, so that they can provide continuity of care and deal with almost any of the clients' needs. Finally, the workers are trained in these programs to acquire a high level of personal and interpersonal sensitivity. Program directors deliberately attempt to select applicants who demonstrate such qualities. The goal is to produce individuals who will have the ability to establish that same kind of strong personal rapport with clients which has traditionally been a hallmark of the good paraprofessional worker.

These findings have emerged from a recent national survey of associate degree program graduates who received their degrees prior to 1972 (Young et al., 1976: their mean age was 30; 83% were female; slightly over half (56%) were married; and minorities constituted only 20% of the sample (blacks, 16%; Chicanos, 3%; and American Indians, 1%). Most of the graduates had had considerable previous experience in the human service field. Another national survey, which was conducted to obtain basic demographic data on students enrolled in programs during 1972 and 1973 (True, Young, & Packard, Note 4; Note 5), reported several important trends. First, the percentage of both younger students and minority students entering associate degree programs is increasing. Furthermore, the proportion of male students enrolled in programs is also rising and was estimated to have increased from 17% in 1973 to 26% by 1976.

These trends are positive signs for the development of associate degree training programs. Traditionally, both males and minorities have been under-represented at the paraprofessional level in the human services system (Alley & Blanton, 1976). The continuation of these trends is important to insure that the associate degree training movement meets its goal of providing a route into the system for previously untapped sources of manpower.

One final trend noted in the most recent survey (Young et al., 1976) was that increasing numbers of students are entering associate degree programs directly from high school. This finding suggests that these programs are beginning to be perceived as a legitimate opportunity to embark on a human services career. Of course, the adoption of a career orientation means that graduates will be more seriously concerned with increasing their opportunities for advancement. Advancement within a service system dominated by professionals depends heavily on academic credentials. Given these realities, some states, most notably Maryland, have developed career ladders which include associate, bachelor, and even masters level "generalist" training programs (Vidaver & Carson, Note 6). Clearly such developments represent a movement toward increasing professionalization for these new human service workers.

A further indication of increasing professionalization is that the Southern Regional Education Board was funded in 1977 to develop models and mechanisms for certification of mental health worker training programs and their graduates. The expansion of associate degree training took place rapidly, resulting in a distinct lack of coherence among existing programs. One consequence of this situation is that the utility of the associate degree worker to potential human service employers varies greatly from one community to another even within a single state. The goal of the Southern Regional Education Board's efforts is to facilitate the development of associate degree programs of a uniformly high quality. Such an outcome would be likely to improve both the respectability and marketability of the associate degree human services worker.

As suggested earlier, the associate degree graduates represent a new breed of human services worker. While they are clearly not highly specialized professionals, their academic degree and formal training also make them distinct from the traditional paraprofessional. Thus, at present they are in some sense a hybrid paraprofessional-professional. As associate degree workers pursue higher academic degrees and greater specialization, however, the balance of their identities may shift more toward that of the professional. Given this trend, it may become increasingly difficult for these new human service workers to retain those special, desired qualities which have long characterized the unique and invaluable contribution of the paraprofessional in human services. Thus, while there are many practical advantages to increasing professionalization of the generalist human services worker, those directing this trend should give serious consideration to the potential negative consequences as well.

Integration of Associate Degree Workers into Professional Service Systems

In spite of the fact that most associate degree programs have focused on training graduates to perform in innovative roles (client advocate, client-community liaison), the majority of graduates are carrying out traditional functions (True et al., Note 5; Young et al., 1976). This fact has been a source of dissatisfaction for many associate degree workers and the administrators of their training programs. It is simply not easy to integrate nontraditionally trained personnel into service agencies which are traditional in orientation.

In keeping with the observation of Levine and Levine (1970) that clinical services are profoundly shaped by their setting, the extent and nature of innovation has varied a great deal, depending on the orientation of the agencies involved. The more traditionally oriented settings (e.g., state hospitals) have tended to utilize the associate degree graduate in traditional roles: interviewer, therapist, and data manager (Drucker & Drag, Note 7; True et al., Note 5). Nevertheless, even these settings have incorporated one aspect of the "generalist" model in that they have typically utilized the new workers in multiple roles. Further, administrators of these programs have indicated that they appreciate the versatility of the associate degree worker and see possibilities for greater innovation in the future. In particular, they have mentioned that the associate degree workers' training in community care would make them especially valuable in providing services to the increasing numbers of individuals being deinstitutionalized by state mental health and mental retardation facilities (Young et al., 1976). Thus, even where the associate degree workers have not always stimulated the development of innovative service delivery, their training seems to have provided them with the potential to play key roles when new service patterns are developed.

In less tradition-bound settings (e.g., community mental health centers) graduates of associate degree programs have reported assuming a number of innovative roles, including those of client advocate, outreach worker, and in-service educator of aides and attendants (True et al., Note 5). Such reports indicate that it is possible to meet both facets of the goal of training generalist workers: (a) providing a source of manpower capable of performing multiple roles in diverse settings, and (b) providing clients with advocates who can help them to receive more comprehensive, continuous care for the human service system.

The ultimate impact of associate degree workers in a human service setting, however, is not determined only by their personal capabilities and the orientation of the setting. It also depends upon how they are integrated into the organization. Depending on how this integration takes place, it is conceivable that in some settings associate degree workers will function as little more than subspecialist assistants to specialized professionals. If this outcome should occur, the generalist-trained graduates will become psychologist or social work "assistants" who are likely to have little innovative impact upon the service delivery patterns of the given agencies.

One excellent example of an agency-based strategy to support the generalist role is the Dayton State Hospital in Ohio (Krauss, 1971). The hospital hired 20 associate degree workers. Rather than splitting them up, it organized these workers into a new Mental Health Technician Department, with an individual from the group of paraprofessionals serving as a department director. In this manner, the workers were better able to maintain their identity as generalists and, consequently, could provide comprehensive and continuous care for clients.

In summary, there is evidence that associate degree workers can be a force for innovation in the human service system. The extent and nature of their impact, however, will vary depending on three interacting factors: training of individual workers, the orientation of the setting in which they are employed, and the manner in which they are integrated into the organization (Intagliata, 1978).

The associate degree training movement has generated implications for the training of professionals. Associate degree workers have typically been trained as generalists in programs that employ faculty members from several disciplines. Given that the boundaries between the helping roles of traditional human services professionals have become increasingly blurred and artificial (Schulberg, 1972), the interdisciplinary, generalist model of training is seemingly more appropriate. Since it is likely that the responsibilities of traditional human service professionals will continue to shift away from the provision of direct client services and toward greater involvement in training, supervision, and coordination, it will become increasingly important for professionals within each discipline to be familiar with the background, capabilities, and perspectives of other professional and paraprofessional care providers. Thus, though they are unlikely to abandon their "specialist" orientation for a generalist model, it would not be surprising to see more graduate level training programs for professionals follow the lead of associate degree programs by incorporating an increasingly interdisciplinary focus (Intagliata, 1978).

ANTHROPOLOGICAL PERSPECTIVES

In order to expand our scope, it is fruitful to look at the functions and utilization of paraprofessionals and nonprofessionals in other cultures. The present discussion will be limited largely to preliterate cultures and developing countries. For the most part, the concept of a paraprofessional is not found in preliterate or developing societies. Specifically, there are few reports of individuals being trained as aides or helpers to professional care givers. However, many societies make extensive use of "amateurs," who function independently of the professional care givers. These amateur care givers will be discussed more extensively below.

In addition to the untrained amateurs, there is also a well-developed system of professional care giving, involving people variously described as native healers, shamans, medicine men, and witch doctors. Although a detailed description of the work of these professionals will not be given here (for a full description, see Torrey, 1972), it must be emphasized that these individuals are professionals. They have mastered a body of knowledge, undergone a specified training sequence, formed professional associations, and established a schedule of fees for services. In spite of these professional characteristics, Western professionals often think of native healers as paraprofessionals and have attempted to use them as auxiliaries in Western-type health care delivery systems. This use, however, is not consistent with the definition of paraprofessional services developed in this chapter; in fact, there is little evidence of the presence of paraprofessionals consistent with that definition in preliterate or developing countries. However, an examination of the use of *nonprofessionals* is relevant to the goals of this chapter.

Amateur Counseling

There are at least two distinct forms of amateur counseling in preliterate and developing societies. The first form involves a type of group, called a "possession cult" (Kiev, 1964; Torrey, 1972) which is similar to self-help groups in the West. An example is the Zar cult of Ethiopia.[4] When an individual (usually a female) is striken with Zar illness (a loosely defined condition generally characterized by apathy, withdrawal, and sometimes by excitement and homicidal impulses), she is initiated into the Zar cult in order to help her deal with what she is told are unfriendly spirits who have caused her illness. Members of the Zar group offer new initiates the feeling of a common bond with peers, "the sympathy of fellow-sufferers" and "opportunities to find interpersonal response and recognition" (Messing, 1959). The following quotation highlights the similarity between the Zar cult and self-help groups in the West:

> By identifying the specific ailment, learning to accept it and live with it, the patient-devotee of the Zar cult perceives and organizes his instinctual impulses into thoughts and language that enable him to function properly in relationship to his environment. His former compulsive behavior is no longer compulsory, once the individual is aware of it and has a genuine feeling that there is an element of choice and manipulation (Messing, 1959, p. 319).

In addition, like Western self-help groups, most notably Alcoholics Anonymous, the Zar cult has a system of peer sponsorship whereby a new member is assigned two "mize," or older members, who serve as "human protectors."

A second form of nonprofessional counseling is exemplified by a system akin to crisis intervention counseling found in rural villages of Ghana. Individuals or families approach selected community members and ask for a meeting the following dawn to discuss a problem.[5] It is believed that dawn is the best time to counsel because after sleep "body and mind become renewed." Thus, if anyone brings up an important problem at another time, the person is told "this is a dawn matter; therefore let us allow the dew to fall on it."

Dawn counselors are nonprofessionals and have no special training. Their selection, however, is based on specific qualities, namely age, "intelligence, diligence, patience, calmness, consideration for others, sympathy and eloquence." Typically an older man in an extended family is the family's counselor. When a family elder is disqualified because he lacks a quality or because he cannot establish a close relationship with those persons who might seek him out, a younger man who stands out in the family is selected. The older man becomes his nominal resource. Other people such as parents, aunts, uncles, spouse, the tribal chief and friends can also be recognized as counselors if they are likely to be the most helpful individuals in special situations.

Dawn counseling is used both to prevent and solve problems. In the area of prevention, counseling takes place regularly at times of transition like childbirth, puberty, leaving home, marriage, or the death of a family member. In premarriage counseling, for example, the couple might be told to anticipate disagreements, to understand that husband and wife will have words with each other, to know that it is not a bad thing to approach elders for help at times of crisis, and, most important of all, to promise to never stop talking to each other and to be honest.

Problem-solving counseling typically follows a specific crisis event, such as a family quarrel or transgression, but sometimes it is requested when an ongoing situation increases in severity (e.g., a husband noticing that his wife is becoming more depressed). Counseling is usually completed in one session, although it is not uncommon to schedule additional meetings for more talking or for what might be called follow-up services.

The purpose of dawn counseling is to communicate to the client the attitudes of the society and to appeal to one's sense of judgment so that the individual will be able to effect significant personal change. Counseling frequently employs short stories to cite examples from the society of solutions or responses to the situation being discussed. Although a detailed description of dawn counseling is beyond the scope of this chapter, it is clear that this type of counseling represents an ongoing, established cultural "institution" involving nonprofessional care givers.

Professionals and Paraprofessionals in Developing Countries

How do the roles of professionals and nonprofessionals in a developing country compare to the roles of these two groups in the United States? An important difference exists. In the United States, nonprofessionals and paraprofessionals have been used mainly to provide service to underserved populations or to provide a vital bridge between those populations and the professional care givers. In preliterate and developing societies, the indigenous *professionals* share the same culture as the vast majority of their clients, and they are reportedly effective as treatment providers. Paraprofessionals therefore are unnecessary. In addition, because there is little likelihood that within the indigenous system the "amateurs" will use their avocation as counselors to acquire higher status or employment, the type of services offered by these people appears to be safe from "professionalization."

As developing countries become modernized, and Western models of mental health care are established, an increasing number of professionals receive foreign training. They are finding that their models for treatment are very different from those of the clients whom they are attempting to treat. Unfortunately, the reaction of many expatriate professionals has too often been to ignore the indigenous conceptions of disease and to utilize their own models (Kreisman, 1975). Competition often develops between these professionals and their indigenous counterparts. Noting the effectiveness of indigenous healers, Wintrob and Wittkower (1968) concluded, "Whether he likes it or not, the psychiatrist in countries progressing through transitional stages of their development has to tolerate the role or function of the native healer and may be forced to cooperate with him." Similarly, Shakman (1969) has reported that Phillipine physicians have labored "to break the power of the indigenous healers." Even what looks like cooperation may, at times, be only toleration. If the native professionals are subsumed into new care giving bureaucracies created by the group trained in foreign countries, they will be "deprofessionalized" and used primarily in an ancillary status. Such use of professionals as paraprofessionals reflects cultural condescension rather than an attempt to improve communication across cultural barriers or to improve service delivery. The frequency of such problems is cause for concern in some developing countries.

Some complementary and cooperative relationships between traditional and modern care givers, however, can be found. Lambo, a Nigerian psychiatrist, utilizes both indigenous care giving systems and Western style methods. He states openly that native treatment centers "do a better job with functional cases, whether neurotic or psychotic," than he can accomplish with his Western methods of psychotherapy (Lederer, 1959). Lambo does not employ the native healers either as aides or as auxiliaries working within the Western treatment context. Rather, these native healers work as professionals in an independent care giving system, thus retaining their autonomy and their identity. Similarly, Dean and Thong (1972) report that shamans and psychiatrists in Bali work together, with each group treating cases that are most appropriate to their training.

What can one learn from these reports that show an extensive use of nonprofessionals and indigenous professionals yet an absence of paraprofessionals in developing countries? Given the relatively homogeneous nature of the societies, the native professional care giver and the nonprofessional counselor are still very much members of their communities. If Westernized professional models of care giving are adopted simultaneously with the occurrence of economic development and changing social relations, Westernized professionals in developing countries may find themselves out of touch with the beliefs, attitudes, and values of many persons in the communities they serve. When that happens, we may see the developing countries inventing paraprofessional roles.

Paraprofessionals in the People's Republic of China

One country that seems to have succeeded in integrating professionals, paraprofessionals, and self-help groups into a single coordinated mental health system is the People's Republic of China. The People's Republic developed an elaborate political and social organization which extends to neighborhood levels. The local groups serve many purposes, among them the provision of health and mental health services. Paraprofessionals diagnose, treat, refer, and help to reintegrate discharged mental patients back into their groups. Recognizing they could not produce a sufficient number of professionals to provide adequate service and also recognizing deficiencies in Western service delivery systems, the Chinese organized and strengthened indigenous self-help groups and natural support systems. Goplerud (Note 8) states that "where self-help groups already existed, they were given responsibilities for a wide range of primary health care activities. Where they did not already exist (e.g., in psychiatric hospitals, prisons, and schools) self-help groups are now used extensively. Examples are: mobilizing mass participation in preventive health activities, treating emotional disturbances of individuals in the local communities, and treating severely disturbed persons in psychiatric wards.

This development of local self-help groups within the context of an extended, decentralized, community-controlled network of paraprofessionals has enabled the Chinese to provide extensive health resources to all people. Historically, this development followed unsuccessful attempts, from 1949 to 1965, to adopt the Western medical model. The Western model did not adequately serve the majority of people, especially those who were poor or living in rural areas. Prior to 1949 China's health system had been similar to those of the preliterate societies described above, and had relied primarily on folk medicine and family welfare support systems.

Along with the extensive paraprofessional system, based in the community, China has utilized native healers and their folk medicine. In fact, strenuous efforts have been directed toward uniting Western and Chinese medical techniques and approaches. Professionals and paraprofessionals alike have become responsible for training and supervising colleagues who lacked their skills and experience. In addition, as they gained experience and further training and education, nonprofessionals and paraprofessionals have been able themselves to become medical doctors. So far observers of the Chinese system have reported neither the mistrust and hostility which has traditionally separated mental health professionals and self-help groups in our country, nor the problems that developed from the "bridging" efforts utilizing paraprofessionals in the United States. There are, however, some signs of dissatisfaction with the system in post-Mao China. Most recently observers report a tendency to rely more on trained professionals rather than on peasant or worker wisdom. It is too soon to say what the effects might be on the overall system.

An American Version

Although the evolution of paraprofessionals in the revolutionary economic and political context of China may not be entirely transferable to other countries, some elements may be appropriate. These elements include the efforts to unite Western and indigenous therapeutic systems; the use of professionals and paraprofessionals alike to train, supervise, educate and provide service; and the use of local self-help groups as a legitimate base for providing curative and preventative health care services, with paraprofessionals and professionals available as needed.

A program in the United States that seems to be utilizing many of these ideas is the Jackson Memorial Community Mental Health Center in Miami (Bestman, Lefley, & Scott, Note 9; Lefley & Bestman, Note 10). At this center, separate teams serve black Americans, Bahamians, Cubans, Haitians, Puerto Ricans, and elderly Anglos. Each team is staffed by indigenous paraprofessionals and directed by social scientists; all members of each team are matched ethnically and culturally to the populations served. Thus, the team is better able to provide culturally appropriate treatment modalities. The community mental health center offers a variety of services, including: a network of culturally homogeneous mini-clinic drop-in centers, group therapy within a social-recreational context, involvement of extended family in family therapy, merger of traditional and scientific techniques in psychotherapy, knowledge and experience with the particular cultural norms as well as such belief systems as Obeah, Vodun, Espiritismo, Santeria, and Rootwork, and consultation with and referral to folk healers. In short, the community mental health center appears to offer a model which in every component incorporates cultural variables and uses indigenous paraprofessionals effectively in providing culturally appropriate psychotherapeutic and environmental interventions.

CONCLUSIONS

The historical and cross-cultural examples direct attention to the relationship among paraprofessionals, professionals and the organization of services. The amateurs who began services in the U.S.A. or those who function as helpers in natural support systems in preliterate or developing cultures entered the work out of a sense of personal calling. They succeeded because of personal traits as well as an ability to understand and participate in the culture and life styles of those who received assistance. Looked at from an historical and cross-cultural perspective, paraprofessionals were not simply cheaper, less thoroughly trained professionals; rather they were individuals who contributed unique skills, perspectives, affiliations, and/or motivations that resulted in the development and delivery of more relevant and accessible services.

Amateurs and paraprofessionals have frequently served a bridging function between those in need and those who controlled the resources of the society. When the bridging function was successful, it led to the creation of a social institution, with a commitment of public resources to do the work the amateurs began. In most instances, particularly in the United States, it was not anticipated that key aspects of a service would change once the service was absorbed into the culture and social organization of the larger society. For example, the new social organization was compelled to employ a different selection process from the one which brought people into the field originally, and it also provided different conditions of work. In the United States, that process led to a separation of workers from those who received their assistance. In China, the process of separation was apparently reversed when Mao became concerned that Westernized social organization was removing services from the control of the people. In Africa, the dawn counselor remains part of traditional village culture and has not yet been separated out. There seems to be some danger that when the paraprofessional function is institutionalized, the individual paraprofessionals themselves become assimilated into the larger culture. Thus, undesired changes may occur during the institutionalization process unless special care is taken to appreciate the unique characteristics and functions of the paraprofessional.

In the United States, service agencies are dominated by professionals who occupy the most powerful, the most prestigious and highly paid positions. Since professional values and practices dominate the service scene, it is not surprising that paraprofessionals would want to identify with and become like professionals. Career ladders, pay structures, and supervisory structures all emphasize, perhaps unintentionally, that the paraprofessional is the low person on the totem pole, and that his or her status can improve only by becoming more like the professional. Training programs may inadvertently teach the paraprofessional to become more like the professional, thereby underscoring the power and status differentials often present in the relationship between the two sets of workers.

This historical and cross-cultural survey suggests that those persons responsible for the development of paraprofessional functions need to give some thought to the conditions of work which would preserve the uniqueness of the paraprofessional in the service system. A paraprofessional should not be thought of as an assistant professional, nor a cheap source of personnel, but rather as someone with a unique contribution to make in the service system. Moreover, the paraprofessional should be able to find rewards for making his or her unique contribution. Career ladders and training should be directed simultaneously toward enhancing the contribution of the paraprofessional as a person able to bridge two cultures, while at the same time making provision for the advancement of the paraprofessional. Picture what would happen to the Ghanian dawn counselor, should the position be supported through a publicly funded village mental health center under civil service and require training from Western schools. Dawn counseling would take place in an office between 9 A.M. and 5 P.M. and be conducted by someone who was removed from the village, educated in Western schools, and trained in Western concepts of the psychological person.

Experiences in working with paraprofessionals demonstrate that high morale and effectiveness are maintained when programs and leaders pay careful attention to the characteristics of the work tasks and the social organization of the service setting, enabling paraprofessionals, thereby, fully to make use of their personal styles and knowledge as helping instruments. At present, some training programs, particularly those in community colleges and other institutions of higher learning, are instilling paraprofessionals with expectations for roles and functions which may not be realized in the work setting. It is as necessary for those persons concerned with the paraprofessional movement to work with employers and professionals to help to construct work situations in which the special contribution of the paraprofessional can be realized, as it is for them to provide appropriate training for the paraprofessionals.

One should also pay serious attention to the recruiting process. Perhaps paraprofessionals should be recruited from among those persons who emerge as leaders in natural support systems, in community organizations, or in other local or self-help groups. The assumption that the best route for entry into the field is through schooling, in the absence of other pertinent life experiences, should not remain unexamined; communication and a deep knowledge of culture, beliefs, and values are particularly important in the mental health field.

The varied historical transformations of human services suggest the need to be very concerned with modification into a formal service of the original impulse to help. The question of how best to preserve the vitality of the impulse to serve is difficult to answer and deserves to be taken very seriously.

NOTES

[1] While mental hospitals and institutions for the retarded always employed aides and attendants, such personnel usually filled custodial roles. Although many had important *de facto* responsibilities, because of the unavailability of professional personnel, aides and attendants were rarely considered part of the therapeutic team. Today's paraprofessionals are supposed to be part of the service team, and they are viewed as fulfilling important and unique functions.

[2] When we speak of "paraprofessionals," we shall mean that the people engaged in the work do not possess graduate (masters or doctorate) level degrees in relevant disciplines and, furthermore, that these people regularly receive salaries for the functions that they perform. Paraprofessionals may or may not have relevant formal training in mental health skills. In earlier years few paraprofessionals were so trained; recently, however, an increasing proportion of paraprofessionals has received formal training. In contrast, "nonprofessionals" (or "amateurs") generally have little or no formal training and do not receive regular salaries for the services that they perform.

[3] Congress recognized the problem of the cultural appropriateness of mental health services in the 1975 Amendments to the Community Mental Health Centers Act. The law calls for treatment to be culturally appropriate. For example, if the center serves a group with poor facility in English, each center must have at least one staff member who speaks the relevant non-English language.

[4] This information was collected by Ms. Sharon Biegen.

[5] This information is taken largely from a course paper written by H. A. K. Nyiplorkpo at University of Cape Coast, Ghana.

REFERENCE NOTES

1. Fort Logan Mental Health Center. *Psychiatric technician training program at the Fort Logan Mental Health Center.* Unpublished manuscript, Denver, Colo., 1965.
2. R. Simon, The paraprofessionals are coming. In *AA and BA associates in professional psychology: Academic, professional and organizational implications.* Sym-

posium presented at the annual convention of the American Psychological Association, Miami Beach, September 1971. (Available from Ralph Simon, Ph.D., Experimental and Special Training Branch, Division of Manpower Training Programs, National Institute of Mental Health, Rockville, Md., 20852.)

3. A. Lubetkin, *Review of associate degree professional training for mental health technicians.* Unpublished manuscript, Harvard University, Laboratory of Community Psychiatry, 1968.

4. J. True, C. Young, & M. Packard, *A national survey of associate degree programs in mental health: Summary data and program description.* Unpublished manuscript, Columbia, Md.: Center for Human Services Research, 1973.

5. J. True, C. Young, & M. Packard, *An exploratory study of associate degree mental health worker programs.* Unpublished manuscript, Columbia, Md.: Center for Human Services Research, 1972.

6. R. Vidaver & J. Carson, *Collegiate practitioners: Maryland's health careers lattice.* Paper presented at the annual convention of the American Psychiatric Association, Washington, D.C., May 1971. (Available from Robert Vidaver, M.D., Department of Mental Hygiene, State Office Building, 301 W. Preston, Baltimore, Md., 21201.)

7. M. Drucker & L. Drag, *Undergraduate or paraprofessional training in mental health fields: The mental health assistants program at Georgia State University.* Unpublished manuscript, 1969. (Available from Dr. Melvin Drucker, Department of Mental Health Assistants, Georgia State University, 33 Gilmer St. S.E., Atlanta, Ga. 30303.)

8. E. Goplerud, *Mental health delivery systems in the People's Republic of China.* Unpublished Ph.D. qualifying paper, State University of New York at Buffalo, 1977. (Available from E. Goplerud, Department of Psychology, 4230 Ridge Lea Road, Buffalo, N.Y.)

9. E. W. Bestman, H. P. Lefley, & C. S. Scott, *Culturally appropriate interventions: Paradigm and pitfalls.* Paper presented at the meeting of the American Orthopsychiatric Association, Atlanta, March 1976. (Available from Department of Psychiatry, University of Miami School of Medicine, P.O. Box 520875, Biscayne Annex, Miami, Fla. 33152.)

10. E. W. Bestman, & H. P. Lefley, *Psychotherapy in Caribbean cultures.* Paper presented at meeting of American Psychological Association, San Francisco, August 1977. (Available from Department of Psychiatry, University of Miami School of Medicine, P.O. Box 520875, Biscayne Annex, Miami, Fla. 33152.)

REFERENCES

Albee, G. *Mental health manpower trends.* New York: Basic Books, 1959.

Alley, S., & Blanton, J. A study of paraprofessionals in mental health. *Community Mental Health Journal,* 1976, *12,* 151–160.

Barnes, H. E., & Teeters, N. K. *New horizons in criminology* (2nd ed.). New York: Prentice-Hall, 1951.

Blanton, J., & Alley, S. Models of program success in New Careers programs. *Journal of Community Psychology,* 1977, *5,* 359–371.

Booth, W. *In darkest England and the way out.* London, England: Corquodale and Company, Ltd., 1890.

Brand, J. L. The National Mental Health Act of 1946: A retrospect. *Bulletin of the History of Medicine,* 1965, *39,* 231–245.

Cohen, H. E. *Social work in the American tradition.* New York: Holt, Rinehart, and Winston, 1958.

Cohen, R. *"New Careers" grows older—A perspective on the paraprofessional experience 1965–1975.* Baltimore, Md.: The Johns Hopkins University Press, 1976.

Danzig, M. Education of the community mental health assistant: Dovetailing theory with practice. *Mental Hygiene,* 1970, *54,* 357–363.

Dean, S. R., & Thong, D. Shamanism vs. psychiatry in Bali, "Isle of the gods": Some modern implications. *American Journal of Psychiatry,* 1972, *129,* 59–62.

Deutsch, A. *The mentally ill in America.* New York: Columbia University Press, 1949.

Felix, R. H. *Mental illness. Progress and prospects.* New York: Columbia University Press, 1967.

Felton, G., Wallach, H., & Gallo, C. New roles for new professional mental health workers: Training the patient advocate, the integrator, the therapist. *Community Mental Health Journal,* 1974, *10,* 52–65.

Foucalt, M. *Madness and civilization: A history of insanity in the age of reason.* New York: Pantheon Books, 1965.

Gartner, A., & Riessman, F. The paraprofessional movement in perspective. *Personnel and Guidance Journal,* 1974, *53,* 253–256.

Genovese, E. D. *Roll, Jordan, roll. The world the slaves made.* New York: Random House, 1972.

Goldenberg, I. I. *Build me a mountain.* Cambridge, Mass.: MIT Press, 1971.

Grob, G. H. *The state and the mentally ill.* Chapel Hill, N.C.: The University of North Carolina Press, 1966.

Grob, G. H. *Mental institutions in America. Social policy to 1875.* New York: The Free Press, 1973.

Hadley, J., True, J., & Kepes, S. An experiment in the education of the pre-professional mental health worker: The Purdue Program. *Community Mental Health Journal,* 1970, *6,* 40–50.

Harrington, M. *The other America.* New York: Macmillan, 1962.

Hollingshead, A. B., & Redlich, F. C. *Social class and mental illness.* New York: Wiley, 1958.

Holzberg, J. D., Knapp, R. H., & Turner, J. L. College students as companions to the mentally ill. In E. L. Cowen, E. A. Gardner, & M. Zax (Eds.), *Emergent approaches to mental health problems.* New York: Appleton-Century-Crofts, 1967.

Intagliata, J. The history and future of associate degree workers in the human services. In K. Nash, N. Lifton, & S. Smith (Eds.), *The paraprofessional: Selected readings* (The Yale Monograph on Paraprofessionalism). New Haven, Conn.: Center for Paraprofessional Evaluation and Continuing Education, 1978.

Kiev, A. (Ed.) *Magic, faith, and healing: Studies in primitive psychiatry today.* New York: Free Press of Glencoe (Macmillan Co.), 1964.

Klein, W. L. The training of human service aides. In E. L. Cowen, E. A. Gardner, & M. Zax (Eds.), *Emergent approaches to mental health problems.* New York: Appleton-Century-Crofts, 1967.

Krauss, M. Mental health technician training program. In National Institute of Mental

Health (Eds.), *Project summaries of experiments in mental health training.* Washington, D.C.: Department of Health, Education, and Welfare, 1971.

Kreisman, J. J. The curandera's apprentice: A therapeutic integration of folk and medical healing. *American Journal of Psychiatry,* 1975, *132,* 81–83.

Lederer, W. Primitive psychotherapy. *Psychiatry,* 1959, *22,* 255–265.

Levine, M., & Levine, A. *A social history of helping services.* New York: Appleton-Century-Crofts, 1970.

Levitan, S. A. *The great society's poor law. A new approach to poverty.* Baltimore, Md.: The Johns Hopkins Press, 1969.

Longmate, N. *The workhouse.* New York: St. Martin's Press, 1974.

Lubove, R. *The professional altruist: The emergence of social work as a profession. 1880–1930.* Cambridge, Mass.: Harvard University Press, 1965.

Magoon, T. M., Golann, S. E., & Freeman, R. W. *Mental health counselors at work: Assessment of non-traditionally trained mental health workers and implications for manpower utilization.* New York: Pergamon Press, 1969.

Marris, P., & Rein, M. *Dilemmas of social reform: Poverty and community action in the United States.* New York: Atherton Press, 1967.

Matarazzo, J. Some national developments in the utilization of non-traditional mental health manpower. *American Psychologist,* 1971, *26,* 363–372.

McPheeters, H., & King, J. *Plans for teaching mental health workers.* Atlanta, Ga.: Southern Regional Education Board, 1971.

Messing, S. D. Group therapy and social status in the Zar cult of Ethiopia. In M. K. Opler (Ed.), *Culture and mental health.* New York: Macmillan, 1959.

Moynihan, D. P. *Maximum feasible misunderstanding: Community action in the war on poverty.* New York: Free Press, 1969.

Myrdal, G. *An American dilemma* (Vol. 2). New York: McGraw Hill, 1964.

Pearl, A., & Riessman, F. *New careers for the poor.* New York: Fress Press, 1965.

Pinel, P. *A treatise on insanity* (D. D. Davis, Trans.). Sheffield, England: Printed by W. Todd for Caddell and Davies, 1806.

Platt, A. M. *The child savers.* Chicago, Ill.: University of Chicago Press, 1969.

Rioch, M. J. Pilot projects in training mental health counselors. In E. L. Cowen, E. A. Gardner, & M. Zax (Eds.), *Emergent approaches to mental health problems.* New York: Appleton-Century-Crofts, 1967.

Rothman, D. J. *The discovery of the asylum. Social order and disorder in the new republic.* Boston: Little, Brown, 1971.

Sanders, R. New manpower for mental hospital service. In E. L. Cowen, E. A. Gardner, & M. Zax (Eds.), *Emergent approaches to mental health problems.* New York: Appleton-Century-Crofts, 1967.

Sarason, S. B., Levine, M., Goldenberg, I., Cherlin, D., & Bennet, E. *Psychology in community settings.* New York: Wiley, 1966.

Schulberg, H. C. Challenge of human service programs for psychologists. *American Psychologist,* 1972, *27,* 566–573.

Shakman, R. Indigenous healing of mental illness in the Phillipines. *International Journal of Social Psychiatry,* 1969, *15,* 279–287.

Sobey, F. *The non-professional revolution in mental health.* New York: Columbia University Press, 1970.

Southern Regional Education Board. *Community college training programs for human service workers: A report of a study.* Atlanta, Ga.: Author, 1975.

Southern Regional Education Board. *A guidebook for mental health/human service programs at the associate degree level.* Atlanta, Ga.: Author, 1976.

Steiner, G. Y. *Social insecurity: The politics of welfare.* Chicago, Ill.: Rand McNally, 1966.

Torrey, E. F. *The mind game: Witchdoctors and psychiatrists.* New York: Emerson Hall, 1972.

Umbarger, C. C., Dalsimer, J. S., Morrison, A. P., & Breggin, P. R. *College students in mental hospitals.* New York: Grune & Stratton, 1962.

Wilensky, H. L. The professionalization of everyone. *American Journal of Sociology,* 1964, *70,* 137–158.

Wintrob, R., & Wittkower, E. D. Witchcraft in Liberia and its psychiatric implications. In S. Lesse (Ed.), *An evaluation of the results of the psychotherapies.* Springfield, Ill.: Charles C Thomas, 1968.

Young, C., True, J., & Packard, M. A national study of associate degree mental health and human services workers. *Journal of Community Psychology,* 1976, *4,* 89–95.

//

GENERAL ISSUES IN SERVICE PROGRAMS INVOLVING PARAPROFESSIONALS

Chapter 3

ACHIEVING ECONOMIC EFFICIENCY WITH PARAPROFESSIONALS

Thomas Marschak*
Curtis Henke†

Because of budgetary constraints and the often overwhelming service needs of consumers, mental health agencies are concerned with providing quality services at the lowest feasible cost. Does the use of paraprofessionals actually increase the economic efficiency of mental health programs? The authors of this chapter answer this question affirmatively, basing their conclusions on a sophisticated economic analysis of 1975 NIMH data gathered from 197 federally funded community mental health centers.

The authors define "productivity" as output per hour of staff members' time, and "economic efficiency" as the selection of the least-cost combination of inputs (including the mix of paraprofessionals and professionals) for the output provided. The data analysis indicates that paraprofessionals complement professionals, by enabling the professionals to be more productive, and that paraprofessionals exhibit relatively high productivity when compared to professionals. Furthermore, the data also suggest that paraprofessionals are especially productive in providing services to populations that are poor, not highly educated, prone to dropping out of treatment and/or referred by "nonprofessional" sources.

*Professor, University of California, Berkeley, School of Business Administration
†University of California, San Francisco, Social Science Research Component, Multipurpose Arthritis Center

The mandate of community mental health centers—to provide services of good quality in a quantity sufficient to meet the needs of their catchment area residents—leads to a difficult and important management problem. Center budgets are limited, and expanding the services provided is not likely to generate enough reimbursement revenue to pay for the extra resources (staff members, physical plant, supplies) needed to provide the expanded services. In fact, the data for 1975 indicate than an average of only 24% of center funds was derived from payments by individuals and third parties for direct and indirect patient services. The problem is to hire personnel with a limited budget so as to come as close as possible to the quality and quantity goals. The evidence presented in this paper suggests that centers vary widely with regard to their success in finding the most efficient personnel combination; that is, that combination of staff members which provides the largest quantity of services of acceptable quality given the budget available. It appears likely that many centers could have increased both the quantity and quality of their services without increasing cost. In particular, altering the number of paraprofessionals used, relative to other types of staff members, affects the quantity and quality of services delivered. Our central concern is, in fact, the role of paraprofessionals in an efficient personnel combination.

The present study attempts to use the only data now available which deal with a very *large* sample of centers and are relevant to the study of alternative personnel combinations. We shall use the data to study the effect of alternative personnel combinations on the quantity and quality of mental health services provided by centers within the large sample. We shall pay particular attention to the effect of changing the paraprofessional component of the combination.

The data come from the most recent (1975) available Inventory of Comprehensive Community Mental Health Centers, from the National Institute of Mental Health (NIMH). The degree to which professionals and paraprofessionals substitute for one another in the production of services by community mental health centers is estimated, and an attempt is made to discover some of the areas in which paraprofessionals are particularly productive. Finally, the data are used to assess how well the typical center has solved the problem of finding the most efficient personnel combination given its budget.

The data have severe limitations, on which we shall comment. But the number of centers included is large, so that there is some hope of finding a statistically reliable relationship between the volume of services which a center provides and the number of staff members of different types which it employs. The issues on which such a relationship could shed light are important enough to justify a careful attempt to find a reliable relationship. Moreover, one important aim of the study is to uncover those kinds of future data gathering which would help us to *improve* our understanding of the relation between personnel combination used and services provided.

This chapter is divided into four sections. The first section introduces some relevant economic concepts and makes precise the notion that paraprofessionals complement professionals; that is, they enable professionals to be more productive.

The second section describes the analysis of the NIMH data and stresses two tentative results: (a) Many community mental health centers appear to have chosen an inefficient mix of paraprofessionals and professionals. (b) Paraprofessionals appear to be especially productive in providing services to populations that are poor, not highly educated, severely disturbed, prone to drop out of treatment, and referred by nonprofessional sources.

The third section suggests future directions for data gathering and research. The final section reviews the existing literature so as to compare the approach used here with others, especially with certain studies in the physical health field.

SOME ECONOMIC CONCEPTS

Certain basic economic concepts are needed in our search for a reliable relationship between the personnel combination a center uses and the services it provides. These concepts are perhaps most easily understood in a hypothetical example, far less complex than a community mental health center. Suppose a drop-in center for parents and children is to be started. Children will receive educational and recreational services while the parents participate in discussion groups and individual counseling. The objectives of the program are (a) to enhance the children's interest in schooling and their ability to learn, and (b) to assist the parents in achieving greater competence as well as a feeling of greater competence in creating a home environment that fosters learning in children. Suppose further that the physical facilities and supplies are already given; only the staffing of the drop-in center remains to be chosen.

A "Production Function" for Services

Before choosing a staffing pattern, we have to recognize that there are many different staffing patterns which can provide a particular group of services without sacrificing quality. Even though each center activity or task may be performed best by a particular type of staff member, other staff members will often be able to perform the same task although they may take more time to do so. Thus, each quantity of center services of acceptable quality may be obtained from many different staff member combinations; and any particular combination of staff members has some maximum quantity of services that it can offer without reducing quality.

Economists use a *production function* to express the relationship between the quantities of the various "inputs" used and the maximum quantity of "output" that can be obtained from these inputs. To apply the production function idea to the drop-in center, assume that the only outputs besides the physical facilities and supplies (which are already fixed) are hours of professionals' time and hours of paraprofessionals' time. Suppose we choose *client-hours* as our unit of output. If a family of four, for example, receives one hour of service, then that counts as four client-hours. The production function can then be expressed as: $S = f (P, PP)$, where P is the number of professional hours per week, PP the number of paraprofessional hours per week, and S the *maximum* number of client-hours of services per week that can be obtained from P and PP. The symbol f denotes a particular mathematical formula which implicitly incorporates the ways that professionals and paraprofessionals can work together. If we have found a particular function f that we believe to be accurate, then f becomes our model of the center's "technology." Using f, we can find the largest volume of services which the center can obtain from any given combination of professionals and paraprofessionals. We can also determine how many paraprofessional hours can be substituted for one professional hour while leaving the quantity of services provided unchanged.

As an illustration, suppose that the relationship governing the drop-in center happens to be: $S = 4 (P^{.6}) (PP^{.4})$.

For this particular production function, Table 3-1 shows the output in client-hours per week of adult and children's services *(S)* that is obtainable from different combinations of professional hours per week *(P)* and paraprofessional hours per week *(PP)*. If the illustrated production function really described the center, then the figures in the S column of the table would correctly show the client-hours obtained when each type of staff member is always used in its most productive way, so that as paraprofessionals are substituted for professionals, the substitutions are made in a way that keeps the staff's total output of services as high as possible. We see from Table 3-1 that there are several staffing patterns that will produce each quantity of

Table 3–1   Output (S), Average Product (AP), and Marginal Product (MP) for Different Staffing Patterns

Staffing pattern	P (hr/wk)	PP (hr/wk)	S (client-hours per week)	AP_P	AP_{PP}	MP_P	MP_{PP}
1	60	38	200	3.3	5.3	2.0	2.1
2	50	50	200	4.0	4.0	2.4	1.6
3	40	70	200	5.0	2.9	3.0	1.1
4	60	105	300	5.0	2.9	3.0	1.1
5	50	138	300	6.0	2.2	3.6	0.9
6	40	193	300	7.5	1.6	4.5	0.6
7	60	215	400	6.7	1.9	4.0	0.7
8	50	283	400	8.0	1.4	4.8	0.5
9	40	395	400	10.0	1.0	6.0	0.4

services. For example, 60 professional hours and 38 paraprofessional hours are capable of producing 200 client-hours of services, but so are 40 professional hours and 70 paraprofessional hours.

Average Productivity of an Input

The attainable quantity of adult and children's services increases as the quantity of either or both types of staff member is increased. The *average productivity* of a given type of staff member is defined as total output of services *per hour* of that type of staff member's time. It depends on the quantity used of *both* types of staff member. For example, the average productivity of professionals when 50 hours of their time are used per week is 4.0 client-hours of services per professional hour (200 divided by 50) when used together with 50 hours of paraprofessionals. However, the figure rises to 6.0 (300 divided by 50) when 50 hours of professional services are carried out in combination with 138 hours of paraprofessional services. So paraprofessionals *complement* professionals; increasing the number of paraprofessionals makes it possible to obtain more services from a given number of hours of professionals' time.

Marginal Productivity of an Input

The marginal productivity of an input is the change in the total output obtained when we slightly increase (say by one unit) the quantity of that input alone and leave the quantity of the other input unchanged. Thus, as shown in the last column for staffing pattern 1, slightly increasing the use of paraprofessionals when the center is using 60 professional and 38 paraprofessional hours per week, allows an increase of 2.1 client-hours per week of services. As with average productivity, the marginal productivity of each type of staff member depends on the quantity of both types used; in our illustration, an increase in paraprofessionals raises both the average and the marginal productivity of the professionals.

If the quantity of one type of staff member is repeatedly increased while the quantity of the other is left unchanged, there will be some level of this changing input beyond which each further unit increase will yield a smaller increase in services than the one preceding it. In our example, as the hours per week of paraprofessionals increase from 70 to 193 to 395, with professional hours unchanged at 40 hours per week, the marginal product of the paraprofessionals decreases from 1.1 to 0.6 to 0.4. This *declining marginal productivity*[1] is widely observed in many kinds of production processes; while not so far investigated in mental health, it has been empirically verified for physical health care (Boaz, 1972; Reinhardt, 1972, 1973, 1975; Zeckhauser & Eliastam, 1974). In the present case, we would certainly expect that if the size of the professional staff is fixed, then adding one extra paraprofessional hour increases services less when there are already many paraprofessional hours than when there are only a few of them: paraprofessionals require supervision from professionals, and we are spreading the fixed professional staff (and other fixed facilities) more and more thinly as we add more and more paraprofessional hours. Similarly, we would expect the marginal productivity of professionals to decline as we add more of them: They need the help of paraprofessionals, and if paraprofessional hours are fixed, then those hours are spread more and more thinly as the number of professionals increases.

As we shall see, it is precisely the declining marginal productivity of each type of personnel that makes the problem of finding the best personnel combination for a given budget a problem of some complexity.

Elasticity of Output with Respect to an Input

A third concept is often useful in measuring the importance of one particular input to the production of output. This concept is the *elasticity of output with respect to a given input.* Elasticity is defined as the *percentage* increase in output derived from a small *percentage* increase (say a 1% increase) in the amount of an input used, while keeping fixed the amount used of the other inputs. Since the elasticity is a ratio of two *percentages,* it does not change if we change the units in which we happen to measure output or the inputs; that is not true for average productivity or marginal productivity. Moreover, suppose the production function has the form we have illustrated—that is, suppose it has the form:

$$S = A \, X_1{}^{b_1} \, X_2{}^{b_2}$$

where S is output; X_1 and X_2 are amounts used of two inputs; and $A, {}^{b_1}, {}^{b_2}$ are numbers. Then, elasticity of output with respect to the first input is *always* b_1 no matter how much of the other input is used,[2] and elasticity with respect to the second input is always b_2. That is a very convenient fact about production functions having this form and is one of the reasons why this form of production function is important in empirical work. (It will be the form we shall use, in a generalized version, in the section, Empirical Analysis.) In our illustration, $A = 4$, $b_1 = .6$, and $b_2 = .4$. We compute that if, for example,

> P is kept at 60 and PP goes from 100 to 101
> (a 1% increase),

then

> S goes from 294.4 to 295.6 (a .4% increase)

so that elasticity of output with respect to paraprofessionals is .4, which (as we claimed) is exactly the power to which PP is raised in our production function. On the other hand, if instead

P is kept at 100 and PP again goes from 100
to 101,

then

S goes from 400.0 to 401.6

which is again a .4% increase. Similarly, if

PP is kept at 60 and P goes from 100 to 101
(a 1% increase),

then

S goes from 326.07 to 328.03 (a .6% increase);

and if instead

PP is kept at 100 and P goes from 100 to 101,

then

S goes from 400 to 402.4 (a .6% increase).

Again, elasticity of output with respect to P is .6, regardless of where we set
PP; and .6 is, as claimed, the power to which we raise P in the production
function.

Redefining Output

The discussion so far has treated output as though it had only one dimension.
In fact, there are many dimensions along which output can be measured
simultaneously. Our hypothetical drop-in center has at least two further output dimensions: the degree to which the children's services and adult services
delivered meet the center's goals; that is, the degree to which children are
interested and succeed in schooling, and adults are able to create, or perceive
themselves as able to create, a home environment which fosters learning in
children. Call these "adult success" and "children's success."

There is likely to be some opportunity for trade-offs among the three
aspects of output (client-hours, adult success, children's success), so that drop-
in centers with the same number of professionals and paraprofessionals could
exhibit different combinations of client-hours, adult success, and children's
success. The particular combination of the three that is, in fact, provided
depends on the characteristics of the people in the catchment area and on the
tasks to which the given numbers of professionals and paraprofessionals are
assigned.

The production function idea remains useful, even with multiple outputs,
if we combine the several outputs into a suitable "output bundle." We then
measure output produced by measuring the number of output bundles pro-

duced. We shall defer a general discussion of how this combination and measurement might reasonably be done until we move beyond the present illustration. For our hypothetical drop-in center suppose that a single output measure has in fact been defined, a unit of output being a suitable "bundle" of client-hours, adult success, and children's success. More client-hours, then, means more output units, and so does higher success.

Finding the Appropriate Staffing Pattern

The goals of the drop-in center are fully realized only when the most successful children's services and the most successful adult services possible are provided to everyone in the catchment area who can benefit from them. The budget limitation will force a compromise between success and numbers of persons receiving services, however; for increasing either the client-hours or the success of services requires the hiring of additional staff members. *Given a budget, a well managed center wants to be sure that its client-hours cannot be increased without decreasing success, and that success cannot be increased without decreasing client-hours.* If that were not so, then the center could be doing a better job with its budget. *But the center must also make sure that the number of units of output which it is providing cannot be provided at lower cost.* If this number of units *could* be provided at lower cost, then doing so would liberate some of the budget, and the portion liberated could buy both more client-hours and more success.

Technical Efficiency

Two distinct types of efficiency are required if the units of output provided are always to be provided at the lower cost. First, whatever combination of inputs is actually employed, that combination must be used efficiently; that is, the maximum output possible with this input combination must be obtained. Economists call this *technical efficiency.* For example, if the drop-in center uses 10 professionals for outreach and 10 paraprofessionals for a literature search for new methods, then very likely the maximum output possible for this manpower combination is not realized. This center would be technically inefficient. Outreach and literature research could both be improved if these professionals and paraprofessionals exchanged roles. Then the center output would increase without changing the size *or* the composition of the staff. A production function assumes that the inputs *are* used with technical efficiency; that is, the production function gives the *maximum* output available from each personnel combination.

Economic Efficiency

A second type of efficiency is *economic efficiency,* or the selection of the least-cost combination of inputs for the output provided, assuming that technical efficiency has already been achieved. Table 3-1 illustrated three of the many different staffing patterns which could be used to produce, with technical efficiency, 200 hours of adult and children's supervision. Suppose that output is now defined to include the success of children's and adult services, as well as the number of hours, and that the production function is still the one previously illustrated. Suppose, also, that the price of paraprofessionals *(PP)* is $5 per hour, and the price of professionals *(P)*, $12.50 per hour. Table 3-2 shows seven possible staffing patterns which provide the identical output of 200 units and the cost of each. As professional hours per week drop from 80 to 60, 13 new paraprofessional hours are needed to replace them to keep output unchanged at 200 units. This reduces the center's cost per week because 13 paraprofessional hours cost less money than 20 professional hours. But the marginal productivity of professionals rises as their hours per week decline, and the marginal productivity of paraprofessionals falls as their hours increase (both implied by declining marginal productivity). When professional hours are further decreased by 18—from 60 to 42—27 additional paraprofessional hours are needed to maintain output at 200 units. If we drop below 42 professional hours, the weekly cost of 200 output units declines a bit further. Two paraprofessional hours are needed to compensate for one further hour's decrease of professional time to 41, with a subsequent saving of $2.50. But beyond this, any additional substitution of paraprofessional for professional time increases the cost since increasingly more paraprofessional hours are required for each hour's decrease of professional time. Thus, $15 of paraprofessional time (three hours) is the cost of saving one hour of professional time, which costs $12.50; decreasing professional time below 41 hours would *increase* the cost of 200 output units. So, if the center wants to provide 200 output units, then the cheapest personnel combination which does so is staffing pattern 4—41 professional hours and 67 paraprofessional hours.

To recapitulate: If too many professionals are being used relative to the number of paraprofessionals, as in staffing patterns 1–3 of Table 3-2, then the marginal output per dollar (marginal product divided by price) is lower for professionals than for paraprofessionals. In other words, one dollar's worth of

Table 3–2 Marginal Products (*MP*) and Costs of
Alternative Staffing Patterns for 200 Units of Output

Staffing pattern	P (hr/wk)	PP (hr/wk)	$\dfrac{MP_P}{Price\ P}$	$\dfrac{MP_{PP}}{Price\ PP}$	Cost/wk ($)
1	80	25	.120	.640	1,125.00
2	60	38	.160	.421	940.00
3	42	65	.229	.346	850.00
4	41	67	.231	.239	847.50
5	40	70	.240	.229	850.00
6	30	108	.320	.148	915.00
7	20	198	.480	.081	1,240.00

paraprofessional time can replace more than one dollar's worth of professional time. As the substitution continues, the marginal-product-to-price ratios become more nearly equal. *At staffing pattern 4 they are approximately equal, and that is why pattern 4 is the cheapest.* Further substituting of paraprofessionals makes paraprofessional time *less* productive per dollar than professional time, as in staffing patterns 5, 6, and 7, where too many paraprofessional hours are used.

The problem which began our discussion of a hypothetical drop-in center is now solved. Many staffing patterns that can provide a given number of client-hours and a given level of success of children's and adult services have been identified, and the one which supplies this output at the least cost has been chosen.

The concepts of production function and of economic efficiency can now be generalized to full-scale community mental health centers.

Generalization to Community Mental Health Centers

An operating community mental health center differs from the hypothetical model of a drop-in center in the greater complexity of its inputs, outputs, and goals. A suitable model of a community mental health center (CMHC) has to be more complex. Intuition alone might possibly have guided the simple drop-in center without our analysis. But the complexity of the CMHC overwhelms intuition and makes an economic model a useful tool for the comparison of personnel combinations.

Not only are there many categories of personnel in a CMHC (e.g., psychiatrists, psychologists, registered nurses, social workers, paraprofessional mental health workers), but there may be appreciable variation in training, experience, and productivity within each personnel category. Because there is such variety in personnel and in the tasks different people perform, there is likely to be greater opportunity for substitution among them than in the example of the simple drop-in center.

This diverse array of staff members provides many types of services to clients with a wide variety of diagnoses and problems. In addition to direct care, many centers offer public education and consultation services. When further dimensions for effectiveness or quality are allowed, the opportunity for variation in output among CMHCs becomes immense.

Yet, finding cost-minimizing staffing patterns for a CMHC is no different in its essentials from doing so for the drop-in center. The production function which models the CMHC contains many more inputs than in the earlier case, but its form is similar. As in the previous case, the production function has a basic property: The marginal product of any input—the amount by which output goes up when one more unit of that input is used—declines as more and more of the input is added. The output for the production function is still a single measure, one which combines in some reasonable way the many components of actual CMHC output. There are many inputs, and the criterion for economic efficiency is that the ratio of marginal product to price be equal for all of them.[3] This is just a straightforward generalization of what we found for the hypothetical two-input drop-in center.

To apply the criterion for economic efficiency we have to settle on a particular function as our best mode of the "technology" of the typical CMHC. In the next section, we use data from many operating community mental health centers to facilitate estimating, statistically, a production function for their services. Before doing so, we reemphasize that the numbers needed to find optimal staff mixes are for the *marginal* products and the prices of each input. The *average* products, figures which are sometimes used in this calculation, are not appropriate and may prove to be misleading guides. It also ought to be clear now that, in order to find the best level for each input, we must *not* study the inputs one at a time. We have to consider all of the inputs together to find the appropriate level of a single one. That is what the production-function framework permits us to do.

EMPIRICAL ANALYSIS

Data

Data collected by the National Institute of Mental Health (NIMH) from 503 federally funded community mental health centers have been used for the analysis. Taken from the 1975 Inventory of Comprehensive Community Mental Health Centers (part of which is included as an appendix), the data contain information about the following: scheduled hours for 13 different categories of staff members; consultation and public education activities; center expenditures and sources of funds; number of persons receiving direct services; clients' utilization of service elements; characteristics of people added to the center rolls during the reporting period; the source of client referral to the center; and the referral after the client is dropped from the center's active rolls. Since the data are derived from the answers recorded on the inventory form, their accuracy is limited by the care taken to complete the questionnaire. There is some indication that the information may not have been carefully reported by all the centers, as there were large numbers of missing responses. Consequently, the sample suitable for the analysis had to be reduced to 197 centers. There are many important variables which the questionnaire did not cover; had they been covered, the results obtained might well have been different. All this has to be borne in mind when interpreting the results which must be regarded as only preliminary and suggestive. We shall address the issue of how future data might be improved in the section, Future Data Gathering and Future Research.

The task undertaken was to find several alternative production functions which, for our sample of 197 centers, fit the observed relation between output and inputs.

Inputs

The community mental health center inputs used in the estimation are the various types of staff hours per year, as well as the item called "other center operating expenditures" in the NIMH Inventory.[4] The use of capital goods (plant and equipment) is also an input in the production of services, but there is no way of estimating this input from the available data. (The center capital expenditures during the survey year, as reported in the inventory forms, do not reflect the value of the current period's capital goods inputs.)

The inventory form contains 13 different categories of staff. Production functions were estimated using the number of hours per year for 11 different types of staff. Ten were taken directly from the inventory classification, and the remaining one—namely, the paraprofessional input—was derived by summing the hours of the remaining three staff categories on the inventory form.

One of the limitations of the Inventory's personnel data is the lack of information concerning the level of *training* of the paraprofessionals. The "mental health worker" category, for example, groups those with years of experience and training with those who are just beginning. This prohibits an examination of a crucial question: What is the effect of training and experience on paraprofessional productivity, and what is the value of the training?

Another shortcoming of the personnel data restricts the examination of the use of staff in specific activities. Staff hours allocated to different activities were requested on the survey form, but the responses proved too unreliable for analysis. When these data limitations are improved, it will be possible to understand much better the effect of using alternative personnel in specific alternative tasks.

Outputs

The community mental health center outputs reported in the inventory are the staff hours spent in consultation and public education, and the patients' use of the various available services: (a) inpatient, (b) residential, (c) partial hospitalization, (d) outpatient, (e) emergency, and (f) home care services. Patients' use is given both in number of service units (patient-days, therapy sessions, or visits) and in number of episodes of each type of service (number of people on each service case load at the beginning of the year, plus the number of admissions to that service during the year).

The output measures we use in estimating production functions are certain weighted sums of the units of each service type provided. Four different sets of weights were used to provide extreme, as well as central, values.

Define *INPT* to be the sum of inpatient, residential care, and partial-care days; *OUTPT* to be the sum of outpatient sessions, emergency visits, and home visits; and *PECON* to be the number of staff hours devoted to consultation, public information, and public education. Then the four output measures used are:

$$Y1 = INPT + OUTPT + PECON$$

$$Y2 = \frac{2}{3} \left(2\ INPT + OUTPT + PECON \right)$$

$$Y3 = \frac{2}{11} \left(INPT + 10\ OUTPT \right) + PECON$$

$$Y4 = \frac{2}{11} \left(10\ INPT + OUTPT \right) + PECON$$

In each of these four measures, the *sum* of the weights given to *INPT* and *OUTPT* is double the weight given to *PECON*.[5] But the weight given to *INPT*, relative to that given to *OUTPT*, varies among the four measures. $Y1$ weights all three types of services equally; it is simply the sum of all services. $Y2$ weights *INPT* twice as much as *OUTPT*. $Y3$ and $Y4$ provide extreme weights; in $Y3$, *OUTPT* is weighted 10 times as much as *INPT*, and in $Y4$, *INPT* is weighted 10 times as much as *OUTPT*.

Each of the output measures expresses a different view of the goals of a CMHC, that is to say, the relative importance attached to inpatient services, outpatient services, and to consultation-information-education. Note that, since inpatient services are measured in patient-days and outpatient services in sessions and visits, $Y2$ may be a particularly appropriate measure if one feels that a patient-day comprises a substantially larger delivery of services than a typical outpatient visit. We estimate a production function for each of the four definitions of output. If the four estimated functions turn out to be close to each other, then we can use any one of them with relative confidence, knowing that the results we get are relatively insensitive to one's view of a CMHC's goals.

For our sample of 197 centers, the means and standard deviations of the output measures, as well as the input numbers, are shown in Table 3-3. This table shows that there is wide variation (large standard deviations) among the centers with respect to all of these variables. Table 3-4 displays the correlation among the four output measures. Each pair among the four is highly correlated, with the pair of extreme-weight measures (Y_3 and Y_4) having the lowest correlation.

Clearly, center outputs have many dimensions other than a count of the services provided. Perhaps the greatest shortcoming of the data is their lack

Table 3–3 Mean Values and Standard Deviations for Outputs and Inputs, 197 Centers

Variable	Designation	Sample mean	Sample deviation
Outputs (service units)			
Variant 1	Y1	46,482	38,545
Variant 2	Y2	45,782	40,135
Variant 3	Y3	48,200	38,643
Variant 4	Y4	44,764	43,879
Inputs			
A. Staff (hours/years)			
1. Psychiatrists	PCHI	10,039	17,147
2. Other physicians	OMD	1,229	4,163
3. Psychologists (MA and above)	PCOL	17,067	12,243
4. Social workers (MSW and above)	MSW	21,256	17,288
5. Registered nurses	RN	17,421	18,152
6. Licensed practical or vocational nurses	LPN	4,119	6,701
7. Other mental health professionals	OMHP	24,839	22,870
8. Physical health professionals and assistants	PHP	1,587	7,449
9. Paraprofessionals (other psychologists—CMA, other social workers —MSW, mental health workers)	PP	44,512	48,112
10. Administrative and other professional staff	AOP	10,212	12,647
11. All other staff	OS	42,151	42,534
B. Operating expenditures ($/yr)	EXP	413,035	427,617

Table 3–4 Correlation Coefficients for Alternative Measures of Output

	Y1	Y2	Y3
Y2	.989		
Y3	.926	.859	
Y4	.943	.981	.746

of any other attributes of output. There is no clue as to the effectiveness of the services supplied, and no record of community work by center staff not included in consultation and public education. Outreach activities are not reported at all.

So, we are forced to ignore important output dimensions. The effect on the estimated production functions is potentially serious. If the excluded components of output are the ones in which some types of personnel are most productive, then the contribution these types of personnel make to a center's output, as reflected in our estimated production functions, will be biased downward, perhaps severely. This is likely to be true for the paraprofessionals in the community mental health centers. Their contribution, as shown in production-function estimates, using the output measures available in the data, may understate their importance to the whole center operation.

Nevertheless, a statistically reliable relation between inputs and outputs —imperfectly measured as output may be—is useful if we can obtain a reliable relation from the sample data. It may well be that a more refined output measure, when it becomes available, will turn out to be highly correlated with our four crude ones, just as the four crude measures are highly correlated with each other. Policy makers who choose not to ignore data from a large sample when they are fortunate enough to have such a sample available, must accept the data's limitations. If there is fairly reliable evidence that many centers can obtain more output from their given budgets—measuring output in one or more of our four imperfect ways—by hiring more of some types of personnel and fewer of others, then that fact is at least something for those who make a center's policy to consider seriously in choosing the center's personnel combination.

Estimating a Production Function Which Fits the Sample

We want, then, to find a production function for each of our definitions of output—a relationship between output obtained and the quantity of each input used. The inputs are the 11 types of personnel—one of which is paraprofessional personnel—as well as "operating expenditures." We want the relation to fit the data well, in a standard statistical sense. The 197 centers differ substantially, as we have seen, with regard to the input combinations they use. *It is precisely this variability* among the 197 centers in the sample which makes it possible to learn something about the way changing the inputs used by a center affects the output obtained. What is learned is expressed in the estimated production function.

The *form* which we choose for the relationship to be estimated has three important properties: (a) It lends itself to straightforward statistical estimation of its parameters from the sample data. (b) Once the estimated parameters are inserted, the result is very likely to be a production function with declining marginal productivities for each input. (c) The elasticity of output with respect to any input can be read immediately from the estimated production function and is a number which remains the same no matter what quantities of the inputs are used.

The form we use for the production function is a generalization to many inputs of the production function we studied earlier in our illustrative two-input example (where we already verified property (c)). It is called the Cobb-Douglas form and has been used in a very large number of empirical studies, including studies in the physical health field (Boaz, 1972; Feldstein, 1968; Hellinger, 1975; Kimbell and Lorant, 1973; Reinhardt, 1973). A production function of the Cobb-Douglas form is

$$S = AX_1^{b_1} X_2^{b_2} \ldots X_n^{b_n}$$

where S is output and $X_1, X_2, \ldots, X_n$ are inputs. In our case there are 12 inputs, and the parameters to be estimated are $A, b_1, b_2, \ldots, b_{12}$. Each of the 197 centers in the sample gives us one value of the 13-tuple ($S, X_1, X_2, \ldots X_{12}$). We seek estimates of $A_1, b_1, b_2, \ldots, b_{12}$ which make the 197 13-tuples come close, in an appropriate sense,[6] to satisfying the equation $S = AX_1^{b_1} \ldots X_{12}^{b_{12}}$. Table 3-5 contains the parameter estimates we obtain, using the four alternative output measures. The standard errors (estimated standard deviations) of each estimate are also shown; the size of the standard error relative to the size of the estimated parameter itself tells us how reliable the estimate is. In addition, the table shows a further measure of the reliability of the entire estimated relationship, namely R^2. This measures the square of the correlation, across all 197 centers, between a center's true value of the output S, and the value of S *predicted* by the estimated relationship—that is, the value of S which we get when we set the inputs ($X_1, \ldots X_{12}$) equal to their values for that center; set the parameters ($A, b_1, b_2, \ldots, b_{12}$) equal to our estimates; and compute the output value $AX_1^{b_1} X_2^{b_2} \ldots X_{12}^{b_{12}}$. The closer R^2 is to 1, the more reliable, in this sense, is the entire estimated relationship.

The standard errors for most of the estimates, and the values of R^2, reveal quite good reliability compared to most production function studies, including those in the physical health fields (Boaz, 1972; Feldstein, 1968; Hellinger, 1975; Kimbell and Lorant, 1973), or at least most studies with a similar number of inputs. (The fewer the number of inputs, the better the standard errors one can expect to obtain.) There are only a few parameter estimates for which the standard error exceeds the (absolute) size of the estimate—which makes it quite unreliable—and for most estimates the standard errors are substantially smaller than the estimates themselves. Reliability does not differ appreciably as between the four production functions (corresponding to our four output measures). Negative parameters are a fairly common occurrence

Table 3–5 Production Function Estimates

Input	Output Y1		Output Y2		Output Y3		Output Y4	
	Parameter	s.e.	Parameter	s.e.	Parameter	s.e.	Parameter	s.e.
PCHI	.1234	.0396	.1129	.0422	.1444	.0396	.0926	.0495
OMD	.0221	.0096	.0208	.0098	.0229	.0092	.0178	.0115
PCOL	.1708	.0541	.1507	.0577	.2258	.0541	.1230	.0676
MSW	.0304	.0236	.0377	.0251	.0112	.0236	.0474	.0294
RN	-.0164	.0182	-.0196	.0194	-.00425	.01822	-.0238	.0228
LPN	.00890	.00825	.0130	.0088	-.00043	.00825	.0198	.0103
OMHP	.0426	.0260	.0496	.0277	.0223	.0260	.0585	.0325
PHP	.00019	.00106	-.00156	.01129	.0380	.0106	-.00491	.01324
PP	.0595	.0271	.0651	.0289	.0487	.0271	.0768	.0339
AOP	.0425	.0185	.0422	.0197	.0430	.0185	.0415	.0231
OS	.2111	.0644	.2144	.0686	.2103	.0644	.2239	.0804
EXP	.0998	.454	.1250	.0483	.0414	.0454	.1683	.0567
Constant	3.4437	.5370	3.3381	.5708	3.5380	.5370	3.0898	.6707
R^2	.652		.637		.628		.587	

Note. Input definitions are given in Table 3–3.
Parameter: Estimate of the exponent in production function.
s.e.: Standard error of parameter estimate.
Number of observations: 197.

91

in production function studies; if taken seriously, they mean that increasing the input in question actually decreases output. In the present case, negative parameters occur for only three inputs—registered nurses (for all four production functions), licensed practical nurses (for two of the four production functions), and physical health professionals (for two of the four functions). But in each case the standard error is large relative to the (absolute) size of the estimate, indicating that the estimate is unreliable and its negative sign is not significant. In any case, these three inputs are not very important, since our central concern is the issue of professional versus paraprofessional mental health personnel.

For all the other inputs, the estimated parameter in each of the four production functions is consistent with our basic requirement that an input's marginal product *declines* as more of it is used if other inputs are kept constant.[7] What Table 3-5 reports, then, are four production functions which the typical center might be willing to accept (and use) as a portrayal of its "technology"; that is to say, the way it can obtain output (as measured in one of our four ways) from alternative combinations of inputs. Though the results reported in the table have many drawbacks, they constitute perhaps the best portrayal of a typical center's technology which one can obtain if one assumes that the 197 centers' reported achievements with the inputs they used accurately reflect what the typical center *can* achieve with alternative input combinations.

The *sizes* of the positive parameters in the estimated production function reflect the contribution of each input to the production of output since, as we saw in the Economic Concept System, a parameter equals the elasticity of output with respect to the input associated with that parameter. That is to say, the parameter associated with an input equals the percentage change in services (output) resulting from a 1% change in the quantity of that input used, with all of the other inputs unchanged.[8] Using output measure $Y2$, for example —a 1% increase in the number of psychiatrist hours alone, with the quantities of other inputs unchanged—would yield a .11% increase in services. On the other hand, the parameter sizes do not by themselves tell us the relative *marginal productivity* of each input, except in the special case where all inputs are used in the same amount. In general, as we saw earlier, the marginal productivity of an input depends on the amounts used of *all* inputs.

In Table 3-5, the size of the paraprofessional parameter *(PP)* relative to the parameters for psychiatrists *(PCHI)* and psychologists *(PCOL)* varies with the output measure used. For $Y2$, the paraprofessional parameter is nearly one-half that of the psychiatrist parameter and one-third the psychologist parameter. The parameters for *PP,* relative to those for *PCHI* and *PCOL,* increase steadily as *INPT* becomes more important relative to *OUTPT* in the output measure; that is, as we move from $Y3$ to $Y1$ to $Y2$ to $Y4$. The same pattern holds for social workers (MSW) and other mental health professionals (OMHP) relative to psychiatrists (PSY). This suggests that the contribution to output of the other professionals and of paraprofessionals, relative to psychologists and psychiatrists, is higher for inpatients than it is for outpatients.

The paraprofessionals appear to be somewhat more productive, relative to MSW and OMHP, than they are relative to PCHI and PCOL. In fact, the *PP* parameter is *always larger* than the parameters for MSW and OMHP. The fact that paraprofessionals exhibit a lower contribution to output (a lower parameter in the production function) than psychiatrists or psychologists is not really surprising, considering the much higher level of training required for these professionals. But, in part, the smallness of the *PP* parameter, relative to PCHI and PCOL, may be due to the bias discussed earlier. If the particular areas to which paraprofessionals contribute most are not well reflected in the service measures used, then paraprofessionals' contribution to output is being underestimated by their estimated parameter.

Another possible explanation for the relatively "low" contribution of paraprofessionals in the estimated productivity functions is simply that paraprofessionals are currently used inefficiently in community mental health centers. For example, they may not be effectively trained or supervised, or the community knowledge they possess may not be fully utilized by the mental health center. Each estimated production function is based, as we have said, on the way paraprofessional-hours and other inputs *are* used in the sample's centers, not the way they *can best* be used.

Although the "true" paraprofessional parameter might, then, be higher than our estimated parameter, the estimated parameter (in the *Y*2 function) is *already notably high.* The fact that paraprofessionals have a parameter one-half that of psychiatrists is in itself evidence that paraprofessionals make an important contribution to a center's output.

Dividing Up the Sample to Learn More About Paraprofessionals' Contribution

There remains one further way to learn about the contribution of paraprofessionals from the 197 center sample. The remaining way is to divide the sample of centers into subsamples according to certain center characteristics which seem likely to affect paraprofessionals' usefulness; to estimate a separate production function for each subsample; and to see how the estimated contribution of paraprofessionals changes as the subsample characteristics change.

Five different characteristics are used to describe the 197 center sample. Table 3-6 shows these characteristics and their mean values for all centers; the definition of low and high values for these characteristics (used to divide the sample into two subsamples); the values of output *Y*2 for the subsamples; and the ratio of number of paraprofessional hours to professional hours in each subsample. The production functions estimated for each subsample are shown in Table 3-7.[9]

Table 3–6 Characteristics Used to Divide the Sample of Centers

Characteristics	Notation	Mean in all centers	Definition of ranges		Mean Y2		Mean PP/PF*	
			Low	*High*	*Low range*	*High range*	*Low range*	*High range*
Ratio of actual to predicted number of drop-outs (based on number of discharges and diagnoses of additions)	DROP	1.006	≤1.00	>1.00	46,154	44,485	.492	.445
Fraction of additions with diagnosis of social maladjustment or no mental disorder	SMMD	.202	≤0.15	>0.15	48,398	42,126	.493	.457
Fraction of additions with at least high school education	EDHS	.655	<0.75	≥0.75	39,400	53,072	.486	.470
Fraction of additions referred to center by other than "Self, Family, or Friend" or "Social or Community Agency"	REFER	.508	<0.50	≥0.50	43,869	47,071	.494	.467
Fraction of additions with family income at least $100 per week	INC	.523	<0.65	≥0.65	51,169	41,584	.508	.459

PP: Paraprofessional hours per year.
PF: Professional hours per year = PCHI + OMD + PCOL + MSW + RN + LPN + OMHP + PHP.

Table 3–7 Production Function Estimates for Divided Sample—Output Y2

	All centers	DROP		SMMD		EDHS		REFER		INC	
Input		Low	High	Low	High	Low	High	Low	High	Low	High
PCHI	.1129†	.1238†	.0347	.1370†	.1122	.1169*	.1123*	.1561*	.0945	.0238	.1764†
OMD	.0208†	.0146	.00573	.0261	.0235	.0224	.0182	.0142	.0226	.0267	.0173
PCOL	.1507†	.1880†	.0854	.1192	.2972†	.1276	.1518*	.1520†	.1571*	.1682	.1051
MSW	.0377	.0230	.0996*	.00119	.1023†	.0321	.0291	.0213	.0412	.0503	.0182
RD	-.0196	.0181	-.1077†	-.553†	.0276	-.0294	-.00353	-.00761	-.0262	-.0469	-.00056
LPN	.0130	.00902	.0263	.0160	.00499	.00262	.0149	-.00950	.0160	-.00904	.0212†
OMHP	.0496*	.0340	.1962*	.0782†	.01189	.02138	.1507†	.0373	.1000	.0186	.1354†
PHP	-.00156	-.00601	.00636	-.266*	.0255	.0548	-.00202	.00577	.00094	.00496	-.00405
PP	.0651†	.0288	.0998*	.1450*	-.00418	.2192†	.0179	.1437†	.0423	.1274†	.0114
AOP	.0422†	.00772	.1023†	.0537†	.0180	.0277	.0285	.0403	.0381	.0497	.0413†
OS	.2144†	.3209†	.0614	.2350†	.898	.1607	.2634*	.1730*	.2493†	.1915	.2190†
EXP	.1250†	.0752	.2331†	.0716	.1835*	.0672	.0843	.0457	.1378†	.2443†	.0766
Constant	3.3381†	2.7484	3.4647†	3.0400†	3.0732†	3.3359†	2.6459†	3.2662†	2.7570	3.3182†	3.1304†
R²	.637	.672†	.696	.704	.649	.578	.731	.726	.595	.663	.665
N	197	130	67	109	88	106	91	91	106	83	114

Characteristic[a]

Note. Input definitions are given in Table 3–3.
[a] Characteristics and their ranges are defined in Table 3–6.
*Significant at 10% level.
†Significant at 5% level.

First, the client drop-out rate is considered. The diagnostic mix of the patients in a center seems likely to be an important determinant of the drop-out rate. Accordingly, for all centers in the 197 center sample, an expected number of drop-outs for a center is estimated, given its diagnostic mix (for the current year's additions) and its number of discharges. Then in one subsample, the centers have a lower drop-out rate than one expects, given the diagnostic mix and the discharges; and in the other subsample, the centers have a higher than expected drop-out rate.[10]

The average center is of about the same size in both of the subsamples (mean $Y2$), but centers in the subsample with a fewer than expected number of drop-outs used a slightly higher ratio of paraprofessionals to professionals than the centers in the other subsample. One can interpret the estimated production functions as follows: Paraprofessionals (and social workers) are more productive, relative to psychiatrists and psychologists, in centers where clients have a high tendency to drop out than in centers where clients have a low tendency to do so. It is possible that the outreach activities in which paraprofessionals engage and their special skills with clients from lower socioeconomic strata, make paraprofessionals relatively productive with client populations whose tendency to drop out is high, and they may keep the drop-out rate from becoming higher still.

The second variable used to divide the centers is the fraction of clients added to the center rolls during the year who had a diagnosis of "social maladjustment" or "no mental disorder." It was thought that paraprofessionals might be used differently in centers with relatively few of these patients than in centers with relatively many. The centers with lower proportions of these patients are generally somewhat smaller than centers with larger proportions (Table 3-6). Table 3-7 shows paraprofessionals to be more productive—as expressed in the parameters of the estimated production functions—in centers in the low range of values of this characteristic. Such centers have a corresponding *larger* proportion of inpatient services, and it may be that they use paraprofessionals rather heavily for these services, even though paraprofessionals are also well suited to serving clients in the "social maladjustment" or "no mental disorder" category.

The educational background of the mental health center clients was also thought to have a potential influence on the use patterns of paraprofessionals. This was indeed born out. The productivity of psychiatrists, psychologists, and social workers was similar in all centers, in both the low and high ranges of the clients' education characteristic. Paraprofessionals, however, were much more productive in centers where fewer than 75% of the new clients had a high school education or more, and less productive in centers where more than 75% of the new clients had a high school education or more. Centers with few of these high educational level patients were smaller and used a higher ratio of paraprofessionals to professionals than the other centers. In the subsample with a low number of high education level patients the estimated paraprofessional parameter was about .2, so that a 10% increase in paraprofessionals would yield (approximately) a 2% increase in output. For psychiatrists, the parameter is only a bit more than .1. Moreover, holding fixed the number of all professionals at their average levels for the subsample, the *output per psychiatrist, psychologist, or social worker,* would decrease by 2%, if the number of paraprofessionals were to decrease by 10%; this illustrates, once again, that paraprofessionals complement professionals (i.e., they help to make professionals productive). It is possible that paraprofessionals are highly productive relative to professionals in serving less educated clients because paraprofessionals themselves share important socio-economic characteristics with the client population.

Next, centers are divided according to the fraction of clients with at least a moderate family income ($100 per week). If paraprofessionals are more effective than professionals with low income patients, but not necessarily more effective with high income patients, this should be exhibited in the production function estimates. Centers with more than 35% of new clients having low income (less than 65% of the new clients have a family income of at least $100 per week) were larger and had a higher ratio of paraprofessionals to professionals than centers with fewer low income people. As expected, paraprofessionals exhibit a much larger parameter estimate in low income centers than in higher income centers, while the reverse is true for psychiatrists. Psychologists and social workers also have a larger parameter estimate for low income centers, but their parameter differences between the low and high ranges of this characteristic are much less than the ten-fold difference for paraprofessionals. Again, the result for paraprofessionals may reflect the fact that they tend to have low income backgrounds themselves.

Finally, referral of new patients was considered. The way that paraprofessionals are utilized in a center may influence the referral agents differently so that different patterns of referral sources reflect different paraprofessional use patterns. The fraction of referrals in the year—derived not from "self, family, or friend" or "social or community agency," but rather from a variety of sources which we may for convenience label as "professional"[11]—was therefore used to divide the sample. Centers with fewer than half of their referrals from "professional" sources were slightly smaller, on the average, and used higher ratios of paraprofessional hours to professional hours than the other centers. Moreover, according to the parameter estimates in centers with few referrals from "professional" sources (and many from "self" and "social agency") the paraprofessional contributions were substantially greater than in the other centers. The psychiatrist parameter is also higher for the first group of centers, but for psychiatrists the parameter difference between the two groups of centers is far smaller. Once again, it is possible that paraprofessionals are especially productive with the client populations likely to be referred by "self" and "social agencies" because they share important characteristics with those clients and those referral sources.

We conclude that while paraprofessionals do contribute significantly to the outputs as measured, their productivity in a center depends on the way that they are used in the center and on the characteristics of the center's client population. Their measured productivity in the whole sample and in the various subsamples may, moreover, be biased downward because our output measured are incomplete, ignoring components of output in which paraprofessionals may be quite productive.

Economic Efficiency

Our discussion of the hypothetical drop-in center in the Economic Concepts section showed one principal application of a production function which adequately describes the transformation of inputs into output. That application is to find how close a proposed input combination, perhaps the personnel combination currently being hired, comes to the basic economic efficiency condition. That is, the production function may be used to assess how close to equal are the various inputs' marginal-product-per-dollar for the particular proposed input combination.

All the preceding cautionary remarks should make one very hesitant to use our estimated production functions for serious policy making as to the hiring of personnel in an ongoing community mental health center. Nevertheless, it is instructive to see how the 197 centers compare with each other in regard to the marginal-product-per-dollar of several key types of personnel which the centers achieve *with the personnel combinations they currently hire.*

Currently, reasonable average annual salary figures for psychiatrists, psychologists, social workers, and paraprofessionals[12] are (in thousands of dollars) 33.6, 21, 14.4, and 9.8 Using these four input prices, and using the Y 2-output variant of our 197 center production function, we compare in three charts marginal-product-per-dollar for paraprofessionals versus that for psychiatrists (Fig. 3-1), versus that for psychologists (Fig. 3-2), and versus that for social workers (Fig. 3-3).

Each cross within a chart corresponds to one mental health center. Economic efficiency for all centers would require that all points lie on the *45-degree line* where the marginal-product-per-dollar is equal for the two inputs.

What we observe is that for all three input pairs there is a *wide dispersion of centers* on *both* sides of the 45-degree line. Taken literally, this means that many centers are currently far from economic efficiency in their hiring of paraprofessionals but that they are far in both "directions": Some centers hire "too many" paraprofessionals relative to psychiatrists, relative to psychologists, and relative to social workers. Other centers hire "too few."

The lesson to be learned is, once again, that different centers appear to use paraprofessionals differently—as part of widely varying personnel combinations and, as we observed before, in different tasks with differing types of clients. The economic efficiency question is too important to rely solely on one of our estimated production functions in deciding whether more or fewer

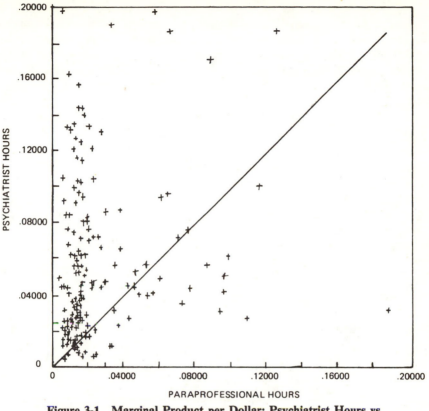

Figure 3-1   Marginal Product per Dollar: Psychiatrist Hours vs Paraprofessional Hours (OUTPUT $Y2$).

paraprofessionals ought to be hired by a given center. It seems abundantly clear, however, that more detailed inquiry into how paraprofessionals are used could help guide hiring policies toward the efficiency goal.

FUTURE DATA GATHERING AND FUTURE RESEARCH

What paraprofessionals in fact contribute to a community mental health center's output of services and what they could contribute when used in the best proportion relative to other staff and assigned to the most appropriate tasks, is clearly a complex question. But if there are indeed regularities in the way paraprofessional use affects the output of services, then the systematic study of *large* numbers of centers has a crucial role to play in discovering these regularities. The larger the sample studied, the more confidence we can place in the relationships we estimate. The analyses just reported seem to go as far as reasonably possible in detecting such regularities from the only large-sample data now available, namely the NIMH Inventory. We have found strong evidence that paraprofessional hours are an important determinant of a cen-

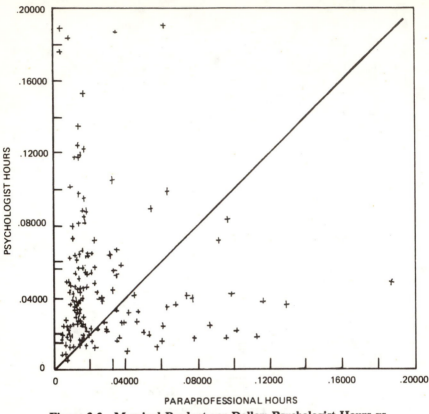

**Figure 3-2   Marginal Product per Dollar: Psychologist Hours vs
Paraprofessional Hours (OUTPUT $Y2$)**

ter's volume of services and that the contribution of paraprofessionals differs significantly between centers with different drop-out rates, referral sources, diagnostic mixes, education and income levels of clients, and inpatient-outpatient ratios.

This suggests that we could learn much more from a national survey more *disaggregated* than the present Inventory. In particular, a useful survey would try to:

1. Separate a center's paraprofessionals and their time used into categories reflecting *level of training, degree of supervision, and indigenous qualities (community residence, socio-economic origins, and the like) which make paraprofessionals resemble the clients they serve.*
2. Identify groups of *tasks* which paraprofessionals in different training, supervision, and indigenous-quality categories are assigned, and to find the approximate number of paraprofessional hours of each category assigned to each task.
3. Identify, at least for a sample of patients, the hours of service by para-

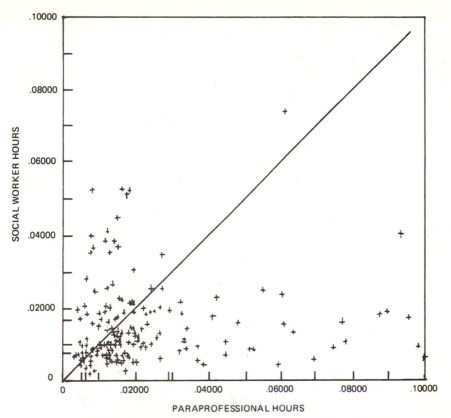

**Figure 3-3   Marginal Product per Dollar: Social Worker Hours vs
Paraprofessional Hours (OUTPUT _Y2_).**

professionals in various training, supervision, and indigenous-quality categories assigned to patients of different diagnostic categories.

4. Examine various *policy* attributes of the mental health center, such as the percentage of staff residing in the catchment area, the types of facilities provided (e.g., satellite clinics), and the working conditions (e.g., pay rates) of paraprofessional staff members.

5. Gather data which will improve *output* measures in future studies. Especially relevant are data concerning client's histories, or at least the initial phase of their histories, once they cease being served by the center—job success, welfare agency support, family status, and so on.[13]

Data from an annual survey of such a disaggregated type, over a succession of years, might help to settle some of the questions which we have raised but left unanswered. The further a new survey of community mental health centers moves in the suggested directions, the more intrusive and burdensome the typical center will find the reporting task. But surely there are many organizations, private as well as public, with internal personnel reporting schemes of the level of detail proposed, who have taken the reporting burden in stride and have learned to live with it comfortably. Manuals written for the purpose might help centers to cope with the additional reporting requirements. There seems little reason, in view of the importance of what we might learn, to rest content with the NIMH Inventory in exactly its present form.

THE EXISTING LITERATURE

The available mental health literature apparently contains no published studies examining the issues we have addressed. While some studies have estimated the total cost of mental illness (Conley et al., 1967; Fein, 1958) or examined the benefits and costs of types of personnel or particular therapies (Karon & Vandenbos, 1976; Weisbrod et al., 1977), quantitative estimates of substitution opportunities, productivity, or the choice of staffing patterns to minimize the cost of client services do not appear to have been published.

The situation is somewhat more advanced in the physical health literature, but the basic contribution of paraprofessionals in mental health differs in some respects from that in physical health. In community mental health, paraprofessionals can both assist the professionals and perform tasks of their own. In physical health, the paraprofessionals are more likely to perform tasks which would otherwise be performed by a physician. As a consequence, it seems likely that the optimal ratio of paraprofessionals to professionals is higher in the mental health field. We shall examine some examples of approaches that have been used in the analysis of physical health staffing and their conclusions regarding professional-paraprofessional substitution and productivity.

The most direct approach to these questions is simply to observe the delegation of tasks from professionals to other health workers, and the increased services resulting from the hiring of more such workers. This approach is illustrated by the results from a survey of pediatricians, reported by Yankhauer, et al. (1970). They found that solo-practice pediatricians who had the services of two other workers experienced 12% to 17% more office visits per hour of physician time than pediatricians who had only one worker to assist them. Similarly, Smith et al. (1972) use observations of task delegation in primary medical care practices in three states to construct a linear model of alternative techniques which are capable of providing the same medical services. They estimate that with efficient task delegation, the employment of a single physician assistant by the average size practice would permit a 49% to 75% increase in the number of visits that could be provided with the same physician time, or permit a reduction of physician patient-contact time in the office by 50% (from 28 to 14 hours per week) while leaving the number of visits unchanged. Golladay et al. (1974) use the same data in a slightly different model to estimate that the introduction of a physician assistant will substantially reduce the cost of a certain combination of medical services.

Reinhardt (1972, 1975) uses an indirect approach to estimate personnel substitution, productivity, and profitable staffing patterns. Using a large sample of office-based, self-employed, American physicians, he estimates statistically a production function, giving the number of office visits that can be obtained as a function of the number of staff hours and other inputs used to provide these services. He estimates that, at the current levels of aide and physician hours (1.96 aides per physician, and 60 physicians-hours per week of practice time), a 10% increase in the number of aide-hours per physician would, on the average, increase the number of visits by 3.1%. Once there are 5.0 to 5.5 aides per physician, however, any further increase in aides would not increase the number of visits provided. Reinhardt estimates further that these self-employed American physicians could profitably employ double the number of aides that they now employ (almost four aides per physician) which would increase the hourly physician output by 25%.

Considering clinic settings rather than physician office practice, Boaz (1972) has studied family planning clinics. As in the other studies we have cited, Boaz finds that, as increasing numbers of paraprofessionals are used with a fixed number of professionals, the additional paraprofessionals make additional services possible but that the increment resulting from each new paraprofessional becomes less with each added paraprofessional. The particular clinics examined by Boaz had hired too many paraprofessionals, with regard to the economic efficiency criterion. In a different clinic setting, Zeckhauser and Eliastam (1974) find that six physicians and four physician assistants working together can provide the same services as eight physicians with no physician assistants. Again, each added physician assistant contributes less to services than the previous assistant.

The physical health literature convincingly shows that paraprofessionals increase professional productivity and permit additional services. While most studies indicate that cost savings could be achieved by increased use of paraprofessionals, others show that it is also possible to use more paraprofessionals than is economically justified. The potential cost savings from shifting present staffing patterns toward economic efficiency appear to be significant in physical health and in mental health as well. Community mental health center directors ought to take economic efficiency seriously in evaluating alternative staffing arrangements.

NOTES

[1]Mathematically,

$$\frac{\partial f(P,PP)}{\partial P} \text{ and } \frac{\partial f(P,PP)}{\partial PP} \text{(two partial derivatives)}$$

are the marginal productivity of P and PP, respectively. To say that they are declining is to say that the corresponding second derivatives are negative; that is,

$$\frac{\partial^2 f(P,PP)}{\partial P^2} < 0 \text{ and } \frac{\partial^2 f(P,PP)}{\partial PP^2} < 0.$$

[2]Suppose the amount used of input 1 goes from X_1 to $X_1 + \Delta X_1$, with the amount of input 2 held at X_2. Suppose that, as a result, output increases from S to $S + \Delta S$. Then, the ratio of the *proportionate* change in output to the *proportionate* change in the amount of input 1 used is

$$\frac{\Delta S/S}{\Delta X_1 / X_1} = \frac{\Delta S}{\Delta X_1} \cdot \frac{X_1}{S}$$

As we let ΔX_1 become small, this ratio approaches a limit, namely,

$\frac{ds}{dX_1} \cdot \frac{X_1}{S}$. But that equals

$$(A \ b_1 \ X^{b_1 - 1} X_2{}^{b_2}) \frac{X_1}{A \ X_1{}^{b_1} X_2{}^{b_2}} = {}^{b_1}$$

So b_1 indeed equals (approximately) the percentage increase in output due to a 1% increase in input, and this is true *no matter what value we choose for* X_2.

[3]Formally, let S denote center output; let $X_1, X_2, \ldots X_n$ denote quantities of n inputs; and let MP_{Xi} and P_{Xi} denote, respectively, the marginal product and price of input X_i. The production function is a relation: $S = f(X_1, X_2, \ldots X_n)$; and if costs are to be minimized, then $X_1, \ldots X_n$ must be chosen so that

$$\frac{MP_{X1}}{P_{X1}} = \frac{MP_{X2}}{P_{X2}} = \ldots \cdot \frac{MP_{Xn}}{P_{Xn}}.$$

[4]The item is defined as "rent, electricity, insurance, travel, employee benefits, etc."

[5]Thus, $Y2$ can also be written as

$$\text{three times} \left(\frac{2}{9} \ INPT + \frac{4}{9} \ OUTPT + \frac{3}{9} \ PECON \right);$$

$$Y3, \text{ as three times} \left(\frac{2}{33} \ INPT + \frac{20}{33} OUTPT + \frac{11}{33} PECON \right); \text{ and}$$

$$Y4, \text{ as three times} \left(\frac{20}{33} \ INPT + \frac{2}{33} \ OUTPT + \frac{11}{33} PECON \right).$$

[6]Taking logarithms on both sides of the equation, one gets the *linear* expression $A + b_1 \log X_1 + b_2 \log X_2 + \ldots + b_{12} \log X_{12}$ on the right side. Each center's 13-tuple is converted to the form (log S, log X_1, log X_2, ... log X_{12}). The estimation consists, then, in performing the usual least-squares regression of log S on log X_1, log X_2, ... log X_{12} so as to obtain estimates of the parameters A, $b_1, b_2, \ldots b_{12}$.

[7]All that is required for this property is that the parameter be (positive and) less than one. This is so since for input i the marginal product is

$$\frac{\partial S}{\partial X_i} = b_i \ X_i{}^{b_i - 1} \underset{j \neq i}{A \Pi} \ \underset{i}{X^{b_j}}$$

and the derivative of marginal product with respect to the quantity of the input used is

$$\frac{\partial^2 S}{\partial X_i^2} = (b_i)\,(b_i-1)\,X_i^{b_i-2}\,\underset{j \neq i}{A\Pi}\,X_j^{b_j},$$

which is negative if b_i is (positive and) less than one.

[8]The demonstration of this fact is a straightforward extension of the argument given in the section, Economic Concept, for the two-input case.

[9]Instead of standard errors, Table 3-7 reports the reliability of parameter estimates by singling out those which are highly significant in the statistical sense.

[10]The actual drop-out rate (drop-outs divided by total discharges) is first computed for each center. Then, using the whole 197 center sample, the actual drop-out rate is regressed on the fraction of additions (new patients) in each of 11 diagnostic categories. The resulting equation is used to predict for each center the dropout rate that would be typical for centers with its diagnostic proportions (of additions). The ratio of the actual rate to the predicted rate (equal to the ratio of the actual number of drop-outs to the predicted number) is the characteristic DROP used for dividing the sample.

[11]These sources are: "clergy"; "private practice mental health professionals"; "non-psychiatrist physician"; "public psychiatric hospital"; "other psychiatric facility"; "medical facility"; "school system"; "court, law enforcement, or correction agency"; "other"; and "unknown."

[12]Based on the data described in S. R. Alley, J. Blanton, R. E. Feldman, G. D. Hunter, & M. Rolfson, *Case studies of mental health paraprofessionals: Twelve effective programs.* New York: Human Sciences Press, 1979.

[13]One prototype study, which collected such data for discharged mental health clients to assess the economic benefits of their treatment, is that of Weisbrod, Test, and Stein, 1977.

References

Boaz, R. F. Manpower utilization by subsidized family planning clinics: An economic criterion for determining the professional skill-mix. *The Journal of Human Resources,* 1972, *7,* 191–207.

Conley, R. W., Conwell, M., & Arrill, M. An approach to measuring the cost of mental illness. *American Journal of Psychiatry,* 1967, *124,* 755–762.

Fein, R. *Economics of mental illness.* New York: Basic Books, 1958.

Feldstein, M. S. *Economic analysis for health services efficiency.* Chicago: Markham Publishing Co., 1968.

Golladay, F. L., Manser, M. E., & Smith, K. R. Scale economics in the delivery of medical care: A mixed integral programming analysis of efficient manpower utilization. *The Journal of Human Resources,* 1974, *9,* 50–62.

Hellinger, F. J. Specification of a hospital production function. *Applied Economics,* 1975, *7,* 149–160.

Karon, B. P., & Vandenbos, G. R. Cost/benefit analysis: Psychologist versus psychiatrist for schizophrenics. *Professional Psychology,* 1976, *7,* 107–111.

Kimbell, L. J., & Lorant, J. H. *Physician productivity and returns to scale.* Paper presented before the American Economic Association Meetings, New York, December 29, 1973.

Reinhardt, U. E. A production function for physician services. *Review of Economics and Statistics,* 1972, *54,* 55–66.

Reinhardt, U. E. Manpower substitution and productivity in medical practice: Review of research. *Health Services Research,* 1973, *8,* 200–227.

Reinhardt, U. E. *Physician productivity and the demand for health manpower.* Cambridge, Ma.: Ballinger Publishing Co., 1975.

Smith, K. R., Miller, M., & Golladay, F. L. An analysis of the optimal use of inputs in the production of medical services. *The Journal of Human Resources,* 1972, *7,* 208–225.

Weisbrod, B. A., Test, M. A., & Stein, L. I. *An alternative to the mental hospital— Benefit and costs* (Working Paper 776). New Haven, Conn.: Yale University, Institution for Social and Policy Studies, 1977.

Yankhauer, A., Connelly, J. P., & Feldman, J. J. rhysician productivity in the delivery of ambulatory care: Some findings from a survey of pediatricians. *Medical Care,* 1970, *8,* 34–46.

Zeckhauser, R., & Eliastam, M. The productivity potential of the physician assistant. *The Journal of Human Resources,* 1974, *9,* 95–116.

APPENDIX: Selected Items from 1975 NIMH Inventory of Comprehensive Community Mental Health Centers

(15) Utilization of the Service Elements During the Reporting Period —Duplicated Count of Clients during Same Reporting Period as used for Question 14.

TREATMENT MODALITY	NUMBER
A. Utilization of Inpatient Services by Center Enrolled Clients *(See Instruction Booklet, Question 7 and 15A1, 2 & 3)*	
1. Number of inpatient care episodes during reporting period Total (lines a + b)	
a. at State or County Mental Hospital *(if used for center enrolled clients)*	
b. at grantee and/or local hospital affiliates	
2. Number of person days of inpatient care provided for above patients Total (lines a + b)	
a. at State or County Mental Hospital	
b. at grantee and/or local hospital affiliates	
3. Number of inpatient beds set up and staffed for priority use by center clients as of December 31, 1975 Total (lines a + b)	
a. at State or County Mental Hospital	
b. at grantee and/or local hospital affiliates	
B. Utilization of Other Residential Care Facility(s) by Center Enrolled Clients *(See Instruction Booklet, Question 7 and 15B1, 2, & 3)*	
1. Number of episodes of other residential care during the reporting period	
2. Person days of other residential care during the reporting period	
3. Number of other residential care beds set up and staffed for use by center clients as of December 31, 1975	

C. Utilization of Partial Care by Center Enrolled Clients

(See Instruction Booklet, Question 7 and 15C1 and 2)

1. Number of partial care episodes during the reporting period
   Total (lines a + b + c)
   a. in day/evening treatment
   b. in day care
   c. in education/training

2. Person days and nights of partial care during reporting period
   Total (lines a + b + c)
   a. in day/evening treatment
   b. in day care
   c. in education/training

D. Utilization of Outpatient Care by Center Enrolled Clients

(See Instruction Booklet Question 7 and 15D1, 2 & 3)

1. Number of outpatient care episodes during the reporting period

2. Of the above, how many were for State Mental Hospital aftercare patients

3. Number of therapy sessions conducted in the center's outpatient facilities during the reporting period
   a. Individual *(excluding medication or drug maintenance)*
   b. Family
   c. Group
   d. Medication or drug maintenance visits

E. Emergency Care

Number of emergency visits recorded during the reporting period
   Total (lines a + b)
   a. Day Emergency visits
   b. Night Emergency Visits

F. Home Visits

Number of home visits recorded during reporting year

108

16 **Diagnostic and Demographic Characteristics of Additions**

CHARACTERISTICS OF ADDITIONS	TOTAL ADDITIONS	SEX AND COLOR			
		MALE		FEMALE	
		White	Nonwhite	White	Nonwhite
	1	2	3	4	5
a. Alcohol Disorder (291; 309.13, 303)					
b. Drug Abuse (294.3; 309.14; 304)					
c. Mental Retardation (310-315)					
d. Depressive & Affective Disorder (296, 298.0, 300.4)					
e. Schizophrenia (295)					
f. Organic Brain Syndromes excluding alcohol and drug. 290, 292, 293-294 (excluding 294.3), 309.0-309.9 (excluding 309.13, 309.14)					
g. Other Psychoses (297, 298.1-298.9, 299)					
h. Transient Situational Disturbances and Behavior Disorders of Childhood & Adolescents (307.0-307.2, 308)					
i. Other Nonpsychotic Mental Disorders (300.0-300.9 (excluding 300.4) 301, 302, 305, 306, 307.3, 307.4)					
j. Social Maladjustment (316)					
k. No Mental Disorder, Deferred Diagnoses, & Nonspecific Conditions (317, 318, 319.0)					
l. Unknown					
m. TOTAL (Should = figure reported in Question 14A2)					

PRIMARY DIAGNOSIS:

(Codes indicated are from the Second Edition of the Diagnostic and Statistical Manual, Amer. Psychiatric Association)

109

AGE:

a. Under 15
b. 15 - 17
c. 18 - 24
d. 25 - 44
e. 45 - 64
f. 65 +
g. Unknown
h. **TOTAL** *(Should = figure reported in Question 14A2)*

WEEKLY FAMILY INCOME:

a. Under $100 including no income
b. 100 - 149
c. 150 - 199
d. 200 - 299
e. 300 +
f. Unknown
g. **TOTAL** *(Should = figure reported in Question 14A2)*

EDUCATION:
Highest grade completed

a. None
b. Grade school (and/or special education)
c. High school (including vocational, business or tech. schools)
d. College or More
e. Unknown
f. **TOTAL**

Chapter 4

THE EFFECTIVENESS OF PARAPROFESSIONALS IN SERVICE DELIVERY

Alan Gartner*

Are paraprofessionals effective in the delivery of services? The author of this chapter reviews the available research and provides an affirmative answer. Well-controlled research supports the contention that paraprofessionals are effective. The research on why paraprofessionals are effective, while limited in scope, suggests that the following factors may be involved: (a) accurate empathy and non-possessive warmth toward clients, (b) procedures for selecting paraprofessionals, (c) training programs, and (d) working conditions. The author also discusses conditions under which paraprofessionals are not effective, dangers to the paraprofessional movement, and additional needed research.

Whatever factors justify the use of paraprofessionals in the delivery of human services, it is the effectiveness of those services which provides the only real criterion for assessing the value of their contribution. Whether the paraprofessionals are meant to offset the shortage of personnel, to increase cost efficiency, to establish closer rapport with the community, or to provide employment for the unemployed, the first goal must be the highest possible degree of effectiveness in the services they provide. To state this goal does not, of course, assure us that data are available to allow an accurate and complete assessment of its attainment. In fact, such is not the case. As with other areas of human services

*Professor, Center for Advanced Studies in Education (CASE), Graduate Center, City University of New York.

work, we cannot easily establish clear cause and effect relationships; we are not able to say that a particular set of paraprofessional behaviors *caused* a specific outcome. Nor are there many studies conducted under rigorous conditions with such trappings as control groups and the like. One analyst (Karlsruher, 1974) reports 9 such studies, while another (Durlak, 1973) reports 14. Furthermore, the few relatively rigorous studies on this subject have neither been conducted by independent researchers nor have they been replicated so as to establish their reliability or validity. These statements are valid, of course, not only for studies concerning the paraprofessional programs, but, to a greater or lesser degree, for programs across the entire range of the human services at all levels of personnel. Indeed, it may well be that paraprofessional programs have been better studied than have other interventions.

GENERAL RESEARCH

Only one book (Gartner, 1971) has assessed the effectiveness of paraprofessionals in a variety of fields. But in the field of education, the work of paraprofessionals has been extensively studied (Bennett & Falk, 1970; Conant, 1973; Gartner, 1976; Gartner, Jackson, & Riessman, 1977). One example is the study made of the Career Opportunities Program (COP), a U.S. Office of Education program, operating in 132 school systems in 48 states during 1969 through 1976. The program involved a total of nearly 20,000 paraprofessionals, and considerable efforts were made to assess their effect upon children and the schools. One finding indicated that in elementary schools, where children were randomly assigned to classrooms within a grade level, the children in those classrooms where COP paraprofessionals were used performed better on standardized reading and mathematics tests than children in classes where paraprofessionals were not used (Kaplan, 1977). Similar results have been reported in other school programs (Gartner, 1976).

Another study of paraprofessional effectiveness in the field of education was a unique study, conducted as part of the national assessment of COP by the New Careers Training Laboratory, Queens College, City University of New York (Costa, 1975). This study involved a comparison of the performance of COP graduates as teachers with the performance of other new teachers, trained in traditional programs. The paraprofessional teachers, trained in the Career Opportunities Program, were participants in a full-blown "New Careers" effort; that is, they received, as part of the program, the training and education needed to prepare them to mount a career ladder, earn a baccalaureate degree, and become eligible for a teacher's license. As a group, these participants were more often than not drawn from the ranks of the black, the poor, and the middle aged. The study (Costa, 1975) compared the teaching of these COP graduates during their first year with the performance of other first year teachers in the same schools at the same grade level. Comparisons were made in 15 communities throughout the country with 10 pairs of teachers in each community. The teachers were compared in terms of attitudes, performance in the classroom, judgment of parents, and effects upon children. The results of the comparison showed that on each of the more than 30 scales and sub-scales where significant differences were found between the two groups of teachers, those differences favored the teachers trained by COP. In short, results indicated that the COP-trained teachers: held more positive attitudes toward the children (including expecting more of them); performed in the classroom in ways which had been identified as more conducive to children's learning; and received more positive judgments from the children's parents. On standardized achievement tests, it was found that the children taught by COP-trained teachers performed better than those in the comparative group. Although this study was not free of methodological complications, the findings, which were confirmed by a smaller, second year follow-up, suggest that paraprofessionals from low-income communities can become effective new professionals, when they are provided with training, education, and the opportunity of employment.

Also within a school setting, but involving counseling rather than teaching, the studies at Southwest Texas State University (Brown, 1965, Brown, 1972; Zunker & Brown, 1966) have tried to assess the effectiveness of paraprofessional service in the lives of their clients. In a number of studies over a 15 year period, the performance of students counseled by paraprofessionals was compared with matched samples of those who did not receive such counseling. The consistent research results led to the conclusion that paraprofessional counseling was an effective, acceptable, practical, and adaptable procedure. This conclusion applies regardless of whether the counseling effort was aimed at the prevention or correction of academic difficulties, whether those counseled were from affluent or poverty backgrounds, and whether the language spoken was English or Spanish (Brown, 1974, p. 260).

RESEARCH IN THE FIELD OF MENTAL HEALTH

Although education is the field most studied, so far, by those interested in assessing the effectiveness of paraprofessional service, it is in the field of mental health where the tradition of paraprofessional use may be the most entrenched. For a long time, the bulk of the staff of mental health institutions has been paraprofessionals. "The old paraprofessional" (Gartner & Riessman, 1971), the psychiatric aide, to use the most common title, can be found in great numbers working a hospital setting, engaged in therapeutic work.

Many studies have been conducted to assess the effectiveness of the variety of vital services delivered by the paraprofessional in the mental health field. One highly significant, well controlled experiment, conducted by Ellsworth (1968), indicates that the old type of paraprofessional, with only very limited training, can play a powerful role in the improved treatment outcome for hospitalized male schizophrenics. In this experiment, for the purposes of the demonstration, aides were assigned to the patients of one building (n = 122) at Fort Meade, South Dakota, Veterans Administration Hospital; patients of two other buildings, who were not assigned aides, served as a control group (n = 214). For patients in both groups, the program was similar in use of medication, use of activity group therapy, the process of reaching decisions as to discharge, assignment of new admissions, and patient characteristics.

The results of this experiment showed that a higher percentage of the experimental group patients were released to the community during the 30-month demonstration period, and a lower percentage had to return to the hospital. Post-discharge outcomes were based upon seven indices: level of behavioral adjustments; median days subsequently hospitalized; released versus not released; percent achieved 12 consecutive months in community; good social adjustment; and discharge status six years later.

Included in this study was a set of 21 pairs of comparisons. For these comparisons, both the experimental and control groups were divided into three sub-groups, each depending upon the type of schizophrenia. Patients in the sub-groups derived from the original experimental group did better on all 21, and in 13, at a substantial level of significance. "Although the chronically hospitalized patients' group profited most by the approach used in the experimental program, the acute group of patients also responded significantly" (Ellsworth, 1968, p. 164).

In another interesting venture beginning in the 1960s, the National Institute of Mental Health sponsored a series of paraprofessional programs. The first of these was Rioch's Mental Health Counselors program (Rioch, 1963), using upper class, well educated women as counselors for adolescents. The program was designed to provide low-cost psychotherapy and at the same time to provide useful work for women with grown children; indeed, their success as parents was seen as an essential job qualification.

In this program, eight women were chosen from among 80 who sought applications. Their median age was 43; seven were married, one widowed; they had an average of 2.4 children; all were college graduates, three with post-baccalaureate degrees; six had held professional jobs; four had been psycho-analyzed; all of their husbands held executive or professional positions. Their upper-class status is further shown by their ability to participate in a two-year training program without pay, with no guarantee of a job at the end.

All eight women completed the four semesters of training which emphasized professional breadth, not technician specificity. It was limited to psychotherapy, and emphasized on-the-job training. Most of the patients of the trainees were adolescents.

Blind evaluation by outside experts of tapes of interviews of trainees (not identified as such) with clients were conducted. On a scale from 1 (poor) to 5 (excellent), the rating of the interviews on eight factors ranged from 2.7

(beginning of interview) to 4.2 (professional attitude), with an overall global impression mean score of 3.4. Evaluation of patient (n = 49) progress showed that none changed for the worse, 19% showed no change; and 61% some change—35% slight improvement, 20% moderate improvement, 6% marked improvement (Rioch, 1963, pp. 683–685). Follow-up evaluation three years later supported the earlier competence judgment (Magoon, Golann, & Freeman, 1969).

Other paraprofessional programs, using mature women in mental health services can be mentioned. One, similar to the Mental Health Counselors program in terms of the background of the women trained as counselors, is the Child Development Counselors program at D.C. Children's Hospital. This program differed from Rioch's in that the counselors worked with patients of a different class background (Eisdorfer & Golann, 1969). A similar cross-class effort was involved in the Albert Einstein College of Medicine Mental Health Rehabilitation workers project which also used mature women (Davidoff, 1969). In each case, evaluation established the effectiveness of the services delivered by the paraprofessional. Other programs have used college students as therapeutic agents, a use of paraprofessionals which crosses both class and age lines (Beck, Kantor, & Gelineau, 1963; Buckley, Muench, & Sjoberg, 1970; Cowen, Zax, & Laird, 1966; Gruver, 1971; Holzberg, 1964; Kreitzer, 1969; Mitchell, W. E., 1966; Rappaport, Chinsky, & Cowen, 1971). There are now more than 500 such programs (Zax & Cowen, 1972), and one study reports that not only did the college students help chronic patients significantly, but they were more effective than trained, experienced mental health professionals, engaged in similar activities (Poser, 1966).

Both students and other paraprofessionals have been used to conduct behavior modification programs, primarily with emotionally disturbed children (Myra, 1970; Ryback & Staats, 1970; Staats, Minke, & Butts, 1970). An evaluative study of one such program reports that improvement in the desired target behavior was achieved in 18 of the 21 cases; no change occurred in 3 cases; and no cases showed any children becoming worse (Suinn, 1974).

In Australia, paraprofessional part-time volunteers (mature adults, successfully married) provide marriage counseling service. Some 270 persons serve approximately 15,000 persons per year. The volunteers receive weekly training for about a year and a half, primarily in a nondirective, client-centered Rogerian approach. Assessments of the results show that in about 15% of the cases the problem was solved, and in another 25% of the cases marital relations were noticeably improved (Harvey, 1964).

Aides trained in Rogerian "play therapy" worked with six Head Start children diagnosed by a psychologist as in need of psychotherapy because of uncontrollable withdrawn and inhibited behavior. "All six children treated by the aide showed signs of improvement during the [treatment] period," as reported by Andronico and Guerney (1969, p. 16).

Research with a different focus, an attempt to assess the aptitude of the proposed trainee for the job of counselor, has been conducted at the Arkansas Rehabilitation Research and Training Center. In this work, led by Carkhuff and Truax, the effort has been made to identify those characteristics which make for more effective counseling, and for the use of lay counselors. Two major experiments are of interest: The first compared the work of lay therapists, clinical psychology graduate students, and experienced therapists (Truax, 1965). It involved 150 chronic hospitalized patients. "The variety of current diagnoses included manic depressive reactions, psychotic depressive reactions, and schizophrenic [reactions]" (Truax, 1965, p. 11). Patients were randomly assigned to lay persons who had received 100 hours of training, to clinical psychology graduate students, and to experienced counselors. "The lay mental health counselors were able to provide a level of therapeutic conditions only slightly below that of the experienced therapists and considerably above that of graduate student trainees" (Truax, 1965, p. 12).

Earlier work of the Arkansas group had isolated three factors as critical to a therapist's effect upon the patient: the ability to communicate a high level of accurate empathy, nonpossessive warmth, and an attitude of genuineness toward the patients. There were no significant differences among the three groups of counselors in the areas of communicating accurate empathy or nonpossessive warmth. On the third factor, communicating genuineness to the patient, however, the experienced therapists showed significantly higher performance.

Truax, the project director, in summarizing the effect upon patients of the work of the lay therapists, wrote:

> Research evaluation indicated highly significant patient outcomes in *overall improvement, improvement in interpersonal relations, improvement in self-care, and self-concern, and improvement in emotional disturbance* (1965, p. 26). (Emphasis in the original.)

The second study conducted at the Arkansas Center addressed more closely the effect of paraprofessional counselors. The paraprofessionals focused on teaching life adjustment skills to clients. Some 400 patients, at the Hot Springs Rehabilitation Center, a large residential center, were randomly assigned in three different groups: (a) to experienced professional MA degree counselors; (b) to experienced MA degree counselors assisted by an aide under maximum supervision; and (c) to aides (former secretaries with little if any college but 100 hours of training), working alone under supervision. Within each of the three patterns, case load was varied at either 30 or 60; thus, there was a 3 X 2 experimental design. Two-thirds of the patients were male; two-thirds white; all had personality or behavioral problems; and a sizable number had speech and hearing defects, or were mentally retarded (Truax & Lister, 1970).

Performance under the three patterns of staffing was measured based upon client work quantity, client cooperativeness, client work attitude, quality of client work, client dependability, client ability to learn, and overall client progress.

On all measures:

> The best results were obtained by the aides, working alone under the daily supervision of professional counselors. The professional counselors working alone had the second best results, while the counselors plus the aide had the poorest effects upon clients (Truax & Lister, 1970, p. 334).

The authors suggest that the paraprofessionals' success may be a result of their probable high level of empathy.

Carrying their conclusions beyond this project, the authors state:

> The findings presented here are consistent with a growing body of research which indicated that the effectiveness of counseling and psychotherapy, as measured by constructive changes in client functioning, is largely independent of the counselor's level of training and theoretical orientation (Truax & Lister, 1970, p. 334).

THREE SURVEYS OF THE RESEARCH ON PARAPROFESSIONALS IN MENTAL HEALTH

Three major efforts have been made to survey the literature which reports assessments of the effectiveness of the use of paraprofessionals in the mental health field. These reports have been authored by Durlak (1973), Karlsruher (1974), and Sobey (1970).

Durlak reports that, based upon over 300 references over the past 10 years, "only six reports were discovered that cited negative results with respect to the clinical effectiveness of paraprofessionals" (Durlak, 1973, p. 301). Durlak identified 14 studies that used various experimental procedures to compare directly the therapeutic effectiveness of nonprofessional and professional personnel; in 7 of the 14 "lay therapists had achieved significantly better therapeutic results than professionals; in the other 7 studies, results for the two groups were similar. *In no study have lay persons been found to be significantly inferior to professional workers*" (Durlak, 1973, p. 301). (Emphasis in the original.)

Among the 27 studies reviewed by Karlsruher (1974) only 5 compared the differential effectiveness of professionals and nonprofessionals as psychotherapeutic agents; in 8 studies the control group received no treatment; and in the remainder there were no controls.[1] Among the 13 studies of programs serving inpatient adults, 12 of the studies report that the nonprofessionals were able to change the behavior of the patients. In 7 of the 8 studies where there was a control of an untreated group, there was "a significantly larger change in the behavior of the group treated by the nonprofessionals than in a no-treatment control group" (Karlsruher, 1974, p. 65). Karlsruher reports that the changes in behavior in the controlled studies included measures of such indices as overt behavior (Appleby, 1963; Carkhuff & Truax, 1965; Verinis, 1970); results of psychological tests (Buckley, Muench, & Sjoberg, 1970; Holzberg, Knapp, & Turner, 1967; Rappaport, Chinsky, & Cowen, 1971); and discharge rate (Carkhuff & Truax, 1965). Only two studies (Anker & Walsh, 1961; Poser, 1966) reviewed by Karlsruher included patient groups treated by professionals as well as by nonprofessionals, "and neither study allows clear interpretation of its findings because of methodological limitations" (Karlsruher, 1974, p. 66).

None of the six empirical studies of outpatient adults compared the therapeutic results of those treated by nonprofessionals with a no-treatment control group or a professionally treated group. While "the behavior of adult outpatients who are treated by nonprofessionals seems to improve . . . it is impossible to determine whether their improvement is greater than the rate of change in an untreated group" (Karlsruher, 1974, p. 67). And in the eight studies of adolescents and children seen by nonprofessionals which Karlsruher reviewed, lack of measures of psychotherapeutic changes, as well as the absence of control groups, lead him to conclude that it is "impossible to determine the psychotherapeutic effectiveness of nonprofessionals with children" (Karlsruher, 1974, p. 68).

Valuable as is the work of Durlak and Karlsruher, the broadest examination of the work by paraprofessionals in mental health is Sobey's study (1970) of over 10,000 paraprofessionals in 185 National Institute of Mental Health (NIMH) sponsored programs. The major finding suggests the most prevalent reason for the use of paraprofessionals:

> Nonprofessionals are utilized not simply because professional manpower is unavailable, but rather to provide new services in innovative ways. Nonprofessionals are providing such therapeutic functions as individual counseling, activity group therapy, milieu therapy; they are doing case finding; they are playing screening roles of a nonclerical nature; they are helping people to adjust to community life; they are providing special skills such as tutoring; they are promoting client self-help through involving clients in helping others having similar problems (Sobey, 1970, p. 6).

The basis for the use of paraprofessionals is illustrated by the responses of project directors to the question of whether, given a choice of hiring professionals, project directors would prefer to utilize paraprofessionals for those functions which professionals had previously performed. In short, 54% preferred to use paraprofessionals over professionals for tasks previously performed by professionals, or to put it another way, only 32% preferred to use professionals (Sobey, 1970, pp. 154–156).

The directors saw paraprofessionals as contributing across a broad spectrum of program activities, including serving more people, offering new services, and providing the project staff with new viewpoints in regard to the project population (Sobey, 1970, p. 159). According to Sobey's report, the paraprofessionals performed three major functions—therapeutic help, special skill training, and community adjustment; and five lesser ones—case finding, orientation to services, screening, caretaking, and community improvement. In 69 projects, the directors reported expanding the professionals' understanding of the client group through association with the paraprofessionals (Sobey, 1970, p. 161). The same thrust is to be seen in the comment that "the introduction of nonprofessionals was perceived as infusing the projects with a new vitality, and forcing a self-evaluation which, although painful, led to beneficial changes for the field of mental health" (Sobey, 1970, p. 175).

The survey also found that the work style and personal attributes of the paraprofessionals were important, as they brought:

> a change in atmosphere within the agency, and more lively and vital relationships among staff and between patients and staff. . . . Improved morale, better attitudes toward patients, definite improvement in overall quality of service were other improvements reported (Sobey, 1970, p. 160).

In summary:

> Nonprofessionals were viewed as contributing to mental health in two unique ways: (1) *filling new roles based on patient needs* which were previously unfilled by any staff; and (2) performing parts of tasks previously performed by professionals, but *tailoring the task to the nonprofessionals' unique and special abilities* (Sobey, 1970, p. 174). (Our emphasis.)

Perhaps because of the breadth of her study, Sobey does not provide empirical data as to effectiveness of the paraprofessionals' work on the client or patient. Unfortunately, most of the studies of indigenous paraprofessionals suffer from a similar absence.

SOME RESEARCH IN COMMUNITY MENTAL HEALTH

The work of paraprofessionals in the delivery of community-based mental health services has been described in a number of reports. Some of the more important reports in this category are described here.

One of the earliest uses of indigenous paraprofessionals was the "Baker's Dozen" project of Fishman and Mitchell (Note 1: Fishman & McCormack, 1969), Mitchell (1968, 1970), and their colleagues at Howard University (National Institute for New Careers, 1968, 1970).

A 1969 survey of 80 community mental health centers found that 42% of all full-time positions were filled by indigenous workers. The figures were higher in drug abuse treatment (60%) and geriatric service (70%) (National Institute for New Careers, 1970, pp. 14–15). A study in the same year of paraprofessionals in 10 community mental health centers in New York City reported that their "actual work as described by administrators varied from unskilled to highly skilled but more often is of the highly skilled variety" (Gottesfeld, 1970, p. 288). The work included interviewing, escort service, home visits, staffing a storefront office, receiving complaints, collecting information, acting as translators, performing individual and group counseling, organizing community meetings, leading therapy groups, assisting patients in self-care, acting as patients' advocates with other agencies, case finding, screening applicants, making case conference presentations, doing casework, giving speeches, planning aftercare services, and giving supportive psychotherapy to ex-patients.

In another key piece of research in the history of paraprofessionals, Hallowitz, the co-director of the pioneering Lincoln Hospital Mental Health Services Neighborhood Service Center program, describes a range of activities for the indigenous worker in such a setting. These include: expediting services, being a friend in need, assisting with sociotherapy, supervised work, services to post-hospital patients, services to the disturbed in the community, and self-help (Hallowitz, 1968).

The Lincoln Hospital Mental Health Services Neighborhood Service Center program began with an Office of Economic Opportunity (OEO) grant January 1, 1965. Three centers were established, each staffed with 5 to 10 aides. They were seen as "bridges" between the professionals and the community. They are expediters of services, advocates, and counselors. Something of the power of their impact and the need for services in a community such as the South Bronx is shown by the service figure of 6,500 persons seen at two of the centers in the first nine months. As the program offered services to the clients' whole family, it was estimated that over 25,000 persons were affected during that period (Riessman & Hallowitz, 1965).

An important example of the early use of paraprofessionals is the program at Harlem Hospital, which has employed indigenous workers in a variety of roles. Harlem residents, interested in working with the aged, provided outpatient, geriatric psychiatric services. They made home visits, provided escort services, observed and reported upon patient behavior, and provided social services. About 30 cases, or half of the study group, were successfully managed. Especially innovative is the Harlem Hospital Group Therapy Program, which used indigenous aides (Christmas, 1966). The aides work in a half-day treatment program for a small group of chronic psychotic post-hospital patients. The aides participate as co-therapists in weekly group psychotherapy sessions, act as participants and expediters of services in the monthly medication group meetings, are members of the weekly therapeutic community meetings, and lead the weekly client discussion groups. In addition, they perform case services, family services, and home interviews; survey patient needs; and provide community mental health education (Christmas, 1966, p. 413). The program was expected to hold one-third of the patients; it has held two-thirds (Wade, 1969, p. 678).

The Temple University Community Mental Health Center has trained indigenous workers as mental health assistants, workers whom they describe as "helpers first, then therapists" (Lynch, Gardner, & Felzer, 1968, p. 428). Over a period of time, a work pattern has developed where the mental health assistants "function as a 'primary therapist' providing ongoing treatment and continuity of care which would include the procurement of ancillary (professional) services whenever appropriate" (Lynch et al., 1968, p. 429). The assistant, a title the workers themselves prefer to "aide," worked with 96% of the patients in the clinic's first year. Two key factors in their work involved "holding" patients, and, by their availability, preventing hospitalization:

> While the percentage of patients' attrition between initial contact and first appointment is still high, it is still a lower rate than that presented for comparable patient aggregates in usual clinic settings. The need to hospitalize patients contacting the crisis center and clinic has decreased by 50% due to the Assistants' availability for immediate outpatient care (Lynch et al., 1968, p. 430).

In summing up his survey of nonprofessionals in mental health, Cowen (1973, p. 448) states, "Collectively nonprofessionals are doing virtually everything professionals do; they are also involved in new activities not heretofore considered part of MH [mental health] services."

EXPLANATORY FACTORS: WHY ARE PARAPROFESSIONALS EFFECTIVE?

As limited as the data are as to the effectiveness of the performance of paraprofessionals in mental health, they are myriad compared to those which address causal explanations. Indeed, there is no study (or set of studies) which allows us to state with any degree of confidence that this or that characteristic —indigeneity, age, sex, race, training, institutional setting, supervision, etc.— *causes* a particular set of outcomes. The best we can do is to identify reports as to types of conditions which appear to conduce toward particular desired outcomes.

Based upon his review of studies of paraprofessional programs, Karlsruher (1974) reports that "no particular group of nonprofessionals appears to be the most effective. That is, whether the nonprofessional is a psychiatric aide, a college student, an adult from the community, a medical doctor without psychiatric training, a medical student, or a student nurse does not seem to influence the outcome of his [sic] treatment" (Karlsruher, 1974, p. 69). He does offer the caveat that the studies which form the bases for this conclusion primarily involve adults as patients. He suggests that other age groups such as "children or adolescents may be more affected by their [the nonprofessionals'] personal characteristics. A disturbed adolescent may be more influenced by another adolescent as a therapist than by an adult" (Karlsruher, 1974, p. 70).[2]

Perhaps the reason that Karlsruher finds no special effect of this or that type of nonprofessional is that, for the most part, his studies involve no special "matching" between client and provider. The qualities of indigeneity stressed in the New Careers effort (Gartner, 1971; National Institute for New Careers, 1968, 1970; Pearl & Riessman, 1965) and the findings as to the success of students as counselors with other students (Brown, 1965, 1972, 1974; Goodman, 1972; Zunker & Brown, 1966) may suggest that among "deprived" populations, that is, the poor, minorities, and youth, shared characteristics between provider and consumer are more critical. Interestingly, the qualities Carkhuff (1969, p. 119) describes as those of an effective lay counselor would apply as well to the indigenous worker. These include: the increased ability to enter the milieu of the distressed; the ability to establish peer-like relationships with the needy; the ability to take an active part in the clients' total life situation; the ability to empathize more fully with the clients' style of life; the ability to teach the client more successful actions from within the clients' frame of reference; and the ability to provide clients with a more effective transition to more effective levels of functioning within the social system.

Reiff and Riessman (1964) emphasize that the ability of indigenous paraprofessionals is "rooted in their background. It is not based on things they have been taught but on what they *are*" (Reiff & Riessman, 1964, p. 6). They are poor; their families are poor; they are peers of the client and share a common language, background, ethnic origin, style, and interests. They can establish special relations with clients, because to the client the paraprofessional "belongs," is a "significant other," is "one of us"; and, along with the clients, there is "the tendency to externalize causes rather than look for internal ones" (Reiff & Riessman, 1964, pp. 9–10).

An alternative explanation for the ability of paraprofessionals has been suggested by Brown (1974). Relying heavily upon Carkhuff's work (Carkhuff, 1969; Carkhuff & Truax, 1965; Truax & Carkhuff, 1967; Truax & Lister, 1970), Brown notes that the criteria for selection of paraprofessionals and the nature of their training may explain the effectiveness of paraprofessionals. Concerning selection, in professional programs the emphasis has been upon highly intellectual indices, such as grade point average, Graduate Record Examination scores, and the like. On the other hand, paraprofessionals are selected for their personal qualities, "a capacity for empathy, warmth, sensitivity in interpersonal relations; high self-confidence and self-regard; and the ability to accept people with values different from their own" (Brown, 1974,

p. 261). And the training of the two groups further accentuates these differences; training for professionals is intellectual and abstract, while that for paraprofessionals is focused upon competencies and attitudes needed to facilitate positive client change.[3]

Addressing the issue of the kind of training as a cause of effectiveness from a research point of view, D'Augelli and Danish (Note 2) note that the most commonly used paraprofessional training programs (Carkhuff, 1969; Danish & Hauer, 1973; Gazda, Asbury, Balzers, Childers, Decelle, & Walters, 1973; Ivey, 1971; Kagan, 1972) "all are concerned with providing to large numbers of potential helpers what might be best termed relationship development skills. . . . The goal of these diverse programs is to enable the helper to create a relationship in which action-oriented change can take place." Carkhuff, basing his work on that of Rogers (1957), identified the qualities of empathy, unconditional positive regard, and genuineness as essential for establishing a helping relationship; and most of the paraprofessional training programs are built around teaching the trainees to respond in these terms (Carkhuff, 1969, p. 3). Similarly, the training programs "employ the integrated didactic-experiential format proposed by Truax and Carkhuff" (Danish & Block, 1974, p. 30).

While selection and training are important, they are only a prelude to performance in the work setting. Unfortunately, we have even less available data as to the consequences of varying work-setting conditions upon the effectiveness of paraprofessional performance. Although limited in its sample and directed toward somewhat different goals, a recent study of 47 paraprofessionals employed in three "exemplary" mental health centers offers interesting insights into the effect of differing work setting conditions on the workers (Alley, Blanton, & Hampden-Turner, Note 3). Among its findings, pertinent to our interests, are the dangers of discontinuity between training ideology and work-site reality; the tendency of paraprofessional workers to drift into work roles which the professionals preferred to avoid, and to find in such roles more freedom, more responsibility,[4] and more pleasure than in others; and the inverse relationship between the growth of the paraprofessionals in the job and the degree of size, structure, and bureaucracy[5] in the work place. It is not surprising that in those work places where the prior "negative" life experiences of the paraprofessionals were regarded as "positive" qualifications for the job by the professionals, where paraprofessionals found ways to integrate their "street knowledge" with more formal educational requirements, and where the formal system of the professionals and the informal system of the paraprofessionals were integrated, the growth of the paraprofessionals was greatest.

Based upon his study of paraprofessional programs, Karlsruher concludes that "neither didactic training nor supervision is necessary to enable the nonprofessional to produce significant behavior change in his [sic] adult patients" (Karlsruher, 1974, p. 70).[6] He also concludes that neither the type of treatment (individual or group) nor length and frequency of treatment, differentiates between more or less successful performance by paraprofessionals (Karl-sruher, 1974, pp. 70–72).

WHEN PARAPROFESSIONALS ARE NOT EFFECTIVE

Of course, the question of effectiveness involves both a question of purpose and comparison. As has been said earlier, Durlak (1973, p. 301) reports that, based upon a survey of over 300 studies, "only six reports were discovered that cited negative results with respect to the clinical effectiveness of nonprofessionals." And Karlsruher (1974, p. 65) reports that of eight studies involving controls, seven "reported a significantly larger change in the behavior of the group treated by the nonprofessionals than in a no-treatment control group"; in the eighth study there was an equal amount of change in the treated and untreated groups.

It is fair to conclude, as Albrecht states, that "if the major goal of the indigenous nonprofessional is solely to render effective therapy and service, then the movement seems able to meet this goal" (Albrecht, 1973, p. 247). However, despite these generally favorable findings, it must be recognized that there are factors which work against the achievement of this goal. These factors lie in two sources: the conceptual bases for the role of the new person-nel; and certain attitudes and actions which they, the paraprofessionals, bring with them to the role. Some of these attitudes or actions might be "excessive dependency, panicking, projecting one's problems onto others, lack of sophisti-cation" (Cowen, 1973, p. 448). However, even beyond the particularities of work behavior, there are the broader issues of contradictory demands within the accepted concept of the paraprofessional's role, including his/her relation-ship to the professional, to his/her community, and to the client. Elsewhere (Gartner, 1970, p. 61), we have said that the paraprofessional is expected to be "worker and consumer, force for change and member of the system, critic of professionalism and aspirant professional." There is role ambiguity (Hal-pern, 1969). Is the paraprofessional to be a "bridge" from the community to the profession (Christmas, Wallace, & Edwards, 1970), to do the professions' menial tasks; or is the task to bring services to the unserved and new services to others? In other words, what are the underlying conceptual bases (Arnhoff, Rubenstein, & Speisman, 1969) for new mental health personnel?

As Minuchin (1969, p. 724) points out, "The inclusion of paraprofession-als in the existing structure of delivery of services brought to a head a bipolarity of approaches to mental illness [the medical model versus the community] which was already incipient in the field." While some see the paraprofessional movement as a cooptive effort (Haug & Sussman, 1969), or pacification (Stat-man, 1970), or "an ill-conceived and unrealistic effort" (Ritzer, 1973, p. 227), Minuchin (1969) argues that the paraprofessional must be both force for and product of a reconceptualization of the very relationship of the individual and society.

NEEDED RESEARCH

Assessing paraprofessional effectiveness is particularly important because the progress of community mental health services may well depend on the effective use of paraprofessionals, considered by many authorities to be the work force of the future. Several researchers in the field stress this important fact:

> The plain and simple truth is that the future delivery of more appropriate mental health services to the general population will be ultimately related to the mental health professional's ability to make maximum and judicious use of nonprofessional manpower [sic] in direct service roles (Durlak, 1973, p. 301).

Cowen (1973, pp. 446–447) goes further; having noted "the now well-recognized fact that standard mental health services have largely failed even to engage the poor," he sees in the paraprofessional movement the "twin potentials for vastly extending helping services and bringing genuine assistance to the many in society who have found prior packaging of MH goods unattractive" (Cowen, 1973, p. 448).

As Sobey (1970) put it, we are in the middle of a "nonprofessional revolution," and to move beyond this stage, we must move beyond "exploring an exciting, challenging new world of usages" to "hard-nosed evaluation" (Cowen, 1973, p. 449). And Goodman (1972) gives further testimony to the growing evidence that the paraprofessional movement is a serious, permanent force for the future.

> As of now, this burgeoning new field appears to be building a conceptual base, testing the administrative feasibility of diverse therapeutic agents and client populations, exploring radical procedures, and just starting the serious business of doing believable research (Goodman, 1972, p. 9).

As the paraprofessional effort continues, there are dangers which must be recognized and countered.

1. The new paraprofessional may be socialized by the professional without influencing the latter very much; in other words, instead of having cross-socialization in which both parties are affected, the impact may be largely one way and the paraprofessional, moving up a career ladder, may by the time he or she arrives at professional status be a replica of the old professional.
2. Movement up the ladder may not occur, and large numbers of paraprofessionals may find themselves trapped at the bottom. There may be ladders with steps that do not reach beyond a very low point; thus, we may have family health aide worker 1, 2, 3, etc., without a new route for moving higher and breaking the credential barrier.

3. The efficiency of the human service system may be increased by the addition of the new personnel, but not really reorganized, so that professionals really perform essentially the same function as they did before, only with more hands assisting them.

4. In moving from an overly academic, abstract, removed training model, there is the danger that the pendulum will swing too far in the other direction so that the workers will largely be trained in a simple type of on-the-job training where they will learn how to perform specific functions, but not really be educated with systematic knowledge of a professional kind. A corollary danger here is that higher education will be vocationalized and rather than having work-study really integrated, work will simply be added on as a substitute for certain courses.

5. Paraprofessionals may be co-opted as a buffer between agency and community rather than being permitted to assist in changing the human service and professional systems.

6. Paraprofessionals may be used to substitute for and compete with professionals in order to save money for agencies.

7. The paraprofessionals may be "compartmentalized," separated off from the professionals, presumably to safeguard their indigeneity, but the effect, of course, will be to limit their effect on the professionals as well as to trap them at the bottom of the ladder.

To counter these dangers, paraprofessionals (and their supporters) can look to at least four overlapping strategies to influence the profession and its practice.

Strategy I: Paraprofessionals may influence professionals by working beside them, changing the atmosphere of their agencies, sensitizing them to the demands of the community as well as by participating in professional organizations and unions.

Strategy II: As paraprofessionals move up a career ladder to become professionals via new combinations of training, work, and education, they may become a different kind of professional at the end of the route. In addition, as paraprofessionals, the latter have the opportunity of performing new kinds of functions—for example, consultation, supervision, training, management, administration, and diagnosis.

Strategy III: Paraprofessionals may change professional practice by performing new work, or new job functions, such as health advocate, expediter, parent educator, program developer. In this way the paraprofessional can provide a whole range of new human service practice.

Strategy IV: Paraprofessionals, in a variety of ways, may improve the performance, efficiency, and productivity of human service agencies, and in so doing, affect the professions.

For whatever else it is that paraprofessionals do, it is doing, and doing well, the tasks that contribute to human service that justifies their presence in the field of mental health and encourages the expansion of their role.

SUMMARY

The most basic criterion for judging the value of paraprofessionals is the effectiveness of the services that they provide. While a number of the research studies on this issue suffer from methodological problems, a growing body of methodologically sound studies supports the hypothesis that paraprofessionals can and do provide effective services.

The largest number of studies concerns the use of paraprofessionals in educational settings. Within the field of mental health, methodologically sound studies suggest that paraprofessionals are effective providers of crisis center responsibilities and various caretaking and educational functions on inpatient wards. While more problematic methodologically, a number of studies also suggests that paraprofessionals are effective as outpatient therapists. Furthermore, the findings of some individual studies (e.g., Poser, 1966; Truax, 1965, Truax & Lister, 1970) and of a comprehensive review of available evidence (Durlak, 1973) indicate that paraprofessionals can on occasion exceed professionals or trained graduate students in their ability effectively to deliver mental health services to clients.

What conditions promote effective performance by paraprofessionals? Some correlational studies provide some clues, if not hard evidence. Research by Truax (1965) suggests that the effectiveness of paraprofessionals depends, in part, on communication of a high level of accurate empathy and nonpossessive warmth toward clients. These qualities may result from the fact that paraprofessionals share characteristics with their clients (Reiff & Riessman, 1964). Additional enhancing factors appear to include carefully designed selection procedures (Brown, 1974), combined with well executed training programs (e.g., D'Augelli & Danish, Note 2). More general work setting factors, although rarely studied, probably also influence the effectiveness of paraprofessionals.

It is important that research on the effectiveness of paraprofessionals be continued. The types of studies needed can be divided into four interrelated categories: First, there is a need for further methodologically sound research on the question of whether paraprofessionals are indeed effective in the delivery of mental health services in general; second, relevant studies are needed for each of the community mental health service areas as well as for typical activities in which paraprofessionals serve, such as involvement in organizing self-help groups; third, there is a need for a series of highly focused studies, singly and in combination, to identify work conditions which influence successful and effective paraprofessional performance. These influencing factors include training, supervision, and the availability of career ladders. Finally, there is a need for research documenting how the skills of paraprofessionals, learned from their life experiences and their adaptation to their environment, can best be used to enhance the effectiveness of services provided by mental health centers.

Whether or not paraprofessionals are here to stay is no longer in question; they comprise a significant and growing component of the present and future mental health work force. Paraprofessionals have been deployed successfully for a number of years in a variety of roles, bringing forth fresh perspectives and new skills to the community mental health movement. Therefore, the important questions for future research in the field must focus on the best ways to tap this new resource, so that the professional mental health worker, the client, and the delivery of services can derive the greatest benefit. A choice must be made between using paraprofessionals as merely a numerically increased force of assistants to professionals, and changing the structure of task assignments in the delivery of mental health services. This reorganization, which would include a redefinition of the roles and functions of both professional and nonprofessional mental health workers, may provide, as its greatest benefit, a mutual exchange of knowledge and experience of incalculable value to the field and to the mental health client.

NOTES

[1]Unfortunately, the studies reviewed by Durlak and Karlsruher differ and, therefore, their reviews are not strictly comparable.

[2]Note in this regard the success of programs involving children teaching children (Allen, 1976; Gartner, Kohler, & Riessman, 1971; Newmark, 1976).

[3]In addition to these characteristics which may affect the positive performance of paraprofessional workers, there is the effect of such work upon the paraprofessionals themselves. Here there is the influence of what Riessman (1965) has called the "helper-therapy principle," that is, the person with a problem is helped (perhaps most) in the process of giving help. Of course, this is a central factor in the entire self-help mutual aid effort (Caplan & Killilea, 1976; Gartner & Riessman, 1977; Katz & Bender, 1976). And the Queens College Mental Health Baccalaureate Program, sponsored by NIMH's Paraprofessional Branch, paraprofessionals are being trained to organize and work with self-help mutual aid groups. (See Chapter 14 by Frank Riessman in this book for a further discussion of these issues.)

[4]In another study (Truax & Lister, 1970), it is reported that faced with high case load paraprofessionals spent more time with clients while professionals spent less. The aides, in effect, appeared to feel that it was necessary to work hard to get to all the cases, while the professionals seemed to feel that with so many clients to see, what is the use? (Truax & Lister, 1970, pp. 331–332).

[5]Based upon a study of paraprofessionals (who were recovering alcoholics) employed as counselors in a mental health center alcoholism rehabilitation program in Indiana (Chalfaut, Martinson, & Crowe, 1975), it is recommended that such persons not be hired unless they have had previous experience in a bureaucratic setting.

[6]The *particular* studies reviewed by Karlsruher support these conclusions.

REFERENCE NOTES

1. J. Fishman, & L. Mitchell, *New careers for the disadvantaged.* Paper presented at the annual meeting of the American Psychiatric Association, San Francisco, May 1970.
2. A. R. D'Augelli & S. J. Danish, Evaluating training programs for paraprofessionals and nonprofessionals. *Journal of Consulting Psychology,* in press.
3. S. Alley, J. Blanton, & C. Hampden-Turner, *Personal and career development: A study of paraprofessionals in three exemplary programs.* Unpublished manuscript, 1976. (Available from Social Action Research Center, 18 Professional Center Parkway, San Rafael, Calif. 94903.)

REFERENCES

Albrecht, G. L. The indigenous mental health worker: The cure-all for what ailment? In P. M. Roman & H. M. Trice (Eds.), *The sociology of psychotherapy.* New York: Jason Aronson, 1973.

Allen, V. (Ed.). *Children as teachers: Theory and research on tutoring.* New York: Academic Press, 1976.

Andronico, M. P., & Guerney, B., Jr. A psychotherapeutic aide in a Head Start program. *Children,* 1969, *16,* 14–17.

Anker, J. M., & Walsh, R. P. Group psychotherapy, a special activity program, and group structure in the treatment of chronic schizophrenics. *Journal of Counseling Psychology,* 1961, *25,* 476–481.

Appleby, L. Evaluation of treatment methods for chronic schizophrenics. *Archives of General Psychiatry,* 1963, *8,* 8–21.

Arnhoff, F. N., Rubenstein, E. A., & Spiesman, J. C. (Eds.). *Man-power for mental health.* Chicago: Aldine, 1969.

Beck, J. C., Kantor, D., & Gelineau, V. A. Follow-up of chronic psychotic patients "treated" by college case-aide volunteers. *American Journal of Psychiatry,* 1963, *120,* 269–271.

Bennett, W. S., Jr., & Falk, R. F. *New careers and urban schools.* New York: Holt, Rinehart, and Winston, 1970.

Brown, W. F. Student-to-student counseling for academic adjustment. *The Personnel and Guidance Journal,* 1965, *18,* 821–830.

Brown, W. F. *Student-to-student counseling: An approach to motivating academic achievement.* Austin: University of Texas, Hogg Foundation for Mental Health, 1972.

Brown, W. F. Effectiveness of paraprofessionals: The evidence. *The Personnel and Guidance Journal,* 1974, *53,* 257–263.

Buckley, H. M., Muench, G. A., & Sjoberg, B. M. Effects of a college student visitation program on a group of chronic schizophrenics. *Journal of Abnormal Psychology,* 1970, *75,* 242–244.

Caplan, G., & Killilea, M. (Eds.). *Support systems and mutual help.* New York: Grune and Stratton, 1976.

Carkhuff, R. R. *Helping and human relations (Vol. 1 and 2).* New York: Holt, Rinehart, and Winston, 1969.

Carkhuff, R. R., & Truax, C. B. Lay mental health counseling: The effects of lay group counseling. *Journal of Counseling Psychology,* 1965, *29,* 426–431.

Chalfaut, H. P., Martinson, L. O. A., & Crowe, D. J. Prior occupational experience and choice of alcoholism rehabilitation counselors. *Community Mental Health Journal,* 1975, *11,* 402–409.

Christmas, J. J. Group methods in teaching and action: Nonprofessional mental health personnel in a deprived community. *American Journal of Orthopsychiatry,* 1966, *36,* 410–419.

Christmas, J. J., Wallace, M., & Edwards, J. New careers and new mental health services: Fantasy or future? *American Journal of Psychiatry,* 1970, *126,* 1480–1486.

Conant, E. *Teacher and paraprofessional work productivity: A public school cost effectiveness study.* Lexington, Mass.: Lexington Books, 1973.

Costa, C. *A comparative study of career opportunities program graduates as first year teachers.* New York: New Careers Training Laboratory, Queens College, 1975.

Cowen, E. L. Social and community interventions. In P. H. Mussen & M. R. Rosenzweig (Eds.), *Annual review of psychology (Vol. 24).* Palo Alto, Calif.: Annual Reviews, Inc., 1973.

Cowen, E. L., Zax, M., & Laird, J. D. A college student volunteer program in the elementary school setting. *Community Mental Health Journal,* 1966, *2,* 319–328.

Danish, S. J., & Block, G. W. The current status of paraprofessional training. *The Personnel and Guidance Journal,* 1974, *53,* 299–303.

Danish, S. J., & Hauer, A. L. *Helping skills: A basic training program.* New York: Behavioral Publications, 1973.

Davidoff, I. F. The mental health rehabilitation worker: A member of the psychiatric team. *Community Mental Health Journal,* 1969, *5,* 45–54.

Durlak, J. A. Myths concerning the nonprofessional therapist. *Professional Psychology,* 1973, *4,* 300–304.

Eisdorfer, C., & Golann, S. E. Principles for training "new professionals" in mental health. *Community Mental Health Journal,* 1969, *5,* 352–359.

Ellsworth, R. B. *Nonprofessionals in psychiatric rehabilitation.* New York: Appleton-Century-Crofts, 1968.

Fishman, J., & McCormack, J. *Mental health without walls: Community mental health in the ghetto.* Washington, D.C.: New Careers Development, University Research Corporation, 1969.

Gartner, A. Organizing paraprofessionals. *Social Policy,* 1970, *1,* 60–61.

Gartner, A. *Paraprofessionals and their performance.* New York: Praeger Publishers, 1971.

Gartner, A. *The utilization of paraprofessionals.* Paris, France: Organization of Economic Cooperation and Development, 1976.

Gartner, A., Jackson, V. C., & Riessman, F. *Paraprofessionals today (Vol. 1): Education.* New York: Human Sciences Press, 1977.

Gartner, A., Kohler, M. C., Riessman, F. *Children teaching children: Learning by teaching.* New York: Harper and Row, 1971.

Gartner, A., & Riessman, F. The performance of paraprofessionals in the mental health field. In G. Caplan (Ed.), *The American handbook of psychiatry.* New York: Basic books, 1971.

Gartner, A., & Riessman, F. *Self-help in the human services.* San Francisco: Jossey-Bass, 1977.

Gazda, G. M., Ashbury, F. R., Balzer, F. J., Childers, N. C., Decille, R. E., & Walters, R. P. *Human relations development: A manual for educators.* Boston: Allyn and Bacon, 1973.

Goodman, G. *Companionship therapy.* San Francisco: Jossey-Bass, 1972.

Gottesfeld, H. A study of the role of paraprofessionals in community mental health. *Community Mental Health Journal,* 1970, *6,* 286–290.

Gruver, G. G. College students as therapeutic agents. *Psychological Bulletin,* 1971, *76,* 111–128.

Hallowitz, E. The expanding role of the neighborhood service center. In F. Riessman & H. Papper (Eds.), *Up from poverty: New career ladders for nonprofessionals.* New York: Harper and Row, 1968.

Halpern, W. I. The community mental health aide. *Mental Hygiene,* 1969, *53,* 78–83.

Harvey, L. V. The use of nonprofessional auxiliary counselors in staffing a counseling service. *Journal of Counseling Psychology,* 1964, *11,* 348–351.

Haug, M. R., & Sussman, M. B. Professional autonomy and the revolt of the client. *Social Problems,* 1969, *17,* 153–161.

Holzberg, J. D. Chronic patients and a college companion program. *Mental Hospitals,* 1964, *15,* 152–158.

Holzberg, J. D., Knapp, R. H., & Turner, J. L. College students as companions to the mentally ill. In E. L. Cowne, E. A. Gardner, & M. Zax (Eds.), *Emergent approaches to mental health problems.* New York: Appleton-Century-Crofts, 1967.

Ivey, A. E. *Microcounseling.* Chicago: Charles C Thomas, 1971.

Kagan, N. *Influencing human interaction.* East Lansing: Michigan State University, 1972.

Kaplan, G. *From aide to teacher: The story of the career opportunities program.* Washington, D.C.: U.S. Government Printing Office, 1977.

Karlsruher, A. E. The nonprofessional as a psychotherapeutic agent: A review of the empirical evidence pertaining to his effectiveness. *American Journal of Community Psychology,* 1974, *2,* 61–77.

Katz, A., & Bender, E. *The strength within us.* New York: Franklin Watts, 1976.

Kreitzer, S. F. The therapeutic use of student volunteers. In B. F. Guerney, Jr. (Ed.), *Psychotherapeutic agents: New roles for nonprofessionals, parents, and teachers.* New York: Holt, Rinehart, and Winston, 1969.

Lynch, M., Gardner, E. A., & Felzer, S. B. The role of indigenous personnel as clinical therapist. *Archives of General Psychiatry,* 1968, *19,* 428–434.

Magoon, T. M., Golann, S. E., & Freeman, R. W. *Mental health counselors at work.* New York: Pergamon, 1969.

Minuchin, S. The paraprofessional and the use of confrontation in the mental health field. *American Journal of Orthopsychiatry,* 1969, *39,* 722–729.

Mitchell, L. Baker's dozen: A program for training young people as mental health aides. *Mental Health Program Reports,* 1968, *2,* 11–24.

Mitchell, L. *Training for community mental health aides: Leaders for child and adolescent therapeutic activity groups; report of a program.* Washington, D.C.: Institute for Youth Studies, Howard University, 1970.

Mitchell, W. E. Amicatherapy: Theoretical perspectives and an example of practice. *Community Mental Health Journal,* 1966, *2,* 307–314.

Myra, M. Results of behavior-modification program for parents and teachers. *Behavior Research and Therapy,* 1970, *8,* 309–312.

National Institute for New Careers. *An assessment of technical assistance and training needs in new careers projects sponsored by the United States Department of Labor.* Washington, D.C.: University Research Corporation, 1968.

National Institute for New Careers. *New careers in mental health: A status report.* Washington, D.C.: University Research Corporation, 1970.

Newmark, G. *This school belongs to you and me: Every learner a teacher, every teacher a learner.* New York: Hart Publishing Co., 1976.

Pearl, A., & Riessman, F. *New careers for the poor.* New York: Free Press, 1965.

Poser, E. G. The effect of therapist training on group therapeutic outcome. *Journal of Consulting Psychology,* 1966, *30,* 283–289.

Rappaport, J., Chinsky, J. M., & Cowen, E. L. *Innovations in helping chronic patients: College students in a mental institution.* New York: Academic Press, 1971.

Reiff, R., & Riessman, F. *The indigenous nonprofessional: A strategy of change in community action and community mental health programs.* New York: National Institute of Labor Education, 1964.

Riessman, F. The "helper-therapy" principle. *Social Work,* 1965, *10,* 27–32.

Riessman, F., & Hallowitz, E. *Neighborhood service centers program: A report to the U.S. office of Economic Opportunity on the South Bronx Neighborhood Service Center,* December, 1965. (Available from F. Riessman, Center for Advanced Study in Education, 33 West 42nd Street, New York, N.Y. 10036.)

Rioch, M. National Institute of Mental Health pilot study in training mental health counselors. *American Journal of Orthopsychiatry,* 1963, *33,* 678–698.

Ritzer, G. Indigenous nonprofessionals in community mental health. In P. M. Roman & H. M. Trice (Eds.), *The sociology of psychotherapy.* New York: Jason Aronson, 1973.

Rogers, C. R. The necessary and sufficient conditions of psychotherapeutic personality change. *Journal of Counseling Psychology,* 1957, *21,* 95–103.

Ryback, D., & Staats, A. Parents as behavior therapy-technicians in treating reading deficits (dyslexia). *Journal of Behavior Therapy and Experimental Psychiatry,* 1970, *1,* 109–120.

Sobey, F. *The nonprofessional revolution in mental health.* New York: Columbia University Press, 1970.

Staats, A., Minke, K., & Butts, P. A token-reinforcement remedial reading program administered by black therapy-technicians to problem black children. *Behavior Therapy,* 1970, *1,* 331–353.

Statman, J. Community mental health: The evolution of a concept in social policy. *Community Mental Health Journal,* 1970, *3,* 5–12.

Suinn, R. Training undergraduate students as community behavior modification consultants. *Journal of Counseling Psychology*, 1974, *21*, 71–77.

Truax, C. B. *An approach toward training for the aide therapist: Research and implications.* Fayetteville, Ark.: Arkansas Rehabilitation Research and Training Center, 1965.

Truax, C. B., & Lister, J. L. Effectiveness of counselors and counselor aides. *Journal of Consulting Psychology*, 1970, *17*, 331–334.

Verinis, J. S. Therapeutic effectiveness of untrained volunteers with chronic patients. *Journal of Consulting Psychology*, 1970, *34*, 152–155.

Wade, R. The view of the professional. *American Journal of Orthopsychiatry*, 1969, *34*, 676–680.

Zax, M., & Cowen, E. *Abnormal psychology: Changing conceptions.* New York: Holt, Rinehart, and Winston, 1972.

Zunker, V. G., & Brown, W. F. Comparative effectiveness of student and professional counselors. *The Personnel and Guidance Journal*, 1966, *44*, 738–743.

RELEVANT READING MATERIALS

Blau, T. H. The professional in the community views the nonprofessional helper. *Professional Psychology*, 1969, *1*, 25–31.

Delworth, V., Sherwood, G., & Casaburri, N. *Student paraprofessionals: A working model for higher education* (American Personnel and Guidance Association Student Personnel Series No. 17). Washington, D.C.: American Personnel and Guidance Association Press, 1974.

Dorr, D., Cowen, E. L., Sandler, I., & Pratt, D. M. Dimensionality of a test battery for nonprofessional mental health workers. *Journal of Consulting and Clinical Psychology*, 1973, *41*, 181–185.

Garber, D. L., & O'Brien, D. E. Operationalization of theory in the training of paraprofessional. *Journal of Education for Social Work*, 1977, *13*, 60–67.

Goodman, G. M., & Dooley, D. A framework for help-intended communication. *Psychotherapy*, 1976, *13*, 106–117.

Magoon, T. M., & Golann, S. E. Non-traditionally trained women as mental health counselors-psychotherapists. *The Personnel and Guidance Journal*, 1966, *44*, 788–793.

Paul, G. L., & McInnis, T. L. Attitudinal changes associated with two approaches to training mental health technicians in milieu and social-learning programs. *Journal of Consulting and Clinical Psychology*, in press.

Porter, L. W., Steers, R. M., & Mowday, R. T. Organizational commitment, job satisfaction, and turnover among psychiatric technicians. *Journal of Applied Psychology*, 1974, *59*, 609.

Reiff, R. Mental health manpower and institutional change. *American Psychologist*, 1966, *21*, 540–548.

Reiff, R., & Riessman, F. The indigenous nonprofessional: A strategy for change in community action and community mental health programs. *Community Mental Health Journal Monograph*, 1965, (No. 1).

Riessman, F. The crisis in new careers. *New Human Services Newsletter*, 1972, *2*, 2.

Riessman, F., & Hallowitz, E. The neighborhood service center: An innovation in preventive psychiatry. *American Journal of Psychiatry,* 1967, *123,* 1408–1413.

Seidman, E., & Rappaport, J. The educational pyramid: A paradigm for training, research, and manpower utilization in community psychology. *American Journal of Community Psychology,* 1974, *2,* 119–130.

Summers, D. A., Fancher, T., & Chapman, S. B. A note on nonprofessional judgments of mental health. *Community Mental Health Journal,* 1973, *9,* 169–177.

Truax, C. B., & Carkhuff, R. R. *Toward effective counseling and psychotherapy: Training and practice.* Chicago: Aldine, 1967.

Varenhorst, B. B. Training adolescents as peer counselors. *The Personnel and Guidance Journal,* 1974, *53,* 271–275.

Zimpfer, D. G. (Ed.). *Paraprofessionals in counseling guidance, and personnel services* (American Personnel and Guidance Association Reprint Series No. 5). Washington, D.C.: American Personnel and Guidance Association Press, 1974.

Chapter 5

THE HUMAN SERVICE GENERALIST: A FRAMEWORK FOR INTEGRATING AND UTILIZING ALL LEVELS OF STAFF

Richard E. Dorgan*
Ronald J. Gerhard†

The "human services generalist framework," a model formulated by the authors, is directly relevant to two frequently occurring concerns within mental health organizations. First, it provides a structure to enable paraprofessionals and master's-level professionals to combine career ladder advancement with continued employment at a mental health agency. Secondly, it assists human service agencies, confronted with increasingly complex service problems, in facilitating the development of "generalist" skills in currently employed staff members.

The framework contains a career grid that gives employees access to opportunities for vertical mobility (increasing responsibility and pay levels) and horizontal mobility (varying job functions). Vertical mobility is made possible through a combination of formal educational curricula, less formal in-service educational training, and practical on-the-job training. People without a high school diploma can enter a career ladder and, if they acquire the relevant competencies, can eventually advance to the top of the ladder. Horizontal mobility can occur across five function areas: services, administration, community participation, research and evaluation, and staff development.

*Richard E. Dorgan is a Human Service Consultant to several health, education and welfare programs and numerous organizations including the Joint Commission on Accreditation of Hospitals. He is a codesigner of the Balanced Service System.

†Ronald J. Gerhard is the Director of the Office of Planning and Budget, Georgia Department of Human Resources, Atlanta, Georgia. He is a codesigner of the Balanced Service System.

Introduction

In the development of a national network of human service programs compatible with a community partnership philosophy, many local community mental health programs have earnestly sought innovative ways to staff new community-based programs—programs for which the supply of competent personnel is very limited. It would appear that a new kind of human service generalist, with an interdisciplinary background, is needed to provide the new array of services. This paper describes one such generalist framework which incorporates paraprofessional and professional staff members into a single integrated "career grid." The career grid framework allows mental health centers (a) to provide competency-based promotions and work assignments to employees, and (b) to enable staff members to receive the training, education, and work experiences necessary to enhance their work-related competencies.

The series facilitates and insures educational and training opportunities, the development of the natural resources of the individual, multiple promotional avenues and maximum flexibility in the deployment and utilization of human service personnel. The series, thus, is not anchored to the formulations of the industrial model. In that model the production process is reduced to small discrete parts, which results in the assignment of individuals to exclusive pieces of the total product or task to be accomplished. The series, on the other hand, is designed to utilize the range of human resources an individual can bring to bear on multifaceted and diversely distributed service programs.

The career grid framework for human services generalists is designed to accomplish seven major objectives: (1) an elimination of the fragmentation of consumer services along rigid lines delineated by the existing professionally oriented civil service classifications; (2) a flexible deployment and utilization of personnel providing human services to all target populations; (3) a recruitment capacity that ranges from the indigenous paraprofessional worker to the professional; (4) a provision of a framework for the development and implementation of an integrative education and training program designed to meet program objectives and functions; (5) an elimination of inequities in salary and career opportunities; (6) a maximization of the opportunity for on-the-job learning; and (7) an insurance of competent delivery of services.

In addition, the framework has four major characteristics which enable it to be utilized as an effective career grid for human service programs.

1. There are entry level openings at every educational level, beginning with no educational requirement and terminating with the doctorate level.
2. Currently employed staff members have upward mobility within the series on the basis of the successful completion of specific work experience and in-service education rather than on the basis of completion of traditional, exclusively formal academic preparation.

3. There are five preparation units ranging from the "introductory" to the "senior" which allow for the completion of prerequisites for career promotion at various stages in the series.
4. The generalist concept permeates the entire series, enabling extensive flexibility in its application and substantial vertical and horizontal mobility.

Varying Definitions of the Generalist Role

The concept of the role of the human service generalist has gradually evolved to include ever broadening responsibilities. This evolution exemplifies a recurrent historical process, in which the role boundaries of personnel are expanded to improve the fit between the services resulting from the roles and the changing needs of clients. Early generalists were "discipline generalists" who performed all of the duties of a particular profession (e.g., psychologists who performed both diagnostic and therapy functions). Later, there evolved "service generalists" whose work encompassed all of the services to be provided, regardless of the professional orientation. Types of service such as individual, family, and group therapy or theoretical backgrounds such as biological, social, or psychological have also been used as a basis for developing "service generalist" concepts. The "service generalist" may also be defined, as in the following matrix (Fig. 5-1), in terms of the target population whom he/she serves.

By examining the following age/disability matrix from a specialist/generalist frame of reference, the issues become clearer. This matrix contains the age and disability groups of most mental health service systems. Rather than representing services per se, each group represents a target population for whom services are to be provided. Service generalists are often defined in terms of the number or types of groups they serve. The broadest application of the term applies to providers who serve all age groups and all disability groups.

The Functional Generalist

The "functional generalist" is a person whose range of activities potentially spans all of the work to be provided by the delivery system. This work consists of five major clusters of activities called functional areas. (For a further elaboration of these areas into specific functions and activities, the reader is referred to an earlier work, JCAH, 1976.) While functional generalists are not prepared to perform all of the functions of the program, their frame of reference is sufficiently broad so that they can see all the elements of each functional area of their own job and can understand the relationships among these various functional areas.

DISABILITY GROUP / AGE GROUP	THINKING AND FEELING (EMOTIONAL)	LEARNING (MENTAL RETARDATION AND OTHER DEVELOP— MENTAL DISABILITIES	DRUG
CHILD			
ADOLESCENT			
ADULT			
ELDERLY			

Figure 5-1 Target Populations Served.

Functional areas are distinguishable divisions of labor. The five functional areas of the system are:

1. *Service*—The process of providing organized activities to reduce or eliminate mental disabilities for a defined population.
2. *Administration*—The process of coordinating the goals, organizational structure and functions of the system.
3. *Citizen Participation*—The process of enhancing the degree and scope of impact of the goals, values and expectations of consumer and citizen groups.
4. *Research and Evaluation*—The process of disclosing needed functions and operating capacities of the system.
5. *Staff Development*—The process of enabling the system to utilize human resources.

The functional generalist approach may be differentiated from other current approaches to classifying personnel in that it *combines* three basic features.

1. The programs in which the generalist is employed are multi-service in nature and are responsible for providing a wide array of activities. A three-tiered career ladder is included. At the basic or initial sequence of the series the generalist performs front-line activities in proximity to designated groups. The intermediate sequence generalist is involved in program planning and implementation. In the third or executive sequence the generalists' responsibilities are divided among policy formulation, comprehensive planning, administration (including coordination and integration of the five functions), and provision of direct services (Table 5-1).
2. The functions performed by generalists require the ability to cope with a wide spectrum of alternatives entailing multiple skills. The generalists are involved in a variety of activities both within and, at times, across functional areas, as well as in work entailing contact with different groups and agencies. Thus, it is necessary for the generalist to perform a combination of roles for one or for several programs; for this reason the generalist is required to be skillful in the application of knowledge and technology that transcends specific disciplines.
3. The functional generalist sees all activities performed as part of a dynamic system of service and support functions, and is able to identify the relationships which exist between those functions.

SEQUENCES OF RESPONSIBILITY

The generalist series is structured to maximize the opportunities for employees to develop their individual capacities for providing functions needed by given programs. The series includes ten skill levels within three sequences of respon-

Table 5–1 The Human Service Generalist Matrix

Sequence of responsibility	Service	Administration	Citizen participation	Research and evaluation	Staff development
1. Basic sequence (HSGT I, HSG I, HSGT II)	Participates in an assistant and/or semi-independent capacity in providing services to consumers.	Participates in an assistant and/or semi-independent capacity in program maintenance.	Participates in an assistant and/or semi-independent capacity in programs entailing citizen involvement; acts as a liaison-monitor of the service network located in the community involving a variety of organizations.	Participates in an assistant and/or semi-independent capacity in record keeping and the collection of data.	Participates in an assistant and/or semi-independent capacity in orientation and high school equivalency program for staff.
2. Intermediate sequence (HSG II, HSGT III, HSG III)	Under the direction of the senior clinician, provides a wide range of highly skilled services.	Under the direction of an executive administrator, develops and plans administrative, business and general operations (both structure and functions) to ensure maintenance of program endeavors.	Under the direction of the comprehensive planner, coordinates and integrates citizen planning through the organization; plans and develops programs involving a variety of organizations to counter gaps in services.	Under the direction of the executive researcher, develops, plans and conducts program evaluation, epidemiological studies, and behavioral science research.	Under the direction of the administrative educator, develops, plans, and conducts ongoing educational programs for the generalist as well as for discipline-specific and program-specific employees.
3. Executive sequence (HSGT IV, HSG IV, HSGT V, HSG V)	As senior clinician, performs highly skilled services and also has supervisory and consultative responsibilities to residential and community programs.	Designs, coordinates, directs and consults to the administration of a comprehensive program of a facility, region or division of department.	Comprehensively plans, establishes priorities and develops strategies for the implementation of a multi-service program and works with citizens' advisory councils and boards of directors.	Designs, coordinates, directs and consults to residential and community service programs, evaluation programs, and research projects.	Designs, coordinates, directs and consults to comprehensive programs of education for staff members, community professionals, and lay groups; integrates all university education for preparation of professionals with the in-service education program for a facility, region, division or department.

sibility; because these ten levels are integrated with the five functional areas, the resulting career grid allows horizontal and vertical routes for individual ascendancy based on demonstrated competence and cognitive skills (Agranoff, Fisher, Mehr, & Truckenbrod, Note 1; Kostur, Note 2).

The generalist series is designed to achieve maximum flexibility, to promote innovation and spontaneity, and to result in responsiveness to consumer needs, program components, and employee potential. Thus, the series avoids rigid and definitive statements regarding boundaries within and between both work levels and functions.

Table 5-1 depicts the three sequences of responsibility and the five functional areas. The horizontal rows represent the three major sequences of responsibility and reflect the generalists' functional-operational relationship to a particular program. The vertical columns indicate the five functional categories which represent the major components of any given program.

It should be noted that the three responsibility sequences in the table contain descriptions of skills learned through classroom and on-the-job experiences. Staff members (especially those who enter at the introductory level) can bring to the job other relevant skills learned through life experiences. For example, an indigenous paraprofessional can be more knowledgeable than his/her professional colleagues about some of the folkways of the local community. Accordingly, paraprofessionals might work in more collaborative ways with their supervisors on tasks that utilize their specialized competencies. Unless recognized for these competencies, the paraprofessional or professional staff member in such instances will be performing functions at a skill level not adequately reflected by the responsibility sequence in which they may be classified. It is important that this fact be recognized and that skills acquired through life experiences be considered at the time of classification of an employee into a given responsibility sequence.

The structure and content of Table 5-1 cover a wide range of programs that are currently described elsewhere in publications concerning the Balanced Service System (Gerhard, Dorgan, & Miles, Note 3; JCAH, 1976; Miles & Gerhard, 1973). The conceptual model depicted describes the structure and provides the function of the generalist series.

The flexibility of the series is further highlighted if one conceives of each of the five functional areas as varying in terms of the proportion it comprises of the individual's total work responsibility. Thus, if a program's administrative and service staff members choose to adopt a truly generalist philosophy and approach, each staff member would be prepared in the five functional components regardless of the level of responsibility. On the other hand, if the choice is to consolidate the functions involved in the familiar broad divisions of labor (service, administrative, etc.), any functional area might then be the focus of staff preparation. It is important to realize that two different definitions and titles are necessary if precise differentiation is desired. The title Human Service Generalist (HSG) is most appropriate for staff members who are educated and trained in all of the functional areas. In contrast, the term Human Service Worker (HSW) might be a more appropriate title to represent one who is competent at a variety of responsibilities within one of the functional areas such as a service provider. Whatever the format adopted, it will obviously have a direct impact on the focus and content of the in-service education program.

Further flexibility can be obtained by the possibility of an individual's performing at responsibility levels that vary across functional areas. Thus, any specific job profile may be versatile, ranging across the level of responsibility and skill in a variety of functional areas. These dimensions are usually untapped in developing employee efficiency-effectiveness ratings.

THE CAREER LADDER[1]

Individuals enter the series as trainees at five possible entry points, as determined by their educational preparation. Movement from a trainee position requires the successful completion of a unit of preparation related to and consistent with the needs of an individual at the given entry level. A given preparation unit consists of education, on-the-job training and at least one year of experience. Promotion to the next trainee level in the sequence (that is, promotion by two steps) requires completion of the relevant preparation unit, as well as a minimum of two years experience and successful mastery of both on-the-job training and in-service education programs. The trainee preparation unit is formal, consisting of a function-related curriculum and tests. This formal curriculum program stands in contrast to the educational components of the nontrainee Human Service Generalist levels. In-service education is informal, generally containing self-selected job-related topic areas. Similarly, on-the-job training is aimed at the trainee's acquiring skills, while work experience is devoted to the employee's application of skills. This alternating structure makes it theoretically possible for an exceptional person entering the series without any formal education to advance to the top position, HSG V. However, it is more likely that most such individuals would finish up somewhere within the intermediate sequence. Mobility of this kind is usually uncommon for most paraprofessionals (Gottesfeld, Rhee, & Parker, 1970).

The intent of this design is *not* to duplicate or replace the traditional university training, but rather to increase staff members' accessibility to the educational and on-the-job training components through the elimination of rigid barriers wherever possible. To accomplish this objective the time requirement for these two components, unlike the time-limited work experience element, is open-ended and may be completed at the pace and capabilities of the trainee.

Once having completed the specified preparation unit for that designated function(s), the individual would be qualified to advance from a trainee position to that of a Human Service Generalist. For example, social workers and nurses are likely, by virtue of their prior training, already qualified to pursue the various service functions at a given generalist level; their choices would be based on their career objective and program needs.

The course requirements within the preparation units may be met by successful completion of function-related waiver examinations, campus-based college and adult education classes, seminars offered by the program, independent studies, and supervised placements at a variety of locations in the health, education, and welfare sectors. No matter what the formal preparation of the trainees, this structure increases their possibility of meeting both education and on-the-job training requirements. The creation of more preparation options and avenues, particularly for the introductory, associate and intermediate levels, makes it possible for the Human Service Generalist Series to provide the paraprofessional with mobility into the higher job levels.

Transferability

It is important to note that without certain safeguards, staff members can end up pursuing jobs rather than careers, despite the paper (theoretical) availability of a career ladder. Perhaps the most important safeguard is to insure opportunities to compete for promotions to the higher level positions. Thus, all staff members should be provided with academic credit for completion of training preparation units, on-the-job training, and qualifying work experience. The opportunities for upward mobility within the employing agency will be limited. If staff members do not have the opportunity to achieve higher academic degrees while receiving additional training, their career mobility can be limited to that possible within the currently limited number of institutions with competency-based (rather than degree-based) career ladders. Training preparation units should be designed to be appropriate to the preference for concrete, applicable examples and experiences often displayed by staff members entering at the introductory level. Finally, staff members would ideally be prepared by pre- or in-service training programs to combine task-related skills with the ability to train and supervise colleagues in these skills; otherwise, on-the-job training programs will not achieve their full potential.

The time may come when trained generalists begin to transfer from agency to agency. When this time comes, issues of reciprocity will arise. In anticipation of this potential problem all education, training, and experience should be carefully documented both in agency records and in individual staff development records (Fig. 5-2).

The Basic Sequence (HSGT I to HSGT II)

Entry level positions in the entire sequence are assigned to match the staff members' skills with the demands of the associated work tasks. The training

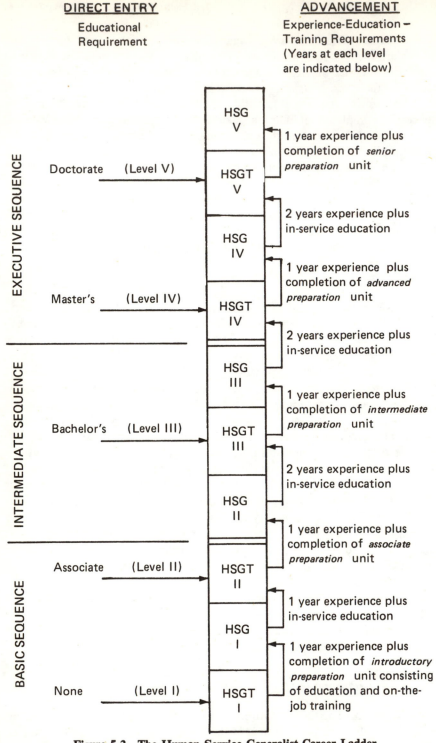

DIRECT ENTRY

Educational
Requirement

ADVANCEMENT

Experience-Education –
Training Requirements
(Years at each level
are indicated below)

EXECUTIVE SEQUENCE

HSG V

HSGT V — Doctorate (Level V)

1 year experience plus completion of *senior preparation* unit

HSG IV

2 years experience plus in-service education

HSGT IV — Master's (Level IV)

1 year experience plus completion of *advanced preparation* unit

INTERMEDIATE SEQUENCE

HSG III

2 years experience plus in-service education

HSGT III — Bachelor's (Level III)

1 year experience plus completion of *intermediate preparation* unit

HSG II

2 years experience plus in-service education

BASIC SEQUENCE

HSGT II — Associate (Level II)

1 year experience plus completion of *associate preparation* unit

HSG I

1 year experience plus in-service education

HSGT I — None (Level I)

1 year experience plus completion of *introductory preparation* unit consisting of education and on-the-job training

Figure 5-2 The Human Service Generalist Career Ladder

program is designed to help the staff members improve skills required in their current job classification level and to acquire skill required at subsequent levels.

An applicant enters as a Human Service Generalist Trainee I. Applications for this trainee-apprenticeship level can be accepted from individuals who may not have completed high school. The decision to accept persons without a high school diploma should remain an option for each program based on its ability to provide the educational resources, related direct service experience, and supervision.

Trainees enter a basic curriculum (Introductory Preparation Unit) to be completed, in most cases, after one year. At the end of this training period, the staff development and supervisory staff should have accumulated adequate information to make a promotional evaluation of the trainee's performance.

At this level (as well as at all other levels of the career ladder), the following procedures are recommended as policy guidelines with respect to employees who cannot or do not successfully complete a trainee position. Educational and supervisory personnel should take the necessary steps to evaluate the various components of the entire program, as well as the performance and overall potential of the trainees during the entire course of the preparation unit. These procedures will result in identification of those individuals who do not demonstrate the capacity to complete the minimum requirements of the program, as well as those components of the educational program which require change. The information accumulated will make an appropriate disposition possible; one option is the extension of the preparation phase and/or a revision of the educational program to increase its match with the learning styles of the trainees. These data may later serve to sharpen the screening process of future applicants.

When individuals presently employed in certified permanent positions enter one of the preparation units to prepare for entrance to the next step of the career ladder, they should remain in their given current job classification until successfully completing the training and receiving permanent classification at the next step. Failure of such employees to complete the new training successfully should not alter their current classification.

Those individuals who have completed the basic training enter employment as a Human Service Generalist I and begin the second year of apprenticeship, which includes a six-month probation period. For these employees, normal promotional procedures are to be followed. It is proposed that a minimum of one year be required at this apprenticeship level (HSG I). At the end of two years of work at the HSG I level (including the HSGT I level), employees are automatically seen by a board of examiners (see below) to determine their eligibility for promotion into the next classification position in the series, HSG II.

The Intermediate Sequence (HSG II to HSG III)

Applicants who have had two or more years of college but who have not received a bachelor's degree will, if accepted for employment, enter one year of preparation training at the HSGT II or associate level. This training program prepares them for employment at the level of HSG II in a six-month probationary status; a minimum of two years of experience at the level of HSG II is also proposed for these employees.

Two sets of employees may be promoted through the Intermediate Sequence by normal procedures. One set consists of employees who originally entered the series with less than two years of college but who have been passed by the board of examiners for advancement into the Intermediate Sequence range. The other set consists of those new employees who have had two or more years of college without obtaining a baccalaureate degree, but who have successfully completed the HSG II preparation unit. This Intermediate Sequence includes Human Service Generalists II, HSGT III, and HSG III, the latter being the top position within the intermediate range; this position may also be referred to as the top of the journeyman phase or the beginning level of the master step. The proposed minimum lengths of experience at each of these levels is two years for the HSG II and III and one year for the preparation position of HSGT III, the Intermediate Preparation Unit.

When staff members in these classes have completed one year at the top of the journeyman phase (HSG III), they are automatically seen by the board of examiners who will determine their eligibility to proceed into the Executive Sequence (HSG IV and V). (This sequence is also referred to as the leadership level.) Eligible persons may be promoted as vacancies occur at higher levels.

Executive Sequence (HSGT IV to HSG V)

The Advanced Preparation Unit is given to new applicants who have acquired a master's degree in an academic field considered directly relevant to the field of human services and for those who have advanced up from HSG III. It is assumed that placement in the HSG IV level will be possible upon successful completion of the training program for all of those persons admitted to HSGT IV. When individuals classified at the HSGT V level have both completed the Senior Preparation Unit and received a favorable board exam rating, they will be eligible for promotion to the last position in the classification series, HSG V.

The training for all existing certified employees who are accepted into the Advanced Preparation Unit should be provided during the periods in which they are working at the levels of HSGT IV and V. These two trainee levels require a minimum of one year each to complete.

Applicants who have acquired the doctorate or the equivalent in a field directly relevant to mental health work enter a Senior Preparation Unit, if they enter the program without the experience that would enable them to be immediately classified as a Human Service Generalist Trainee V. After a successful board exam rating they are eligible for promotion to the HSG V position. The classification HSG V at the top of the series covers highly responsible positions for a total operation of an agency, program, region, or statewide position.

The Degree Waiver: The "waiver" applies to those applicants who have received an accredited academic degree in human service; this training includes at least one year of practicum experience consistent with the functions the person will perform. The rationale for adopting this recommended policy is based on the realization that some nontraditional universities, such as those "without walls," are beginning to offer programs containing this practicum feature. Applicants may enter the next position beyond that of a trainee for the respective level when their credentials warrant a waiver for specific preparation unit(s).

THE STAFF DEVELOPMENT CONTINUUM

The success of the career grid depends on a well developed and coordinated staff development program that makes use of function-related education and training features to integrate the levels of responsibility carried out by staff members both within and among the five functional areas. This program is called a "staff development continuum." Each unit of the continuum differs in content to allow for variations in the background and sophistication of the trainees admitted. In the higher units (III and IV) of the continuum, the content becomes progressively more sophisticated in all five of the functional areas. In these upper levels a sixth dimension involving leadership and executive preparation is added. The preparation units oriented toward staff members at specific responsibility levels are supplemented by continuing staff development programs for all employees, regardless of their career ladder position. This combination of programs gives every staff member the opportunity for eligibility for advancement into the leadership and executive sequences.

THE BOARD EXAM[2]

An evaluative board would determine the eligibility of each generalist for classification at each level of the 10-class series. The board should be comprised of individuals with an understanding of the functions to be performed at the next level and the individual's performance at the current level.

The board would review the emotional stability and intellectual curiosity of employees, as well as their accomplishments throughout the different phases of their educational and employment histories. After collecting the information, the members would make a formal appraisal of the candidate's potential for performing more advanced functions. The board's decision should be based on the individual's cognitive abilities, demonstrated competence in the preparation units, and performance outcome of the various functions involved in the generalist role (Berger, Kostur, Lowenthal, & Wells, Note 4). The individual's capacity for further growth is of crucial importance in the final determination.

To accomplish this evaluative objective, the board would need to assess the candidate's preparation unit records, case reports, staff participation, and overall effectiveness of job performance; the assessment of job performance would be objectified by research and supplemented by the supervisors' appraisal. The major goal is the compilation of a comprehensive and objective profile of the employee.

After being evaluated, each candidate would be given a score. One possible formula is illustrated by the following set of possible components: (a) 50% devoted to the candidate's job performance; (b) 25% based on the oral and written examinations conducted by the board; and (c) 25% derived from performance in completed preparation units.

FUTURE STRATEGIES

The discussion, to this point, has been confined to the conceptualization of the various aspects of the generalist series. It is now appropriate to note that several more practical steps must be taken to achieve legitimacy for the series with funding and accreditation bodies. The first step involves strategies for bringing about acknowledgement of the mounting evidence, that with education and training, individuals varying widely in backgrounds can perform functions that have traditionally been viewed as the exclusive domain of specific professions (Gartner, 1971; Hansell, 1976; Platman, Dorgan, & Gerhard, 1976; U.S. Department of Health, Education, and Welfare (1965).[3] The second step involves beginning to determine objectively for funding sources (particularly third party) the cost effectiveness of services rendered by staff members of the different levels of Human Service Generalist career ladder.[4] If the cost effectiveness is identical or superior for the staff member combinations involving the lower levels, it will be possible to use appropriate proportions of staff from these levels while containing costs without losing the desired quality of services. The third step involves deployment of bachelor and sub-bachelor level paraprofessionals into the four functional areas that support service delivery. These functions, it should be noted, are ones that each program must perform if it is to achieve its service mission and its related goals and objectives.

Historically, one of the more prominent accreditation bodies, the Joint Commission for Accreditation of Hospitals, has displayed professional focus in terms of defining standards (JCAH, 1971, 1973a, 1973b, & 1974). However, in one of its most recent publications (JCAH, 1976) this traditional insistence on professional preparation has been modified in favor of an emphasis on competence and outcome performance. The intent of these standards is to enable community programs to utilize a wide range of staff members, varying both in terms of their formal education and experience. This approach makes it possible for community programs to negotiate with third party payers (who usually require accreditation) for reimbursement for service functions performed by staff members regardless of their formal educational preparation. This arrangement is consistent with the spirit of the legislation that gave birth to these community programs, as well as with the philosophy and design of the Human Service Generalist Series.

A CAUTIONARY NOTE

The Human Service Generalist career grid can be adopted and used as an effective tool for staff planning and development geared to future priorities and program strategies. Since in-service education and training are a vital and essential ingredient of the series, it is recommended that implementation should parallel the development of means to utilize the series and to provide the necessary educational resources. Appropriate educational resources can be provided by a mental health center itself, by area institutions of higher learning, or by a consortium involving one or more mental health centers, educational institutions, or other human service agencies.

NOTES

[1] Chapter 10 by Tarail and Chapter 11 by Pattison, Kuncel, Murillo, & Mandelian contain sections relevant to the conceptualization and implementation of career ladders within existing specific community mental health centers.

[2] Chapter 4 of a companion volume (Alley, Blanton, Feldman, Hunter, & Rolfson, 1979) contains a description of a competency-based system for evaluation of employee performance.

[3] Chapter 4 of this source book by Alan Gartner presents an up-to-date literature review of the effectiveness of paraprofessionals.

[4] Chapter 3 of this source book by Thomas Marschak and Curtis Henke presents a relevant economic efficiency framework, supplemented by data.

REFERENCE NOTES

1. R. Agranoff, W. Fisher, J. Mehr, P. Truckenbrod (Eds.), *Explorations in competency module development: Relinking higher education and the human services.* Center for Governmental Studies, Northern Illinois University, 1975, De Kalb, Ill. 60115.

2. W. Kostur, *Task analysis-key to competency training.* Unpublished manuscript, Elgin, Ill.: Center for Human Potential, Inc., 1975.
3. R. Gerhard, R. Dorgan, D. G. Miles, *The balanced service system: A model of social integration.* Manuscript submitted for publication, 1977.
4. M. Berger, W. Kostur, J. Lowenthal, S. Wells, *A competency based approach to mental health management in a state hospital* (Working Paper No. 8). Elgin, Ill.: Center for Human Potential, Inc., 1972.

References

Alley, S. R., Blanton, J., Feldman, R. E., Hunter, G. D., & Rolfson, M. *Case studies of mental health paraprofessionals: Twelve effective programs.* New York: Human Sciences Press, 1979.

Gartner, A. *Paraprofessionals and their performance: A survey of health, education and social service programs.* New York: Praeger Publishers, 1971.

Gottesfeld, H., Rhee, C., & Parker, G. A study of the role of paraprofessionals in community mental health. *Community Mental Health Journal,* 1970, *6*(4), 285–291.

Hansell, N. *The person in distress: On the biosocial dynamics of adaptation.* New York: Behavioral Publications, 1976.

Joint Commission on Accreditation of Hospitals. *Standards for residential facilities for the mentally retarded.* Chicago: Author, 1971.

Joint Commission on Accreditation of Hospitals. *Accreditation manual for hospitals* (Rev. ed.). Chicago: Author, 1973. (a)

Joint Commission on Accreditation of Hospitals. *Standards for community agencies serving persons with mental retardation and other developmental disabilities.* Chicago: Author, 1973. (b)

Joint Commission on Accreditation of Hospitals. *Accreditation manual for psychiatric facilities serving children and adolescents.* Chicago: Author, 1974.

Joint Commission on Accreditation of Hospitals. *Principles for accreditation of community mental health service programs.* Chicago: Author, 1976.

Miles, D. G., & Gerhard, R. *Toward a balanced service system for New York state.* Albany, N.Y.: New York State Department of Mental Hygiene, 1973.

Platman, S., Dorgan, R., & Gerhard, R. Psychiatric medication: The role of the non-physician. *International Journal of Social Psychiatry,* 1976, *22*(1), 9571–9574.

U.S. Department of Health, Education, and Welfare. *Pilot project in training mental health counselors* (Publications No. 1254). Washington, D.C.: National Institute of Mental Health, Public Health Service, 1965.

Chapter 6

TRAINING, SUPERVISION, AND EVALUATION OF PARAPROFESSIONALS IN MENTAL HEALTH

Harold McPheeters, MD*

This chapter describes strategies for selecting and preparing paraprofessionals for future employment, as well as methods useful in facilitating continued effective performance after paraprofessionals are hired. Three interrelated approaches are involved. Training activities teach relevant skills to workers, both prior to (pre-service) and subsequent to (orientation; in-service) employment. Supervision activities provide the workers with information about performance, whether as a trainee or as a paid agency employee. Finally, evaluation strategies focus on the success of training and service programs in meeting stated goals.

Agency professionals are not necessarily prepared by graduate education to carry out training, supervision, and evaluation functions. These functions, however, are very important to effective performance by paraprofessionals. For these reasons, this chapter should be especially important reading for agency professionals responsible for programs or activities involving paraprofessionals.

Within the paraprofessional mental health/human services manpower movement, the training and development of persons to become effective paraprofessional workers in the mental health system have received considerable attention. Only a small portion of these workers (e.g., some alcohol and drug abuse counselors) have been employed without plans for some kind of special

*Director, Commission on Mental Health and Human Services, Southern Regional Education Board, Atlanta, Georgia.

training beyond a simple orientation to the agency's rules and procedures. The variety of training programs in both pre-service and in-service is remarkable. There clearly are many alternative ways in which paraprofessional workers can be trained, but there are several common characteristics that appear to be helpful in making these training programs most effective. This chapter reviews some experiences gained in the many training programs and the ongoing staff member development activities of supervision and employee evaluation; these programs and activities are being used to develop the full potential of paraprofessional workers.

RELEVANCE OF LIFE EXPERIENCE

In the paraprofessional manpower movement far more emphasis has been given to life experience as a factor in both the selection and training of workers than has been given in the professions. This experience has been most notable in the case of alcohol counselors and drug abuse counselors, many of whom have been selected because they had previously had a personal problem with alcohol or drug abuse. It was felt that persons with such life experience would have a greater rapport and credibility with clients who have these problems; but, even more, it was recognized that such candidates already had a firsthand knowledge of the problem, the culture, and the kinds of rationalizations used by these clients. In effect, they already had life experiences that had prepared them to work with their clients better than any training program could do.

While this recognition of life experience as a crucial selection and training dimension has been especially characteristic of alcohol and drug abuse counselors, it has also been widely recognized in many other areas of paraprofessional manpower development. A considerable part of the literature of the paraprofessional human service worker movement has been concerned with the concept of the "indigenous nonprofessional" worker (Riessman & Popper, 1968); the basis of the concept is that neighborhood persons who had experienced the problems of being poor, of having lived in the ghetto, or of having been on welfare had already obtained an education about the culture and problems of the persons they would serve. Special efforts were made to offer priorities in the selection process to those persons who were indigenous to the neighborhoods and clients they would serve; this was done in part because such persons already had this life experience which would not have to be repeated in a training program. This pattern was widely used for social welfare nonprofessionals, for homemakers, for youth workers, for community development workers, for parent aides, and for a variety of mental health workers in ghettos, barrios, and neighborhood storefront programs.

Perhaps the predominant reason for hiring indigenous nonprofessionals was that they could establish a high degree of credibility with the clients they were to serve. This enhancement of credibility certainly has been shown to be true, but the reason for this outcome was largely that the life experiences of paraprofessionals had trained them in the culture of the community and for a style of working that enabled them to relate quickly to their clients.

In addition to selecting people who were indigenous to the neighborhoods they were to serve, people with some expertise in the program's area were sought; that is, reasonably good home managers, though not compulsive cleaners, were hired as homemakers; parent aides were hired who previously had children in school; and community development workers were employed who had some experience in leading formal or informal groups. Here, too, it was felt that persons with related life experiences would already have considerable skill in the program area in which they were to work.

Pre-Service Formal Education

There has been great variety in the kind and amount of pre-service formal education. For some of the New Careers programs where the message was "hire now, train later," there was virtually no pre-service training beyond an orientation program which prepared the workers for the rules and procedures of that particular agency. More commonly, the new paraprofessionals were given some kind of pre-service training program after they were employed, but before they actually began their work; most often this was a period ranging from 6 to 12 weeks in length. These pre-service programs were usually conducted by the agency in which the workers were employed, but occasionally there were contracts for the actual training to be provided by technical schools, private training groups, or by local community colleges. These pre-service training programs generally placed heavy emphasis on practice skills and on learning by doing. While there were usually some classroom lectures, films, and discussions, theory was generally played down in favor of more immediately practicable skills. Frequently, there was a heavy dose of practicum training in which the new students worked with the clients of the agency in learning to apply their skills.

At a much more formal level were the pre-service training programs that were initiated by technical schools and community colleges to train workers in certificate programs or in associate degree programs for eventual employment. These programs usually lasted from one to two years and included a full range of classroom and field training courses; they usually had more traditional selection criteria based on previous academic achievement, and they tended to follow the familiar academic pattern. This was especially true for the programs in community colleges which usually required general studies courses such as English, history, and physical education in addition to the courses more specifically related to mental health knowledge and practice.

In most of the associate degree programs there was no specific job opening in which the workers were to be hired. Thus, the training programs tended to be broadly based in knowledge and skills in the hope that such a broad base would open up more job opportunities. There were always questions about the model of worker being trained: Was the worker to function only in narrow roles as an outreach person or an advocate; was the worker to be an assistant to one or another of the existing professionals; was the worker to be only a psychotherapist; or did the role offer an entirely new conceptualization? In general, the pre-service programs that had specific jobs in sight were better able to answer these questions than were the community colleges. It was the result of this uncertainty that led most of the community colleges to adopt the "generalist" model which has assumed that the worker's job focuses on helping a small number of clients with all aspects of their work; this model involves calling for consultation when needed, but essentially it is concerned with maintaining a parent surrogate relationship to a small number of clients (McPheeters, 1969).

When mental health agencies employ graduates of community college programs who have not been specifically oriented to the agency, it is important to find out from the graduates themselves or from the college program from which they have graduated just what model of worker was the focus in the training period. If it was different from the model expected by the agency, a period of special orientation to the agency's needs is required. This should not ordinarily require the graduate to repeat the full pre-service training program of the agency, but the graduate should participate in certain parts of it.

Ideally, all of the major mental health agencies in a given geographic area should be involved with the advisory committee of any local community college's mental health/human service program so that they can help shape the curriculum model that they want the graduates to learn. Not all community colleges have such ongoing advisory committees, although it has been strongly recommended that they do so (Southern Regional Education Board, 1976). In addition, it is recommended that if any agency knows that it is likely to employ graduates of a local college program, it should seek to provide some of the field training within the agency. This would offer the opportunity to prepare the graduates for the specific model of worker which the agency wants.

ORIENTATION ON THE JOB

When the new workers arrived on the job, it was necessary to provide some basic orientation to the rules, policies, and procedures of the agency. The on-the-job orientation programs included all of the usual material related to working hours, vacation time, sick time, pay day, and typical items involving agency forms and requirements. These programs also included information about the law and state regulations, the goals and objectives of the employing agency, and various programs offered there. However, in the case of para-professional workers, such programs also required information about the roles the workers were expected to play in relation to clients and to the other staff members. It included an orientation to the role of the supervisor, to the possibility of making entries in the clinical records of clients, and to the kind of activity reports they were to keep. Particularly for those workers who were not indigenous to the area, there might also be some orientation to the local geographic area; in addition, there would be information about the gatekeeping practices and eligibility requirements of the other community agencies with which the mental health center worked.

THE NEED FOR SUPERVISION OF NEW EMPLOYEES

An important aspect of the introduction of new paraprofessional workers to their jobs was the matter of close supervision for the first several months. Close supervision at the beginning of employment was desirable for several reasons, but chiefly because it was at this stage that problems were likely to arise about the roles of the new workers themselves or of other staff persons. Such misunderstandings could lead to gaps or conflicts with other staff in the delivery of services. There needed to be close supervision of the new worker to assure expected outcomes and to intercept and correct any misunderstandings in their early stages before they became irreconcilable conflicts. (Supervisors can be reluctant to explore problems of this kind at their early stages, in the hope that the underlying conflict would resolve itself.) In the case of paraprofessionals, it has been especially desirable to maintain a close supervisory relationship and make corrections as soon as problems become apparent.

In addition to its role-related function, close supervision of new employees was important to teach the paraprofessionals skills which they had not been taught in their pre-service training or else which they had not yet fully mastered. Such supervision also enabled the new workers to refine skills and learn how to adapt them to the specific clientele of the agency. In all of these respects supervision was actually an extension of the training for the new employees.

THE NATURE OF SUPERVISION FOR NEW EMPLOYEES

There were two kinds of supervision that were offered to employees. One was a simple monitoring to assure that the worker was complying with preordained work standards; the other was a much more developmental kind of supervision in which the worker was offered consultation and education to assure that his or her performance was continuing to improve and the range of competencies was expanding. In the case of paraprofessionals it proved particularly desirable that the supervision be of the developmental kind, especially if there was some expectation that the worker would continue to grow in a career sense (Nash, 1975).

A probelm that sometimes faced paraprofessionals in mental health agencies was that the supervisors were unclear of just what was expected of the paraprofessionals. This was especially likely when the worker was assigned as a generalist, but was then given supervision by one of the professional departments. The worker was then judged by the standards of a single profession rather than by the total needs of the clients served in the generalist role. However, in many instances paraprofessionals were supervised by the service chief of the unit or service to which she or he was assigned. At other times there was a supervisor who had formerly been a paraprofessional but who had moved up the career ladder into a supervisory position. These latter two arrangements were both satisfactory, given that provision was made for the supervision to be both frequent and sensitive in the beginning stages. The new worker needed reassurance and assistance in entering the world of work with clients and professionals. It was awesome and frightening without help.

It should be noted that supervision resulted in the worker learning patterns of behavior that would likely remain for the rest of his career. Thus, close supervision at the start was especially helpful to assist the paraprofessional in acquiring these patterns. Many paraprofessionals started off wanting to give advice, to be directive, and to demand action on the part of their clients. With supervision they learned rather quickly to become more supportive and less directive and demanding; this, however, required a sensitive supervisor to help in the transition.

TRAINING

In-Service Training

The largest amount of training for paraprofessional workers resulted from the in-service training provided at the initiative of the employing mental health agency during the early period of employment as well as over time in their employment. This was especially true for the New Careers workers who were employed, immediately began work, and then soon entered into a part-time, in-service training program. However, during the past decade in-service training became more important for all levels of paraprofessional and professional workers; it has become increasingly evident that much of the preparation of staff for the delivery of service must be done in the service situation, as an addition to the pre-service training the worker may have received. Most mental health centers and mental hospitals now have a staff development or training officer whose full-time responsibility is the development and administration of in-service training programs for all levels of staff.

While there are many variations, the formal in-service training for paraprofessional workers generally began soon after the workers were employed. There may have been some delay resulting from the fact that there were not sufficient candidates to make up a class; however, in such cases, the workers were given close supervision until the next regularly scheduled in-service program could be undertaken.

A question that had to be addressed by the staff development officer and the administrator of the mental health program was whether the in-service training programs should be conducted by the staff of the mental health agency or by the staff of a local community college or a technical institute on a contract basis. Just a few years ago, there would have been little question about this issue, for in-service training was carried out by the agencies themselves. But today there is a strong likelihood that in-service programs will be planned and conducted through a local college or technical school. There are several advantages to such an arrangement: (1) the students can receive academic credits and academic degrees for their study; (2) the academic institutions are likely to have greater expertise in such areas as educational technology and student evaluation techniques; (3) the colleges are likely to have access to greater training resources such as libraries, videotape machines, and audio-visual departments; and (4) the colleges already have qualified faculty persons for many of the areas of knowledge that may be required for the in-service training program. In many cases the community colleges and technical institutes have been willing to conduct some of their classroom training at the mental health agency for the convenience of the learners.

While the trend is growing to arrange for the in-service training of para-professionals to be conducted by local educational institutions, this arrangement has not always been feasible or desirable; because of this fact, the staff development offices often had to make arrangements for the entire in-service program to be planned and carried out by the agency. Unfortunately, an agency-based program was unable to offer academic credits, and often the certificate from such an agency-based, in-service training program carried little weight if the worker wanted to transfer to another agency. Often, however, there was no alternative available.

In either case there had to be considerable negotiation between the service administrators of the mental health agency and the persons who would actually carry out the in-service training. This negotiation involved scheduling, objectives, content, and practicum training. At first glance the scheduling should have been a minor problem, but in fact, it was often difficult for the service chiefs to allow any substantial number of employees to be away from their service obligation for sustained periods of in-service training time. The usual solution to this problem was to schedule the classroom instruction on a part-time basis, frequently halftime. The work assignments were then correlated with the classroom teaching and closely supervised so that the work assignments were the equivalent of the practicum training. This arrangement had the advantage of assuring that the practical training was congruous with the style of service delivery used in that specific agency.

It must be noted, however, that it was not uncommon for the faculty of the community college to have had no previous practical experience in certain skills. In such cases arrangements were usually made for agency practitioners to be given faculty appointments or at least to be named as field instructors to provide the clinical instruction and skill training for the students. In some cases the classroom faculty also came out to the agency to receive practical training along with their students. In rare cases practitioners were brought in from nearby universities to provide this training.

The length of basic in-service training programs most commonly seems to have been in the range of 8 to 16 weeks; however, there are examples of programs that lasted as long as 9 months or a year. A number of mental health agencies have scheduled in-service training programs at intermediate and advanced levels for workers who had completed the basic programs and proven to be good employees. The advanced programs were likely to feature specialized skills or knowledge and were scheduled for any interested employees, professional as well as paraprofessional.

The content of the training programs has been quite variable; however, the classroom instruction has tended to be weighted toward knowledge about personality growth and development, interpersonal processes, psychopathology, and techniques of intervening with clients. In all in-service training the content has been strongly oriented to application and practical skills. This has been especially true in the practicum training which has been related to the clients and services offered by the agency day by day. Because the practicum part of the training has been offered in the regular agency setting, there has been a heavy emphasis on the overall delivery of services rather than just on one-to-one counseling or therapeutic work with clients. Thus, while the classroom instruction may have focused on the techniques of intervention with individual clients, the practicum or field portion was likely to be broadened to include the use of technical terms, case management, case reporting, and client evaluation. The requirements of the community mental health centers legislation demanded that staff be competent in a variety of service delivery skills such as: consultation, education, rehabilitation of the chronic patient, and prevention. In addition, the staff members must possess the traditional skills of diagnosis and treatment of individual clients which have always been stressed in basic professional and paraprofessional training.

The basic content of the in-service training programs has varied according to the philosophies of the program director and the training faculty regarding mental disabilities and their treatment. Some programs were oriented to a medical-psychiatric model, others to behavioral-psychological models, others to social learning models, and still others to educational-counseling models. They also varied according to the job descriptions of the specific agency which sponsored the training program. Thus, some programs included information about physical development and first aid while others provided virtually nothing about physical care. Some programs focused exclusively on interpersonal processes with individuals while others included training in social and group processes. Virtually all programs included at least some training in certain basic interpersonal skills such as interviewing and helping skills.

Competency-Based Training Versus Other Approaches to Training

In all of education there has been great interest in competency-based approaches to learning. While this thrust has been variously interpreted, it generally refers to an identification of very specific skills which the learner must master together with the specific criteria and measures by which the instructor and the learner would know when the learner has attained passable proficiency in the given competencies. It has been an especially appropriate approach for teaching the specific skills of intervention in mental health and the human services; many programs, in fact, have made considerable use of competency-based techniques for at least part of the training. (For example, competency-based training was used in the Elgin State Hospital program in Illinois and in the College for Human Services in New York City. The "crystals in competence" identified by the College of Human Services comprises an especially unusual and creative approach to competency determination [Sunderland, 1977; Wells, 1977].) Because of the required rigorous definition of the competencies and precise measures of performance, competency-based education has not appealed to all instructors, especially those who felt that they are more psychodynamically oriented and more concerned with the personal growth of their students. It also had limitations for some of the more complex aspects of working with troubled clients.

The competency approach is especially appropriate for in-service training in which the agency knows exactly which skills it wants its workers to have. In addition, competency-based training has several general advantages in both pre-service and in-service training for paraprofessionals:

1. It provides specific competency goals which the learner can achieve with measurable success; this provides motivation to move on to the next competency.
2. It offers flexible scheduling so that persons who have already achieved proficiency in certain competencies are able to demonstrate this proficiency and then move on to other competencies without unnecessary repetition of course work.
3. It allows learners to move through the program at their own rate; some can achieve overall competence in a few weeks while others will take several months to do so.

Other more traditional approaches to learning have been used more frequently than competency-based approaches; there has been a strong tendency to use traditional lectures, films, and classroom discussions in the presentation of information about such topics as personality and psychopathology. Overall, however, the content of in-service training programs has tended to stress the skills of intervention and the practical applications of knowledge rather than knowledge and theory for their own sake. This thrust differs from that frequently carried out by traditional, pre-professional academic programs.

Experiential Learning Approaches

Because of the stress on the learning of skills, there has been a strong emphasis on various forms of experiential learning; several training programs have used the stimulus films developed by Kagan (1972). In addition, Danish and Hauer (1973) have described a Helping Skills Program that makes use of active trainee participation, modeling by the instructor, and immediate feedback to the trainee concerning the appropriateness of responses. Many instructors have used the interpersonal skills training program of Carkhuff (1967). Many others used case demonstrations, audiotape and videotape playbacks of trainee performance, simulations, microlabs, as well as individual and group counseling. The emphasis in all of these experiential learning techniques is on trainee involvement and performance. The techniques require the trainee to act either in a simulated or in a real case situation; then his or her performance is reviewed and critiqued. The trainee learns from practice and feedback to perform the skills at a creditable level of competence. (This approach is very much like that of training athletes in the performance of the specific skills of their sport.)

Field Training

The ultimate test of an in-service training program has been how well the trainee has ultimately been able to work with clients and with other staff persons of the mental health agency to bring about the desired results with clients and communities. Effective performance in this domain required an amalgamation of all of the knowledge and individual skills of the trainee, as well as certain personal values and attitudes about clients, the agency and its purposes. This kind of amalgamation has been best learned in the field, where the trainee worked with real clients in a real agency setting and under supervision of the agency's professional staff. The field training component of in-service training was relatively easy to develop since the trainee was already an employee of the agency and, most likely, was already working part time with clients and professionals. In some in-service training programs the trainee was required to have field placements in a different service from the one to which he was assigned for his regular work, but in most programs the regular work assignment was structured as the field training site. Thus, the field training took place step by step along with the classroom instruction. This was in contrast to the typical pattern of academic professional training in which field training followed the classroom instruction and the total curriculum was divided into pre-clinical and clinical segments. This form of training in which the field training progressed *pari passu* with the classroom instruction seemed to be especially appropriate for paraprofessional workers when the emphasis was on skill development and when the total training period was relatively short. There is some evidence that with paraprofessionals, this blending of field and classroom training was more effective than having the components separated (Vanderkolk, 1973).

Goal Setting

The goal setting for the use of paraprofessionals had two major elements: the goal setting for programs which used paraprofessionals, and the goal setting for individual workers. In regard to overall goal setting for programs that used paraprofessional workers, there was a need for high-level attention to be given to the roles in which workers were to be used. There were several possible choices for the ways in which paraprofessional jobs might be focused:

1. Around specific tasks or activities (e.g., administering and scoring tests, doing intake interviews).
2. Around specific professions (e.g., social work case aide, psychological assistant).
3. Around administrative needs of the agency (e.g., the worker might be assigned to various duties which needed to be done at certain times. Examples are: escort duty, chauffeur duty, mail room duties, and messenger duty).
4. Around major functions (e.g., outreach, treatment, rehabilitation).
5. Around a small group of target clients and families for whom the worker retained a kind of parent surrogate responsibility for all aspects of their treatment and rehabilitation.

The jobs of paraprofessionals have been structured in all of these ways in various settings. However, there were serious implications for both clients and workers depending on which was chosen. The first three were more sensitive to the needs of the agency and of the professions while the latter two were more sensitive to the needs of programs and clients.

A surprising number of paraprofessionals have been promoted to positions of relatively high administrative responsibility. Among these are directors of satellite clinics, a director of a geographic unit of an inpatient service, a director of a hotline program, a chief of an outreach service, a director of a community support system for chronic mental patients, and a director of a local mental health association. At least one has become the director of in-service training, and one has become director of a community college mental health training program.

More and more mental health agencies have been organized into functional interdisciplinary units in which professional identities have been deemphasized. The paraprofessional was then used as a generalist worker with a small group of clients for whom he kept major responsibility. The overall unit team then set the major goals and plans for its clients, and each worker was responsible for carrying out that program for those clients for whom he had primary responsibility. Of course, the worker had access to the various professionals for consultation or referral when needed.

In agencies that placed considerable stress on the professions, the paraprofessionals were more likely to be used as aides to one or another of the professions and thus to carry out specific tasks of that profession and to be closely supervised by that profession. Some of these workers found frustrations in the limitations of such jobs as well as times when they had "nothing to do" because no work had been assigned.

In a few mental health agencies the paraprofessionals were assigned to functions such as outreach, advocacy, or aftercare that were not clearly the responsibility of any of the established professions in order to avoid any conflicts. It must be noted that all of these patterns of utilization were possible program alternatives. There is no research to show the advantages of one over another although some persons believe that the generalist orientation is more productive and more rewarding for both workers and clients.

It was important that the agency's leadership firmly agree on what model of paraprofessional use was to be adopted before the paraprofessionals were introduced into the system; furthermore, this decision had to be clearly understood by *all* staff. There had often been misunderstanding and conflict between professionals and paraprofessionals when there was ambiguity about models or when the staff had not had the decision fully explained to them (Boyette, Blount, Petaway, Jones, & Hill, 1972).

The goals for individual workers varied greatly depending on which of these job orientations was used. If it was a generalist orientation, the goals were set in terms of numbers of clients to be restored or maintained in a community adjustment. If the job orientation was to tasks, the goals were in terms of the numbers of tasks (e.g., tests administered or intake interviews completed). If the job was oriented to being an aide to one of the professionals, the goals were set by the professional supervisor.

In the past there was little conscious goal setting for individual staff persons in mental health agencies, but this has been rapidly changing as administrators are being required to make the organization more productive, to generate more reimbursable hours of work, and generally to be more efficient. A few programs such as the Huntsville-Madison County (Alabama) Mental Health Center have extensive job contract programs for each worker in order to set worker goals and in order to have a specific mechanism for evaluation of workers (Turner & Lee, 1976a, 1976b).[1]

SUPERVISION

Techniques

Once paraprofessionals come into an agency, the method of supervising them varied depending on the organizational structure of the agency and the orientation of the job. If the worker was assigned as an aide to a professional, the supervision came from that professional or from the head of that professional department. If, however, the worker was assigned to a functional team, the supervision would most likely come from the leader of the team regardless of professional discipline. A few agencies have created a department of paraprofessional mental health workers, parallel in the organization to the traditional professional departments. In such a case, the paraprofessionals received supervision from a senior person with training and experience similar to their own.

When supervision was ongoing (rather than periodic), there were at least two types of expectations concerning the goals to be accomplished by supervision. In some agencies, supervisors were simply to assure that the workers were meeting predetermined standards; in other agencies the supervisors were to foster the workers' overall growth and development, as well as to detect and correct deficiencies from standards. From the perspective of the paraprofessional the objective of supervision was generally to foster overall growth and development; but accomplishment of this outcome required more consultation, education, and counseling from the supervisor than some were prepared to give.

A very typical format for supervision was to have a single supervisor who periodically filled out an employee rating form which was then discussed with the employee and placed in the files. This procedure was most likely required once every six months or once a year, and differed considerably from ongoing supervision. It was better than nothing, but it was often a formal process that focused more on social adaptive skills (e.g., whether the worker was on time, whether he kept up to date with paper work) rather than performance with clients. In many agencies supervisors were instructed to couple this formal evaluation process with more personal evaluation and counseling regarding ways in which the worker might improve his performance. The supervisory sessions were held much more frequently than the required employee ratings.

Another approach to supervision was to have periodic sessions of the unit team that were focused on the performance of the team and of its individual members. Such sessions provided for inputs from more individuals and provided for a wider understanding of individual strengths and needs. A further method of supervision was for the supervisor to review and discuss individual client cases with the paraprofessional. This approach included a review of the clinical record and a discussion of the processes and problems being encountered by the worker. It was an excellent teaching mechanism as well as a supervising mechanism. There was also the informal conversation, a method which allowed the supervisor to assess how well the worker was doing and to advise and counsel the worker on strategies for achieving greater growth and productivity. This approach was very useful, but its success depended on a good relationship between the two staff members and on the regularity of the meetings.

Terminations

Occasionally it became evident that it was necessary to terminate an employee whose performance was not adequate. The most frequent causes for dismissal of all kinds of employees in mental health agencies have been social adaptive disorders which are not related to competence in the performance of professional skills. These problems show up in the supervisory process and include personality conflicts, erratic work habits, and irresponsible behavior. They have been brought to the attention of the employee and documented in his or her record. The employee has usually been given a definite period of time within which to correct the deficiencies and only then would be dismissed if he or she failed to do so.

Dismissals regarding difficulties in professional practice were handled in much the same fashion except that there would be more explicit counseling and education regarding the problem. If it turned out that the worker was still unable to satisfactorily perform certain critical work with clients despite diligent effort and goodwill, the employee was often counseled and reassigned to another position in the agency which did not require the competence which he or she was unable to attain. In some such cases workers were dismissed when there was no such position available. When an employee would be dismissed for lack of competence, it was important that this employee be told that an inability in a specialized area of competence does not mean that he or she is a total failure as a human being. The employee should be counseled to pursue work in the areas of his strengths rather than to seek repeatedly a position in which he is unable to compete.

EVALUATION

Evaluation of the training, use, and effectiveness of paraprofessional workers is still in its infancy. There are many dimensions of evaluation. Perhaps the simplest level of evaluation has focused on evaluation of the process itself. Basic data were often kept regarding the numbers of paraprofessional trainees, their demographic characteristics, the training experiences, the problems encountered, and the numbers graduated, employed, and terminated. When this kind of process data was aggregated and analyzed, it told a great deal about the overall program. Such records could be correlated with cost data and could be observed over time to detect changes that could require modification in the programs. Unfortunately, this kind of process evaluation was not done on every program even though it required little technical expertise or cost; however, it was very useful when done.

Evaluation of the outcome of training was more difficult, but not impossible. If the competency-based approach was used, there were specific criteria and measures employed to evaluate when and whether the trainees had attained the competencies. Pencil-and-paper tests were often used for evaluating the knowledge learned.

When data were kept regarding the employment, retention, promotion, and productivity of workers, these data provided measures of outcome of the whole paraprofessional manpower development program. When goal attainment scaling was used for the treatment program, it was possible to judge how well the paraprofessional workers attained the goals set for their clients. This was a measure of outcome for both client and worker.

Special research studies, such as one recently conducted by Liberman and True (1977), showed that paraprofessionals were approximately as effective as professionals in brief psychotherapy. Studies such as these are in the nature of evaluative research rather than evaluation. They are not appropriate for every agency, but it is important that they be done to further document outcomes and the relative effectiveness of paraprofessionals.

The findings from such evaluation efforts have been fed back into both the training programs and the agency's operating procedures. Perhaps certain skills needed to be redefined or taught in a different way; perhaps the patterns of job orientation or supervision needed to be changed. Evaluation should have helped decide where the programs needed to be modified or emphasized, and there should have been a great deal more evaluation done. Hopefully, more will be done in the future.

NOTE

[1] The Child and Parent Service of the Huntsville-Madison County Center is described in Chapter 4 of the case study source book, a companion to this volume (Alley, Blanton, Feldman, Hunter, & Rolfson, 1979).

REFERENCES

Alley, S. R., Blanton, J., Feldman, R. E., Hunter, G. D., & Rolfson, M. *Case studies of mental health paraprofessionals: Twelve effective programs.* New York: Human Sciences Press, 1979.

Boyette, R., Blount, W., Petaway, K., Jones, E., & Hill, S. The plight of the new careerist: A bright horizon overshadowed by a dark cloud. *American Journal of Orthopsychiatry,* 1972, *42,* 595–599.

Carkhuff, R. R., & Berenson, B. G. *Beyond counseling and therapy.* New York: Holt, Rinehart and Winston, 1967.

Danish, S. J., & Hauer, A. E. *Helping skills: A basic training program.* New York: Behavioral Publications, 1973.

Kagan, N. *Influencing human interaction.* East Lansing, Michigan: Michigan State University, 1972.

Liberman, B., & True, J. E. *Evaluation of the comparative effectiveness of professionals, mental health associates, and other paraprofessionals in therapeutic intervention with psychiatric outpatients.* Submitted for publication, 1977.

McPheeters, H. L. *Roles and functions for mental health workers.* Atlanta: Southern Regional Education Board, 1969.

Nash, K. B., & Mittlefehldt, V. A. Supervision and the emerging professional. *American Journal of Orthopsychiatry,* 1975, *45,* 93–101.

Riessman, F., & Popper, H. L. *Up from poverty.* New York: Harper and Row, 1968.

Southern Regional Education Board. *A guidebook for mental health/human service programs at the associate degree level.* Atlanta: Author, 1976.

Sunderland, S. C. *Performance based education and the human service profession: The four major structures of the college for human services.* Paper presented at the Southern Regional Education Board Symposium on Human Service Competencies, Atlanta, Georgia, May 1977.

Turner, A. J., & Lee, W. E., Jr. Motivation through behavior modification, part I: The job contract. *Health Services Manager,* 1976, *9*(9), 1–5. (a)

Turner, A. J., & Lee, W. E., Jr. Motivation through behavior modification, part II: Evaluation. *Health Services Manager,* 1976, *9*(10), 1–3. (b)

Vanderkolk, C. J. Comparison of two mental health counselor training programs. *Community Mental Health Journal,* 1973, *9,* 260–268.

Wells, S. *Competency: Practical wisdom.* Paper for the Southern Regional Education Board Symposium on Human Services Competencies, Atlanta, Georgia, May 1977.

RELEVANT READING MATERIALS

Allen, D. (Ed.). *A humanistic definition of human service performance.* Syllabus for a graduate program in human service performance based assessment for human service professionals. New York: College for Human Services, 1974.

Carkhuff, R. R., & Berenson, B. G. *Beyond counseling and therapy.* New York: Holt, Rinehart and Winston, 1967.

Combs, A. W., Avila, D. L., & Purkey, W. W. *Helping relationships: Basic concepts for the helping professions.* New York: Allyn and Bacon, 1971.

Danish, S. J., & Hauer, A. E. *Helping skills: A basic training program.* New York: Behavioral Publications, 1973.

Dugger, J. G. *The new profession: Introduction for the human services/mental health worker.* Monterey, California: Brooks/Cole, 1975.

Holler, R., & DeLong, G. *Human services technology.* St. Louis: Mosby Co., 1973.

Schulman, E. D. *Intervention in human services.* St. Louis: Mosby Co., 1974.

Sobey, F. *Nonprofessional revolution in mental health.* New York: Columbia University Press, 1970.

Southern Regional Education Board. *Roles and functions for mental health workers.* Atlanta: Author, 1969.

Southern Regional Education Board. *A kit for review of mental health worker training programs.* Atlanta: Author, 1974.

Southern Regional Education Board. *A guidebook for mental health/human service programs at the associate of arts level.* Atlanta: Author, 1976.

III

SPECIALIZED ROLES FOR PARAPROFESSIONALS

Chapter 7

A GUIDE FOR THE INDIGENOUS CHANGE AGENT

Louis G. Tornatzky*

The probability of successfully inducing social change in mental health (and other) organizations is greatly enhanced by a well-planned set of strategies which takes into account specific features of the organization. This chapter describes practical procedures and a conceptual framework useful for agency staff members, whether paraprofessional or professional, who wish to act as change agents in the organization by which they are employed.

The author begins by describing the "classic bureaucratic" and "human relations" schools of organizational theory and discussing the relevance of these two approaches to the understanding of mental health organizations. Next, the author explains the resistance to change within organizations in terms of organizational theory principles and points out the importance of group processes for bringing about change. Then he describes the four vital stages in social change.

The author emphasizes the importance of knowledge and skills developed outside of a local organization. His stance is that it is inefficient to try to reinvent the wheel when other parties may have already created and refined the innovations relevant to the needs of an organization and its clients. He highlights the relevance of assistance from an outside consultant, the need to identify relevant innovations that have been developed and evaluated, and various sources of relevant information for the budding change agent.

*Associate Professor of Psychology and Urban and Metropolitan Studies, Michigan State University, East Lansing, Michigan.

COMMUNITY MENTAL HEALTH CENTERS AS ORGANIZATIONS

How can you as a paraprofessional or professional staff member bring about change in your community mental health center? For example, how can you help to introduce a new service program or to change the jobs performed by paraprofessionals? Before focusing on these questions, you should first be convinced that change is both possible and manageable.

This chapter describes potential blocks to change and outlines strategies for dealing with these obstacles. The practical suggestions are based both on research findings and on personal experiences in creating change in mental hospitals across the nation. As in many sets of practical suggestions, we might begin with a cautionary note.

Mental health paraprofessionals and professionals have distinct disadvantages in entering the arena of organizational change. Much of their on-the-job activity involves interaction in which there is a heavy concern with the individual idiosyncrasies of people, particularly clients. All of the underpinnings of therapeutic activity—modern personality theory, psychoanalysis, assessment and testing—have as their premise the notion that individual differences are the key to understanding human behavior. Unfortunately, when paraprofessionals or professionals become self-styled change agents they inappropriately carry this conceptual bias into that activity. The budding change agent must begin to look at his/her community mental health center as something other than the sum of the personalities who work there. S/he must begin to view his/her center as an *organizational* entity, with various sub-groups, cliques, peer relations, all interacting in a complex buzzing system. Most of the resistances to programmatic change in community mental health centers can be explained in terms of organizational and group concepts. Understanding these concepts is the first step in understanding the concept of organizational change.

BUREAUCRACIES AND NON-BUREAUCRACIES

What type of organization is the community mental health center (CMHC)? Some aspects of a CMHC approximate a rational-legal bureaucracy as described by such classical writers as Weber (1947). The purpose of a classical bureaucracy, or formal organization, is to rationalize the world of work and task accomplishment. Several assumptions are made in this model of organizational functioning.

One premise is that the world itself *is* rationalizable, understandable, and reducible to well-defined categories of knowledge. A second premise is that individuals participate in organizations largely for material gain, security, and extrinsic rewards. Given these assumptions, an organization of the work to be done logically follows. The task confronting the organization is dissected into sub-tasks so as to permit the creation of specialists. Thus, all members of the organization concentrate on one specific area of work, becoming more skillful and knowledgeable about the sub-task than they are about the whole task. In this way the organization can increase its amount of focused expertise directed towards task accomplishment.

In a large organization where specialization occurs, there is a corresponding necessity for some means to coordinate specialist activities. Thus, we have such things as a chain-of-command and a hierarchical decision-making structure such that individuals higher in the hierarchy control and coordinate those below their station. Another way of enhancing the coordination of specialists in a classical bureaucratic structure is to have written rules and procedures and well-defined job descriptions. As a finishing touch to the rational-legal bureaucracy, there is a heavy emphasis on impersonal communication, so as not to allow individual idiosyncracies and personalities to intrude upon the accomplishment of the overall task. Typically this goal is achieved by the use of written memoranda and other types of formal internal correspondence.

An examination of the operation of many community mental health centers often reveals features which correspond roughly to the classic bureaucratic model that has just been described. For example, the organization of treatment activities into various categories of services[1] is based on the premise that intervention activities can be assigned to convenient conceptual boxes. Similarly, the notion of the "treatment team," with each of the professional disciplines ostensibly engaging in quite different types of activities, indicates an attempt to achieve some degree of bureaucratic job specialization. Finally, although CMHCs pride themselves on their apparent staff equality, a *de facto* hierarchy does exist, and is used to achieve coordination by fiat. This is particularly so when decisions involve "medical" considerations.

However, members of most CMHCs will find that their organization differs greatly from the classic model. The typical human service organization, of which the community mental health center is an example, usually deviates significantly from the rational-legal bureaucratic structure that has just been described. Despite persistent attempts for decades to fulfill the dream of the "ideal" bureaucracy, it remains nothing more than a vision. As Perrow (1972) points out so aptly:

> The problem is that even if the interest of the organization is unambiguous, men do not exist just for organizations. They track all kinds of mud from the rest of their lives with them into the organization, and they have all kinds of interests that are independent of the organization.

In short, members of organizations often have the propensity to be whimsically, unpredictably human. Similar observations have repeatedly been made in the organizational literature in the past few years. What has developed is a contrary view of how organizations should or do function, which has been labeled as the human relations school of organizational theory. Its early advocates include such individuals as McGregor (1960) and Likert (1967).

The human relations argument is that the functioning of people in organizations can best be understood in terms of emotional-affective dynamics, rather than by considerations of material gain or the rational demands of the task. Of historical interest in the development of these notions are the famous Hawthorne studies (Roethlisberger & Dickson, 1947). Here it was found that productivity in an assembly plant was predicated more on group cohesion, group norms, and morale than on manipulating material rewards, or on restructuring the physical aspects of the work setting. For example, it was found that teams doing electrical wiring increased their production primarily because of the attention paid to them as members of a research project. As an outgrowth of this study, and others like it, there has been a significant movement to humanize and "soften" modern organizations. There is an increasing emphasis on more open communication among organizational members, and on developing the human potential of members of the organization, with a decreasing emphasis on unilateral decision making and intra-organizational power politics.

What is the "correct" model of organizational functioning for a community mental health center, and what do these issues matter for the indigenous change agent? The answer to the first question is that there probably is no single most appropriate model for an organization such as a community mental health center. As an outgrowth of the conceptual dilemmas alluded to above, what has emerged in recent years is a *contingency* approach to the understanding of organizations. Under this model (Lawrence & Lorsch, 1967; Litwak, 1961; Perrow, 1971), the consensus is that some tasks are more appropriate for bureaucratic organizations and other tasks are more appropriate for the more informal, human relations type of organization.

As Litwak (1961) has argued, perhaps the best way to understand these phenomena is to talk about the differences between *uniform* and *non-uniform* tasks. Uniform tasks are those which are understandable, predictable, rationalizable, repeatable, and thus appropriate to the type of work organization implicit in the classic bureaucratic model. In contrast, the term non-uniform describes those task areas in which limited knowledge exists, things happen very fast, events are quite unpredictable and non-repetitive, and idiosyncracies are the rule. When we look at the tasks performed by community mental health centers, we can see that many of them fall into the latter category and therefore are more appropriately handled by informal group processes.

The therapeutic process itself, with the built-in complexities of human functioning, is a task that is difficult to imagine as being handled by specialists in the classical bureaucratic sense. Perhaps in a nightmare world we might find an Id Therapist IV who coordinates his activities with a resident Ego Specialist IV, who in turn consults periodically with the Super Ego Interventionist VII; luckily such civil service classifications do not exist. Also, in most community mental health centers, there is a great deal of planning and development activity that is typically done in the context of fairly informal group meetings such as *ad hoc* committees, workshop planning sessions, and so forth—and justifiably so. Many of the activities should be, and are, done in an unstructured manner.

What do these considerations imply for the paraprofessional or professional who desires to be the internal change agent of a CMHC? If we look at some of the resistance that is typically encountered by individuals trying to make changes within such organizations, we see the relationship between resistance and certain group processes more clearly. One source of resistance to programmatic change in centers is the fact that new programs often are contrary to the implicit or explicit treatment norms of professionals. The attempt to change individuals' values and norms is almost by definition a *non-uniform* task, and thus appropriately handled by the human relations approach and by informal group processes. When people feel their values are being confronted, they often experience anxiety and uncertainty and behave quite defensively. As has been pointed out by Zaltman, Duncan, and Holbeck (1973), several other attributes of new programs may produce recalcitrance on the part of the staff. For example, if a program is incompatible with existing professional *roles* and *status,* there is a likelihood that it too will produce pangs of uncertainty and resistance, thus producing a non-uniform task situation. Similarly, the more *complex* a new program is, the more likely it is to produce at least initial resistance, misunderstanding, and uncertainty on the part of the center staff.

In order to deal with these phenomena the internal change agent must use *group processes* to make the path of change more inviting. The flexibility, openness and fluidity of informal group processes are appropriate for the task situations created by the change process. Consider a few suggestive research findings. It has been found (Fairweather, Sanders, & Tornatzky, 1974; Havelock, R. & Havelock, M., 1973) that staff involvement in decision making about new programs is likely to increase the chances of their adoption. In a classic study of this phenomenon, researchers in a pajama factory (Coch & French, 1948) found that involving production line workers in the planning and implementation of new practices significantly increased the likelihood of their acceptance. In a comprehensive survey of industrial organizations, Burns and Stalker (1961) found that a non-bureaucratic organizational climate was more conducive to successful innovation. All of these findings provide grist for what follows.

The point to be remembered throughout is that changing a community mental health center is not an act of individual heroism. First, an effective change agent is one who can manipulate "the system" in a cooperative effort to move in a new direction for the good of the organization and its clients. Second, to the extent that one can mobilize supporting group processes, participative decision making, and appropriate task structuring, one can move the change process through the stages from an initial awareness of need to a successful and stabilized adoption of an innovative program.

THE CHANGE PROCESS

Let us assume for a minute that you, as the neophyte CMHC indigenous change agent, have come to the realization that a new program is needed, for example, for the outpatient treatment of alcoholic clients. You are aware of a few program alternatives which have been piloted successfully in other centers, and are willing to look at a range of possible alternative programs. You find yourself somewhat alone, however, in this perceived need for internal social change. What are the steps that you must go through in order to move your colleagues in the center through the process of change?

As we and others[2] see it, there are four stages of the innovation adoption process. These include:

1. Creating an awareness of the need for change
2. Searching for a solution
3. Implementing the chosen alternative
4. Stabilizing and evaluating the new programmatic change

Let us now consider what type of activities the paraprofessional change agent might engage in as s/he moves through this process.

Creating an Awareness of the Need for Change

Typically, most staff members working in mental health facilities are not terribly objective about the effectiveness of their therapeutic efforts or about the value of strategies for using paraprofessionals. In short, there is usually a singular lack of awareness of any need to make programmatic changes. There are several ways in which the indigenous change agent can pique staff members' curiosity about possible program alternatives.

One activity in which you as an indigenous change agent may engage is a lengthy process of intensive interpersonal re-education. For example, if you work on the alcoholic unit in question, you may, over a period of several weeks, try cornering your fellow staff members and pointing out what you see as rather glaring shortcomings in the current services offered. Since you are a peer, and *homopholous* (Rogers & Shoemaker, 1971) with your fellow staff (similar to them), your comments on program frailties might be more acceptable than those coming from an uninvited outside critic. It is also probably desirable to carry out this interpersonal persuasion process in a highly *informal* context. Often, when the attempt to make staff members aware of the need for change is made in an informal setting (such as a lunch or a party) there is less defensiveness, anxiety, and resistance.

Another possible way of heightening the awareness for change on the part of fellow staff members is for the indigenous change agent to become a close friend of the CMHC program *evaluator.* In recent years, program evaluation has been used increasingly as a tool to push for programmatic change. A robust methodology has emerged (Campbell & Stanley, 1966; Fairweather & Tornatzky, 1977) which has enabled program directors to obtain quite useful information about the degree to which their efforts are successful. With some persuasion and cajolery, perhaps you as an indigenous change agent can get your local program evaluator to do a follow-up study on some of the clients who have gone through the alcohol program as it currently exists. If your hunches are right, what will emerge is a picture of negligible program effectiveness. If you can further press the program evaluator to present this information to your fellow staff members, this tactic can also heighten the *awareness of the need for change*.

A way in which this awareness can be more systematically stimulated is by the use of an *outside change agent* consultant. In fact, there is some evidence to suggest (Fairweather, Sanders, & Tornatzky, 1974) that not much change will occur unless an outside change agent provides at least a partial stimulus to change. In many organizations an internal push for change on the part of the staff is looked upon with a jaundiced eye by administration, thus necessitating the use of a "credible" outsider. Fortunately, as an outgrowth of the human-relations concepts described above, a movement of *planned change/organizational development* has emerged (Argyris, 1972; Bennis, 1966; Huse, 1975) with a full cadre of professional change agents for hire. One of the tenets of the planned change/organizational development method is that it should serve a facilitating function in assisting organizations in the self-identification of problem areas. Therefore, organizational development consultants, after being invited by your center director[3] or the director of your alcohol unit, would work with staff over a period of days or weeks in order to stimulate interest in looking at current organizational functioning. In fact, if the need for an approved outsider is particularly strong, this consultant might be involved throughout the entire change process. A variety of different techniques and tactics might be employed (Huse, 1975). Typically, these organizational development activities are done in the context of a fairly informal setting where free and open communication occurs between staff members and their supervisors.

All of the above activities are designed to change a shared perception on the part of the staff members in your program. The typical perception of your peers will be that everything is okay. It is hoped that at the end of this process of building awareness, a bit of uneasiness about current practices will emerge, coupled with a motivation to look at alternatives.

Searching for a Solution

Given that you and your fellow staff members have all arrived at the conclusion that something new must be done, the next question to be answered is, "What is 'new'?" There are two schools of thought about how one should proceed in identifying new program options. One view, largely held by organizational development practitioners, is that the collective wisdom of staff should be mobilized to generate their own solutions to what they see as program deficits. Through a process approximating that of brainstorming, a new program wrinkle is thought out and then put into operation. In fact, many organizational development consultants are quite uncomfortable about being directive, or forcefully suggestive, in the selection of new program options.

This writer strongly objects to this point of view. When mental health workers depend exclusively on their own resources for resolving program difficulties, they very often do little more than reinvent the wheel. In considering the real utility of ostensible "innovations," we might do well to recall the observations of another student of human behavior: "I have seen all the works that are done under the sun; and, behold, all is vanity and vexation of spirit" (Ecclesiastes, 1:14). Unless a new program is established in such a way that its effectiveness can be determined empirically, it is better, albeit not ego-enhancing, to make use of others' experiences. There *are* resources to which one can turn for new program alternatives, and the indigenous change agent —or the external consultant—should be familiar with them.

In recent years several government agencies have funded projects designed to compile information about new treatment modalities. For example, the DOPE Project (Wilmer, Greathouse, Wilton, Ershoff, Foster, & Hetherington, 1976) has compiled a computer bank of evaluated programs across a variety of different client populations. For a minimal cost, one can request information about existing programs in the area of alcohol treatment, for example, and even specify the sophistication of evaluation data desired. Another resource, with a lesser emphasis on supportive data, is the *Source Book of Programs for Community Mental Health Centers,* published by the American Institute for Research (Arutunian, Kroll, & Murphy, 1976). This book is a compendium of several hundred programs for community mental health centers, all of which have been tried in other locales. The BAM Project, operating out of the UCLA Neuropsychiatric Institute, is currently in the process of disseminating to community mental health centers data-based information about behavioral treatment techniques (King, Note 1).

These items do not exhaust the potential sources of information about new programs available to the indigenous change agent. Similar listings of exemplary programs have been developed by the Department of Justice, the Department of Labor, and the Social and Rehabilitation Service in the Department of Health, Education, and Welfare. The point is that in a search for new program alternatives, much of the work has already been done by others at considerable expense. It is logical and invaluable to become familiar with these information sources. Once again, this area is one with which your local CMHC evaluator can assist you. An attempt should be made to select a new program that has the most convincing evidence of its effectiveness. If you are unfamiliar with evaluation methodology and statistical concepts, find someone, such as your CMHC evaluator, to help you make an informed choice based on available data.

The actual choice and decision about a specific new program direction should be a *group-participative* one. As we have indicated, decisions reached unilaterally by unit directors or center directors often meet with resistance from staff members such as yourself. Thus your role as an indigenous change agent is to attempt to get your fellow staff members to meet on several occasions, discuss the different program alternatives that you or others have searched out, and finally reach consensus about what program alternative should be attempted.

One cannot overestimate the degree to which the change agent must be patient during this process of choice. This period is likely to be highly anxiety-provoking for all concerned. Professional futures will be perceived to be at stake, existing job descriptions may be altered, and professional roles may be changed. All of these shifts are likely to produce considerable discomfort for the unit staff. Bear with it. If possible, it may be desirable for the group members to try to form closer relationships with each other during this time. Often it is desirable for the group that is making the new program decision to meet off the center grounds, perhaps for lunch and/or drinks at a local restaurant. Once again, the more that interpersonal trust and participation can be enhanced during this period, the more likely it is that the implementation of the new program itself will be successful. In a real sense the group of staff members involved in the change process should have a *group identity* independent of the particular sub-roles of its members. It should consider itself to be an *ad hoc* planning group, perhaps giving itself a name. One may often find that people play quite different roles in this context. For example, the leadership of the *ad hoc* planning group may not at all correspond to the formal leadership of the CMHC unit most directly involved, and may in fact consist of a person of nominally low professional status.

In the process of selecting a new program alternative, one often can make use of an outside consultant. However, the cautionary note previously indicated still holds true. If the consultant enters your organization and attempts to help the staff group to generate its own "innovation" through discussion alone, then a different kind of consultant may be needed. The role of the effective outside consultant during this stage would be that of assisting staff in gaining access to information sources such as have been described. S/he should have at his/her fingertips a range of proven program alternatives, from which your staff group can make a rational choice. Once again, the consultant should be facilitative, but not entirely non-directive. S/he should help the group to make a choice, but the consultant should insist that the choice be an *informed* one, based on the best program alternatives available.

Implementation and Adoption

Discussion is now transformed into action. This period is the one when staff members actually begin to do things differently in their work with clientele. Paradoxically, it is also a period when some of the informal processes, open communication, and broad-based participation described above need to be *constrained* and dampened a bit. Implementing a new program usually involves a number of discrete and specific tasks. As the staff group moves toward the actual beginning of the new program, a more structured set of activities is called for.

As Zaltman and Duncan (1977) have pointed out, the period in which a new program is actually put into operation is one in which a clear delegation of responsibility and the presence of a more centralized authority are necessary. For example, when one begins a new program it may be necessary to alter existing procedures for interviewing and evaluating clients referred to an alcohol-treatment program. A person, or persons, from the *ad hoc* planning group should be delegated to accomplish this task, with the obligation to report back to the larger group on their activities. Similarly, new types of forms, or testing materials, that are more appropriate to the new treatment program, may need to be created. Once again a person or persons should be delegated this responsibility with clear expectations as to when and where the task should be completed. Another important area in which responsibility should be assigned is that of staff training and development. In any new program there will be significant changes in the nature of the interaction between treatment personnel and clients. This may necessitate training exercises such as role playing, discussion problem scenarios, reviewing program procedures, and so on. Coupled with this renewed emphasis on structure, the indigenous change agent should see that a time schedule of activities and expected completion dates is developed. Setting objectives and clear dates for completion serves as a continuing stimulus for staff involved in the tasks of implementation.

The role of structure need not be over-emphasized in this implementation phase. There is still a continuing need for people to let off steam and to resolve their uncertainties about the impending change. Thus, not only must the indigenous change agent have structured, task-oriented meetings, but he must also continue to provide free-floating, unstructured settings in which group dynamics and human relations issues can be dealt with. It is hoped that by this time the members of the staff group will have formed a unit more cohesive than that which existed at the onset of this process. This outcome should be reinforced by informal gatherings both on and off the work site.

Sometimes it is extremely valuable to have an outside change agent or consultant to assist the group in the implementation phase as well as in the earlier stages. It has been found by Fairweather, Sanders, and Tornatzky (1974) in a national study of change in mental hospitals that the outside change agent is particularly important during the implementation process. However, the importance of the external change agent to these hospitals was not due to his technical expertise or knowledge, but to his role in facilitating task accomplishment and allaying group concerns and uncertainties. Once again, if your center has had the opportunity to work with a change agent or consultant throughout the process described thus far, it is probably a good idea to continue his/her involvement during this final implementation phase.

Stabilizing and Evaluating the New Program

By the time you have reached this phase of activity, you have probably used up several months of your time. Also by this time, you will have seen the establishment of a new program that hopefully is more responsive to the needs of your clientele. There are two things that need to be emphasized now for the achievement of a successful closure of your activities. One involves shutting off the change processes, and the other is getting some internal feedback about how well you have done.

Throughout this discussion we have stressed the notion that the indigenous change agent must facilitate informal group processes, group decision making, and so on. One of the disadvantages of successfully accomplishing this objective is that it is often difficult to turn people off after they have become enamored with the notion of change and renewal. "Change junkies" can be found in many organizations. We are assuming that the new program that you have adopted has some relative advantage over the one that it replaced. Give it a chance to prove its worth. You need not immediately involve yourself in another search for program alternatives, and so on. The goal should be to make the new program a stable and routine part of center activity.

To keep yourself honest, it is also recommended that the effectiveness of your new program be evaluated rigorously. As pointed out previously, there is utility in gathering program evaluation information, and this also holds true when one has established a new and more effective program. Parenthetically, if you have decided to "phase in" the new program over a period of time, you might have the opportunity to do a highly sophisticated, truly experimental comparison of the new and the old programs (Fairweather & Tornatzky, 1977). If you decide to engage in this activity, rather convincing data—positive or negative—can be obtained about relative program effectiveness.

OTHER RESOURCES FOR THE BUDDING CHANGE AGENT

This short chapter is not designed to be an encyclopedic review of knowledge that is available to the person interested in effecting change. Some of the references that we have cited are classics in the field of innovation and change. Some works with which the reader may wish to become more familiar are given below. Havelock (1973) has developed a fairly comprehensive guide for the change agent interested in innovation in education; this book is also likely to be quite helpful to the mental health innovator. For those who wish to become the complete change agent, one publication developed through the auspices of the National Institute of Mental Health (Human Interaction Research Institute, 1976) can be of considerable value. This publication attempts to summarize the literature and concepts relevant to change. One should also become familiar with the classic work of Rogers and Shoemaker (1971), which reviews several hundred studies in the innovation diffusion area.

However, aside from all the resources in the form of knowledge, concepts, guidelines, and tips that can be offered to the potential indigenous change agent, the principal resources that s/he possesses are more personal and internal. Change agent activity requires a certain passion of the spirit, and a supply of stamina and patience. The writer of this chapter has been involved for several years in attempting to achieve programmatic innovation in a particularly recalcitrant group of state and federal mental hospitals. Throughout this largely discouraging activity, one of the convictions that has sustained the endeavor is the belief that change *can* occur, and that given a certain amount of persistence, it *will* occur. With any luck, the aspiring change agent should find his task difficult, but interesting.

NOTES

[1]At the time of this writing, the typical range of services offered by CMHCs includes: services to the aging; alcoholic services; children's services; consultation-education; drugs; partial hospitalization; emergency services; follow-up; inpatient services; outpatient services; and transitional care.

[2]See Rogers and Shoemaker (1971) for a different, but analogous description of the stages of the innovation process.

[3]Throughout this paper we will de-emphasize the role of higher administration in the change process. We see that role primarily as that of a "gatekeeper"—while administrative authority can surely *stop* change, it cannot make it happen by fiat. The change process can only take place if the change agent concentrates on nurturing the supportive group process described here. For a discussion of the relationship between administrative authority and change, see Fairweather, Sanders, and Tornatzky (1974).

REFERENCE NOTE

1.   L. King, *Summary progress report.* Unpublished report. Oxnard, California, 1976.

References

Argyris, C. *Interpersonal competence and organizational effectiveness.* Homewood, Ill.: The Dorsey Press, 1972.

Arutunian, C., Kroll, J., & Murphy, S. *Source book of programs: 1976 community mental health centers.* Palo Alto, Calif.: American Institutes for Research, 1976.

Bennis, W. *Changing organizations.* New York: McGraw-Hill, 1966.

Burns, T., & Stalker, G. *The management of innovation.* London: Tavistock Publications, 1961.

Campbell, D., & Stanley, J. *Experimental and quasi-experimental designs for research.* Chicago: Rand McNally and Co., 1966.

Coch, L., & French, J. Overcoming resistance to change. *Human Relations,* 1948, *1* (4), 512–532.

Fairweather, G., & Tornatzky, L. *Experimental methods for social policy research.* New York: Pergamon Press, 1977.

Fairweather, G., Sanders, D., & Tornatzky, L. *Creating change in mental health organizations.* New York: Pergamon Press, 1974.

Havelock, R. *The change agent's guide to innovation in education.* Englewood Cliffs, N.J.: Educational Technology Publications, 1973.

Havelock, R., & Havelock, M. *Educational innovation in the United States, Vol. 1: The national survey: The substance and the process.* Ann Arbor, Michigan: Institute for Social Research, the University of Michigan, 1973.

Human Interaction Research Institute, in collaboration with the National Institute of Mental Health. *Putting knowledge to use: A distillation of the literature regarding knowledge transfer and change.* Los Angeles, California: Human Interaction Research Institute, 1976.

Huse, E. *Organization development and change.* St. Paul, Minnesota: West Publishing Co., 1975.

Lawrence, P., & Lorsch, P. *Organization and environment.* Cambridge, Massachusetts: Harvard University Press, 1967.

Likert, R. *The human organization.* New York: McGraw-Hill, 1967.

Litwak, E. Models of bureaucracy that permit conflict. *American Journal of Sociology,* September 1961, *57,* 173–183.

McGregor, D. *The human side of enterprise.* New York: McGraw-Hill, 1960.

Perrow, C. *Complex organizations: A critical essay.* Glenview, Illinois: Scott, Foresman and Co., 1972.

Roethlisberger, F., & Dickson, W. *Management and the worker.* Cambridge, Massachusetts: Harvard University Press, 1947.

Rogers, E., & Shoemaker, F. *Communication of innovations.* New York: Free Press, 1971.

Weber, M. *The theory of social and economic organization.* A. M. Henderson & T. Parsons (Ed. and trans.) New York: Oxford University Press, 1947.

Wilner, D., Greathouse, V., Wilton, R., Ershoff, D., Foster, K., & Hetherington, R. Inside DOPE—The custom research databank in the analysis and transfer of information. *Evaluation,* 1976, *3*(1–2), 11–14.

Zaltman, G., & Duncan, R. *Strategies for planned change.* New York: Wiley-Interscience, 1977.

Zaltman, G., Duncan, R., & Holbeck, J. *Innovations and organizations.* New York: Wiley-Interscience, 1973.

Chapter 8

PARAPROFESSIONALS IN PSYCHOSOCIAL REHABILITATION PROGRAMS: A RESOURCE FOR DEVELOPING COMMUNITY SUPPORT SYSTEMS FOR THE "DEINSTITUTIONALIZED" MENTALLY DISABLED

Julius Lanoil*
Judith Clark Turner†

This chapter focuses on the role of paraprofessionals in working with discharged mental patients in the community, with particular emphasis on "psychosocial rehabilitation" programs. It also describes the "Community Support System," which is being developed by the National Institute of Mental Health. Designed to foster more workable arrangements for serving the severely mentally disabled, this approach draws heavily on the experience of the psychosocial rehabilitation movement.

Psychosocial rehabilitation programs provide an array of basic opportunities and services to participants and take the approach of building strengths instead of removing pathologies. The chapter contains practical guidelines on the selection, training, and use of paraprofessionals in psychosocial rehabilitation programs. In addition, it describes the basic characteristics of these increasingly popular programs and their relationship to current federal community mental health legislation. The chapter concludes by highlighting the issues central to the development and retention of an effective paraprofessional workforce to meet the emerging needs for psychosocial rehabilitation. (The psychosocial rehabilitation program di-

*Director Habilitation Service and Assistant Clinical Professor, College of Medicine and Dentistry of New Jersey, Rutgers Medical School, University Heights, Piscataway, New Jersey 08854.

†Chief, Community Support Systems, Mental Health Service Support Branch, Division of Mental Health Service Programs, Room 11C–20, 5600 Fishers Lane, Rockville, Maryland 20852

rected by the first author is described in more detail in chapter 6 of a companion volume, *Case Studies of Mental Health Paraprofessionals: Twelve Effective Programs.*)

This chapter will focus on the role of paraprofessionals in working with discharged mental patients in the community, with particular emphasis on experience gained from the "psychosocial rehabilitation" movement. The material is particularly relevant to follow-up, transitional, and day care service areas of a community mental health center. First, we will briefly describe the nature of psychosocial rehabilitation programs and the role that paraprofessionals play in agencies providing such services. Second, we will discuss what has been learned by various psychosocial rehabilitation agencies about effective selection, training, and deployment of paraprofessional workers. This section will draw particularly on the experience of the first author in two such agencies, Fountain House in New York and The Club at Rutgers Community Mental Health Center in New Jersey. Third, we will discuss the increasing need for and importance of psychosocial rehabilitation programs in the service delivery system. In this section, we will consider the relationship of psychosocial rehabilitation to current Community Mental Health Center (CMHC) legislation and to the National Institute of Mental Health's (NIMH) pilot Community Support Program (CSP). Finally, we will identify and briefly discuss issues we believe must be addressed in developing and retaining an effective paraprofessional work force to meet emerging needs in the field.

THE NATURE OF PSYCHOSOCIAL REHABILITATION PROGRAMS

The term "psychosocial rehabilitation" as it is now commonly used in the United States refers to programs for the mentally and emotionally disabled that provide certain basic opportunities and services—socialization, living arrangements, educational and work opportunities and advocacy—in the context of a supportive, normalizing group in the community (Dincin, 1975; Glasscote, Cumming, Rutman, Sussex, & Glassman, 1971; Lanoil, 1976). A particular feature of psychosocial rehabilitation programs that distinguishes them from more traditional mental health services for the chronically mentally disabled is the emphasis on "personhood," rather than on "patienthood." Whereas traditional mental health agencies tend to conceptualize their task as treating pathological conditions, psychosocial programs emphasize strengthening abilities to deal with everyday life. As a part of this emphasis, clients of psychosocial rehabilitation programs are regarded as "members" of a rehabilitation club, rather than as recipients of treatment or other services.

The social structure of the club, unlike that of a traditional mental health program, is such that clients or members are actually *needed* to assist staff to keep the agency functioning smoothly (Lehrer, & Lanoil, 1977). Thus, members perform such necessary tasks as typing and distributing newsletters and fund-raising materials, cleaning and decorating the facility, preparing food, collecting attendance or other research data, operating the transportation system, and giving tours to new clients and visitors. These jobs are structured to provide prevocational and vocational opportunities, and are an integral part of the rehabilitation program.

Psychosocial rehabilitation methods have developed somewhat spontaneously over the past 25 years, without reference to a particular body of theory. It has been noted, however, that current practices in the field are usually consistent with "normalization" theory as recently articulated by Wolf Wolfensberger (1970; 1972) and others. The normalization principle was developed initially in Sweden but has had a great impact on the mental retardation field in the United States as well. This principle implies programmatic characteristics such as the following:

- Offering normative social roles such as worker or club member to people with disabling conditions
- Providing age-appropriate, culturally-appropriate daytime and evening activities
- Dispersing living arrangements widely throughout the community to avoid clustering large numbers of disabled persons in a given residential setting
- Separating the residential setting from the place in which daytime opportunities and services are provided
- Status enhancement of disabled people through careful attention to language, names of service settings, etc.
- Offering real work opportunities, not "make-work"
- Minimizing distance between "clients" and "staff"

All of these characteristics, and others elaborated by Wolfensberger, typify the psychosocial rehabilitation approach.

As an example of this emphasis, community living arrangements of psychosocial agencies frequently involve cooperative apartment programs, in which the agency holds the lease and client-members share apartments and split the rent. Eventually, clients may take over the lease on their own. No live-in staff is necessary, but the psychosocial agency provides a range of advocacy, rehabilitation, and support services. Other types of living arrangements, such as halfway houses, etc., may also be provided—all of them in small groups dispersed through the community.

A number of psychosocial agencies also offer "Transitional Employment Programs." Through such programs, the agency arranges with business and industry for a number of work slots to be set aside for client-members. These jobs are used as on-the-job training and work-conditioning experiences, with each job being shared by two clients. Clients work half time, for approximately three months in a given placement. In this way, clients are able to test and improve their skills in a "real world" environment, before eventually applying for regular work (Bean, & Beard, 1975; Schmidt, Nessel, & Malumud, Note 1).

THE ROLE OF THE PARAPROFESSIONAL IN PSYCHOSOCIAL REHABILITATION

The relatively small numbers of professionals currently involved in psychosocial rehabilitation (primarily social workers, psychologists, and rehabilitation counselors) tend to assume clinical, research, intake, or administrative and leadership functions in the programs. People directing such programs, therefore, have turned to "paraprofessional" workers—that is, persons with a bachelor's degree or less formal education—to fill a large proportion of the direct service functions.

The normalizing philosophy and social structure of the programs has significant implications for the roles and functions of both professional and paraprofessional workers. For example, unlike more traditional mental health programs in which staff tend to specialize both by discipline and by function, staff of psychosocial agencies tend to act as "generalists." Jerry Dincin (1975), director of a psychosocial program in Chicago, underlines this point:

> In most agencies there is a generalist approach to the staff. It is expected that all staff members will be involved in all areas of the agency. While there are some exceptions to this in some professional areas of expertise, in most agencies the staff plays interchanging roles. For example, case workers do group work, vocational counselors do case work, and psychologists do job placements. Something may be lost in this process, but a lot more is gained. The compartmentalization inherent in making "referral" from one department to another is mitigated (p. 133).

The generalist role of staff is further elaborated by Beard and Schmidt (Note 2) in describing the use of staff at Fountain House. They emphasize that "the primary function of *all* staff at Fountain House is identical—that is, to function in a manner which is supportive of the responsibilities being assumed by members in the program." For this reason, they emphasize, "staff do not regard support personnel as 'aides' to professionals, where the significant input comes from the person with 'greater professional status.' " Instead, they maintain, the field of psychosocial rehabilitation "has not yet reached a level of effectiveness where role or function of the expert can be clearly identified."

The day-to-day content of staff activity in a psychosocial agency also differs dramatically from the functions of staff in more traditional mental health programs. Psychosocial workers are seldom found in their offices doing counseling or therapy in the usual sense of the word. Instead, they may be found working side by side with their "clients": frying hamburgers as part of a prevocational program; riding a bus or visiting the laundromat to teach skills of daily living; visiting the welfare or food stamp office to perform the much-needed advocacy function; or helping clients paint and furnish their apartments as part of a cooperative apartment program.

To understand the significance of these activities in the rehabilitation process, it is important to emphasize that the activities are carried out in the context of a strong, somewhat subjective relationship with the client. According to Dincin (1975):

> This type of relationship is not often duplicated in other settings. It includes a strong element of reaching out to the client, of helping him overcome his reluctance to participate, and of taking an active role in persuading him to participate in the program (p. 132).

A high degree of staff-client involvement is encouraged, and the distance between clients and staff is minimized. In many ways staff relate to clients more as friends and/or co-workers than as people with mental health problems. As Dincin (1975) puts it:

> Since the lack of motivation is endemic among schizophrenic clients, a particular attitude concerning motivation has evolved: one that usually does not include a heavy reliance on the more traditional casework and psychotherapeutic interview. Staff members in the rehabilitative centers believe that motivation can be created by such characteristics as:
>
> 1. A strong professional desire to influence the member
> 2. An ability to develop a feeling of "dynamic hopefulness" in the member
> 3. Creativity that enables the member to use the center for the member's involvement
> 4. Professional tenacity in the face of symptoms, regression, hostility, and resistance
> 5. The genuine ability not to be fearful of the member's illness
> 6. Great frequency of interpersonal contact
> 7. A deep-seated investment in all areas of the member's current life situation (p. 132).

ADVANTAGES OF PARAPROFESSIONAL WORKERS IN PSYCHOSOCIAL REHABILITATION

There are important advantages to staffing psychosocial programs with a high proportion of paraprofessional workers. First, paraprofessionals are less likely to have conflicts which stem from professional self-image. They therefore feel freer to engage in such untraditional programmatic activities as working with clients on jobs in the community or living with clients in residential situations. They regard these activities as appropriate to the goals of the rehabilitation program. This is reinforced when professional staff spend at least part of their time doing the same kind of work with clients.

Second, paraprofessionals are often better able to relate to clients as people—an important part of the normalizing process. Paraprofessionals tend to come into the field with fewer preconceived notions about the nature of schizophrenia as an illness. If the setting supports normalizing relationships, paraprofessionals will respond to client behaviors directly, spontaneously, and genuinely. This provides clients with opportunities to learn about the likely effects of certain behaviors in the world outside the agency.

Perhaps for the reasons cited above, it has been noted that at Fountain House (Glasscote et al., 1971)—and many other psychosocial agencies—that:

> There is an ambivalence ... about formal training. Some of their most valuable, and indeed charismatic, staff members have only a high school education. Some of the products of highly reputed training facilities have been unable to accept the untraditional ways of Fountain House, where social workers have no desk of their own, interviews with members are conducted in the course of preparing lunch, cleaning the common rooms, or sorting clothes for the thrift shop. Fountain House emphasized to us repeatedly that it has nothing *against* the professionally trained person, and having such people on the staff gains fundable positions. ... But it was emphasized that training in itself does not assure that a person will be able to relate in the personal and involved manner that characterizes the services of Fountain House—indeed, that the training may be antithetical (p. 49).

In addition to the philosophical and programmatic advantages of using paraprofessionals for direct service roles, there are obvious financial advantages: well-selected, trained and supervised paraprofessionals can extend service dollars farther than would otherwise be possible.

ISSUES IN SELECTION OF PARAPROFESSIONAL STAFF

The paraprofessional staffs currently employed in psychosocial rehabilitation programs have come to the field from a variety of backgrounds. This includes former mental hospital staff retrained on the job for community work; former patients who possess the necessary attributes and skills; people with associate degrees in rehabilitation from community colleges; people with high school diplomas, relevant life experiences, and rich work histories; and people with bachelor's degrees in psychology or sociology who wish to work in mental health, but do not necessarily wish to pursue graduate work.

No objective methods have been developed to predict who will become an effective psychosocial rehabilitation worker. The director of one agency observed that "it appears to be a matter of trial and error." He also pointed out, however, that the trial period need not be long. After about three months, "if the new staff worker has not begun to grasp the rationale and catch the spirit of [the program], he is helped to realize that he would probably be better off in a more traditional agency" (Beard, 1976, pp. 393–413).

In selecting people with high school diplomas, many psychosocial agencies pay particular attention to the combination of relevant life experiences and work skills in areas needed for the agency program. Experience in other fields often brings a fresh outlook. In addition, skills in food service, business, clerical work, sports, photography, or other areas can often be directly applied to the social or vocational activities of the agency.

In selecting and hiring former patients, different agencies have different policies. For example, at Fountain House the rule used to be that a former patient would have to work one year on an independent job before being considered for a staff position with the agency. This rule changed as the transitional employment program became more sophisticated, giving supervisory staff the opportunity to observe client leaders performing a variety of staff functions. The Club notifies rehabilitated mental patients when staff positions become available and allows open competition. In fact, there is a slight bias in favor of hiring former patients, since they have proved extremely valuable as staff members. Often the sensitivity and commitment of former patients is unique, and they can contribute to many phases of the rehabilitation process.

Regardless of the particular combination of training and experience a prospective paraprofessional worker may have, there seem to be certain personality characteristics that are important. Among these are flexibility, the ability to work under stress, an appreciation of people who are different, the desire to work as part of a group in a therapeutic milieu, and a general disinterest in working in a traditional office-based job eight hours a day. In addition, effective workers often possess certain qualities of personality that can best be described as charismatic—a certain "something" that attracts others to follow their lead.

Many successful psychosocial rehabilitation workers also have in common a dissatisfaction with former jobs in which roles were too rigidly defined or opportunities to express caring were too limited. Beard (1976) sums up this issue:

> People, whether professional or paraprofessional, want to feel significant. To do so, they must get into a setting whose purpose is conducive to feeling significant. Because we are working with clients who are the least promising, our staff feels that any success of accomplishment is significant (pp. 393–413).

In-Service Training of Paraprofessionals

Despite the advantages of employing paraprofessionals in this field, it must be recognized that those without previous related experience initially lack a number of types of knowledge that are important in the rehabilitation process. First, they may lack necessary mental health knowledge, such as a general understanding of the nature and effects of psychotropic medications, an ability to distinguish between degrees of psychopathology, an ability to deal with crisis situations, and an awareness of how and when to make use of psychiatric consultation. If they are unfamiliar with mental illness, they may initially be overly concerned with what they may or may not say to clients. This usually dissipates, however, as they learn that the former mental patient is not as fragile as first appearances would suggest.

In addition, they are likely to lack a number of specific skills that are important in the rehabilitation process. One such skill, for example, is the ability to develop rehabilitation plans and to maintain adequate case records. Another important area relates to interviewing, group process, and counseling. These skills are required in certain areas of the agency's functioning, such as intake, working with parent groups, interagency liaison, goal planning, social skills groups, activity area meetings, and employment meetings.

Because of these limitations, a great deal of time and energy must be devoted to in-service training. Assuming that the person hired has appropriate personality attributes, the agency must be ready to accept the fact that one to two years of experience will be necessary before the person feels capable—and in fact, *is* capable—of performing at a high level of competence.

To minimize the training time required, some agencies (for example, the Harlem Rehabilitation Center in New York) use paraprofessionals in more limited, specialized roles. This approach has the advantage of getting a specific activity accomplished without extensive investment of training time, but it also has the disadvantage of limiting the amount of learning. At the same time, this way of using staff causes a problem in creating continuity of care within the agency, making it difficult to maintain a therapeutic milieu. In addition, it creates a cadre of paraprofessional specialists, rather than the generalists who are so much needed in holistic, normalizing programs.

Training Opportunities Presently Available

Since no formal training programs exist in the field, most agencies have developed extensive, but informal training programs for new staff. This usually involves a combination of methods and experiences that will help the worker develop both the skills and the attitudes required to perform effectively in the psychosocial setting.

Attitudes are particularly important. The new staff member must come to understand and agree with the rehabilitative goals, philosophy, and methods of the program:

> He must be able to adjust his self-image with the kinds of activities required. He must find the program consistent with his abilities and predilections. "He must like to work this way." In short, the staff worker coming to a psychosocial center must undergo the involvement and influencing process same as a client, since there is no formal training he might have had to prepare him (Lanoil, Note 3).

The degree to which the psychosocial program is successful in orienting and training all new professionals and paraprofessionals is the degree to which the program can be rehabilitative.

Although the in-service training usually goes on through a combination of techniques in different settings, including formal one-hour-per-week supervision, the process is most effective when personal relationships develop between experienced staff and the new worker. These relationships usually develop when the new staff worker seems to have "good potential." The worker's potential is determined first by commitment to clients, second by openness to learning, and third by the assumption that program development skills can be acquired.

In addition to socializing new workers into the agency milieu, most psychosocial programs also provide some on-the-job didactic training, focusing on particular skills and knowledge required. For example, in settings planning special programs—such as transitional employment, goal planning, or parent groups—consultants from the field are often brought in to train staff. When a program director becomes aware of a special staff need (for example, a need for greater understanding of psychiatric medications and their side effects), a lecture series on the subject may be initiated. In addition, some psychosocial agencies, such as Places for People (connected with St. Louis Hospital) and The Club at Rutgers Community Mental Health Center, have relationships with junior or senior colleges to assist with in-service training of paraprofessional workers.

In most psychosocial agencies, the in-service training process is assumed to be an ongoing one, in which the staff worker develops greater depth through staff meetings, learning from clients, listening to more experienced staff, and risking himself by taking on various assignments rather than forever specializing in one area. In addition, most psychosocial programs are open environments which deal with landlords, employers, and many other people in the community whose input—both structured and informal—helps staff to gain a realistic understanding of client needs. This, in turn, affects the direction of the program.

THE ROLE OF PSYCHOSOCIAL REHABILITATION IN THE SERVICE SYSTEM

The psychosocial rehabilitation approach originated with the private, non-profit facility, and we expect that such agencies will continue to give major leadership to the field. There are, however, reasons to predict that the psychosocial rehabilitation approach will increasingly become a part of the public sector—that is, state or county operated mental hospitals or community mental health centers—as well. Current deinstitutionalization trends and growing federal and state recognition of the need for more extensive community service networks point in this direction.

For example, in the past two years two major Congressional studies (Senate Special Committee on Aging, 1976) and many other articles and reports have documented the fact that thousands of mentally disabled persons have been released from institutions *before* adequate community programs were developed, and they now can be found in the community with nothing to do and no place to go. At the same time, thousands of people who continue to enter or reenter institutions do so primarily because of the lack of rehabilitation and support systems. Clearly, this is a problem of major proportions for which more substantial resources must be mobilized in the future. The Congressional studies and other developments have stimulated intensified interest and activity in this area in both the legislative and administrative branches of government.

RELATIONSHIP OF PSYCHOSOCIAL REHABILITATION TO FEDERAL MENTAL HEALTH LEGISLATION

In thinking about the future of this field, it is important to note that federal mental health legislation enacted in 1975 gives increasing attention to issues related to psychosocial rehabilitation. Title I of Public Law 94–63 requires that state mental health agencies applying for federal resources under Section 314(d) of the Public Health Service Act develop a new type of state plan, designed not only "to eliminate inappropriate institutional care of people with mental health problems," but also "to assure availability of appropriate noninstitutional services" for such people. Clearly, such noninstitutional services for many of those being diverted or discharged from mental hospitals *must* involve rehabilitative programs, if the emphasis on appropriateness is to be fulfilled.

The same law also amends the community mental health center requirements to specify that in the future federally funded centers must provide, in addition to the original five essential services, seven other services. Two of the newly mandated services are "follow-up care" for persons discharged from mental health facilities, and "programs of transitional halfway house services," designed both as an alternative to admission to an inpatient facility and as a transitional living arrangement for people moving to a more independent living arrangement.

The complexities of implementing these legislative mandates prompted the National Institute of Mental Health to convene during 1975 and 1976 a series of working conferences designed to clarify the service needs of the adult mentally ill as well as the responsibilities of state and local mental health agencies (and other human service agencies) for meeting these needs (*Community living arrangements* . . . Note 4). One outcome of these conferences is a conceptualization of a "comprehensive community support system" for adults with severely disabling mental health problems (Turner, 1977). This concept draws heavily on the experience of the psychosocial movement in defining both the services required and the principles for developing such systems.

What Is a "Community Support System"?

As conceptualized by the National Institute of Mental Health, a community support system must be designed "to guarantee . . . that appropriate forms of help are available . . . to meet the needs and develop the potential of the population-at-risk." In the working conferences, an effort was made to delineate the essential functions that such a system must perform for a specific population, that population being: "adults with a severe or persistent mental or emotional disorder that seriously limits their functional capacities relative to primary aspects of daily living such as personal relations, living arrangements, work, recreation, etc." (*Definition and guidelines* . . . Note 5).

Ten basic functions of a community support system for this population as currently conceived by the National Institute of Mental Health include:

- Identification of the population-at-risk, whether in hospital or in the community
- Assistance in applying for entitlements
- Crisis stabilization services in the least restrictive setting possible
- Psychosocial rehabilitation services, including transitional living arrangements, resocialization and vocational rehabilitation
- Supportive living arrangements, employment opportunities and other supportive services of indefinite duration
- Adequate medical and mental health care
- Backup support, consultation and assistance to family, friends, and community agencies in coping with problems
- Involvement of concerned community members in planning community support programs, befriending mentally disabled persons, and offering housing and job opportunities

- Clearly defined grievance procedures and mechanisms to protect client rights, both in hospital and in the community
- Case management, to facilitate continuing availability to clients of appropriate opportunities and services (Note 5)

Since this conceptualization emphasizes service *functions* rather than type of service *provider,* it makes it possible to view both hospitals and community mental health centers as part of a community support system. Such a system includes agencies responsible for rehabilitation, social services, housing, income maintenance, and other such services. A diversity of arrangements in local communities must exist to assure that the necessary functions are performed. Specific roles of hospitals, community mental health centers, psychosocial rehabilitation centers, and other public or private agencies in a given community must be worked out through a process of interagency collaboration, and they will vary greatly from place to place and from time to time.

The NIMH Community Support Program

In an effort to stimulate states and communities to establish more workable arrangements for serving the severely mentally disabled, the National Institute of Mental Health is developing a pilot program—the Community Support Program (CSP). The program, being initiated in the fall of 1977, involves contracts with state mental health agencies for two types of special projects: Statewide Community Support System Strategy Development Projects and State/Local Community Support System Demonstration and Replication Projects. Both types of contracts attempt to translate the community support system concept (of which psychosocial rehabilitation is an important element) into practice on a systematic basis.

Thirty states responded to the initial NIMH request for proposals, which was issued in July, 1977. About half of the states responding were able to meet the stringent review criteria, and have been or will be funded in the near future. The response from the states indicates a high degree of recognition throughout the country of the importance of more normalizing and rehabilitative community service systems. The response also indicates substantial efforts on the part of a number of states to move mental health system resources in this direction.

Issues in Developing and Retaining a Well-Trained Paraprofessional Work Force to Meet Future Needs

As program development proceeds in the community support system area, the experience of the relatively small number of "psychosocial rehabilitation centers" throughout the country will have considerable influence. Effective program development will also require larger numbers of appropriately qualified professional and paraprofessional workers, both for leadership and direct service roles.

At present, the number of professionals and paraprofessionals who are thoroughly trained (on the job) and experienced in psychosocial rehabilitation practice is very limited. As of 1971, Glasscote and his associates were able to identify only 13 comprehensive psychosocial rehabilitation centers in the entire country, when comprehensiveness was defined as including socialization training and socialization opportunities, work, and living arrangements. Since that time, similar service clusters have been developed by a variety of types of agencies. St. Louis State Hospital, for example, developed an extensive psychosocial rehabilitation program using redeployed hospital staff in the community (Sandall, Hawley, & Gordon, 1975). The Club, as mentioned earlier, provides a comprehensive psychosocial rehabilitation program at a community mental health center *in place of* the traditional "day care/partial hospitalization" program. Many other agencies throughout the country are moving in this direction. Nonetheless, there are relatively few seasoned staff available now at either the leadership or direct service level.

This shortage of appropriately trained personnel will severely limit the extent and quality of future program development efforts. One reason for current shortages is the fact that current professional training programs for psychiatrists, social workers, rehabilitation counselors, psychologists and nurses offer little of practical value for potential organizers and administrators of psychosocial programs. Indeed, as mentioned earlier, professional training tends to discourage people from becoming involved with the chronically mentally disabled, since the skills they have acquired often are not relevant to the challenges of working with chronic patients in a community setting.

At present, no long-term training opportunities exist that are specific to psychosocial rehabilitation. It is encouraging to note, however, the emergence of a new organization, the International Association of Psycho-Social Rehabilitation Service (IAPSRS), which held its first annual conference in Philadelphia in 1975. One of the major purposes of this organization is exchanging information among all levels of personnel active in the field. This is being done through annual conferences, special meetings and workshops, and other channels.[1]

In addition, Fountain House in New York has an NIMH grant to provide short-term training to people from community mental health centers or other local agencies developing psychosocial rehabilitation programs. This project provides a three-week practicum in concepts and practices of the program, preceded and followed by on-site consultation from Fountain House staff.[2] It is expected that the availability of this training will prove particularly valuable in developing leaders who can initiate new or expanded community support programs at the local level.

RETRAINING HOSPITAL STAFF

The single largest pool of potential paraprofessional workers for the future is state, county, and private mental hospital employees. These people can be a particularly valuable resource because, as the director of the St. Louis psychosocial program points out, "they are not frightened by odd behaviors; they have a solid foundation of specialized psychiatric knowledge; they are familiar with commonly used medications and their side-effects; and they are trained and willing to take responsibility for a particularly difficult group of clients" (Sandall, Note 6).

In addition to the programmatic advantages of bringing more hospital staff into the field, there are compelling administrative and political reasons for doing so. Hospital employee unions have in some instances blocked efforts to phase down hospitals and move toward community care because of the threat of loss of jobs (Santiestavan, 1975). If hospital staff members are viewed as a resource for developing community service systems, a commonality of interest emerges between hospital employee unions and administrators seeking to update service systems. A number of successful experiments throughout the country have demonstrated that hospital staff can be retrained to work effectively in community settings (Baron, 1975). Providing such training can thus meet two needs: the need to provide the community services and the need to keep hospital workers employed.

There are, however, certain problems inherent in the effort to retrain hospital staff, the most serious of which is the difficulty of changing the attitudes and role concepts that have developed over years of hospital employment. Often the social structure and administrative practices of the hospital have created insensitivity to patient needs and have developed staff who view themselves as custodians of patients rather than as members of a therapeutic milieu.

In the experience of the first author, it is almost impossible to have any long-term effect on these attitudes and behaviors *unless* hospital staff members who are trained in psychosocial rehabilitation have an immediate opportunity to apply their learning. This means working in an environment that reinforces different types of staff behaviors and different role relationships to mentally disabled people. One way to provide this would be to create psychosocial programs on hospital grounds, to serve both as a transition for the more disabled patients preparing for discharge and as a retraining site for hospital staff moving into the community. In addition to new types of working environments, the new skills and behaviors taught when retraining hospital staff should be reinforced through appropriate promotion policies.

THE PROBLEM OF CAREER LADDERS

Another important issue for the future is the need to find better ways to retain well-qualified workers, both those already in the field and those who may enter it from hospitals or other settings. Because of the lack of formal training and credentialing, opportunities for advancement of competent staff are limited, and retention of highly capable persons often becomes a problem.

One way to deal with this problem is to develop special career ladders for psychosocial staff. Advancement should be related to the role and responsibilities of the paraprofessional worker and to experience specific to psychosocial rehabilitation. This has been done at The Club in New Jersey, with good effects both on staff morale and on the program itself.

Nevertheless, in a degree-oriented society, paraprofessional workers face very real limitations in advancement opportunities, regardless of their expertise and ability to take on responsibility. In view of this, those who wish to make careers in the field are often ambivalent as to whether to continue working or to seek graduate degrees. Those employed in state- or county-operated agencies may tend to move to the private sector, where advancement opportunities are usually greater because of more flexible personnel policies. Others may enroll for full-time academic work in order to improve career prospects. Those who continue working while going to graduate school tend to stay in the field, while those who enroll in graduate school full time seem more likely to seek clinical jobs after receiving their degrees.

Since traditional professional degrees tend to discourage people from working with the severely mentally disabled, it may be time to think about developing more formal training opportunities (including possibly AA, BA, and/or MA degrees) with a specific focus on psychosocial rehabilitation. The advisability of this and the appropriate level for such training is an issue requiring considerable debate. Questions arise, for example, as to whether such training should be viewed as a subspeciality of rehabilitation, social work, or some other established profession. In any case, it seems particularly important to recognize the need for more well-qualified program leaders. Neither new services nor new training programs can develop fully without the leadership of people who are both trained and experienced in the complexities of planning, implementing, and maintaining quality in psychosocial programs.

SUMMARY AND RECOMMENDATIONS

In this chapter, we have tried to describe the nature and relevance of psychosocial rehabilitation services in an era of "deinstitutionalization." We have emphasized the growing need for such services on a nationwide basis, and we have predicted that federal, state, and local agencies will increasingly try to move programs for the mentally disabled in that direction. We have also reported the vital role that paraprofessional workers can and should play in such services, emphasizing both philosophical and pragmatic reasons for thinking that there will be increasing opportunities for paraprofessionals in this field.

If our understanding is correct, it is important to begin now to initiate thoughtful long-range planning to deal with training, retention, and career development issues. In so doing, we will be better able to use the talents of paraprofessionals, to provide them with more satisfying and upwardly mobile career opportunities, and at the same time to assure delivery of the highest quality services to the thousands of clients who need them.

NOTES

[1] For further information, contact International Association of Psycho-Social Rehabilitation Services, 501 South 12th Street, Philadelphia, Pennsylvania 19147.

[2] For further information, contact Mr. James Schmidt at Fountain House Foundation, 425 West 47th Street, New York, New York 10036.

REFERENCE NOTES

1. J. Schmidt, J. Nessel, & T. Malumud, *An evaluation of rehabilitation services and the role of industry in the community adjustment of psychiatric patients following hospitalization* (Final Report SRS-RD-1281-T). New York: Fountain House, July 1969.
2. J. H. Beard & J. R. Schmidt, *The use of support personnel in the rehabilitation of the psychiatrically disabled.* Paper presented at Research Utilization in Rehabilitation Facilities, Proceedings of an International Conference of June 1–18, 1971. N. Pacinelli (Ed.). Social and Rehabilitation Service of Health Education and Welfare (Grant No. 22-P-55091/3-01), Washington, D.C., October 1971.
3. J. Lanoil, *A sociological definition of the psychosocial rehabilitation center.* Unpublished manuscript, 1976. (Available from Julius Lanoil, Rutgers Community Mental Health Center, The Club, P.O. Box 101, Piscataway, New Jersey 08854.)
4. *Community living arrangements for the mentally ill and disabled: Issues and options for public policy.* Proceedings of an NIMH working conference, September 1976. (Available from Judith Turner, Community Support Program, Division of Special Mental Health Programs, National Institute of Mental Health, 5600 Fisher's Lane, Room 11–103, Rockville, Maryland 20857.)
5. *Definition and guidelines for community support systems* (Request for proposal NIMH-MH-0080 & 0081). Washington, D.C.: National Institute of Mental Health, July 29, 1977.
6. Hilary Sandall, personal communication, August 1977.

REFERENCES

Baron, R. State hospitals in transition: Impact on staff. *Currents,* July 1975, *2*(2), 3–19.
Bean, B., & Beard, J. Placement for persons with psychiatric disability. *Rehabilitation Counselor Bulletin,* 1975, *18*(4), 253–258.

Beard, J. H. Psychiatric rehabilitation at Fountain House. In J. Meislin (Ed.), *Rehabilitative medicine and psychiatry.* Springfield, Ill.: Charles C Thomas, 1976.

Dincin, J. Psychiatric rehabilitation. *Schizophrenia Bulletin,* 1975, (13), 131–148.

Glasscote, R. M., Cumming, E., Rutman, I. D., Sussex, J. N., & Glassman, S. M. *Rehabilitating the mentally ill in the community.* Washington, D.C.: The Joint Information Service of the American Psychiatric Association and the National Association for Mental Health, 1971.

Lanoil, J. Advocacy and social systems networks: Continuity of care for adult schizophrenics. *Psychosocial Rehabilitation Journal,* 1976, *1*(1), 1–6.

Lehrer, P., & Lanoil, J. Natural reinforcement in a psychiatric rehabilitation program. *Schizophrenia Bulletin,* 1977, *3*(3), 297–304.

Returning the mentally disabled to the community: Government needs to do more. Washington, D.C.: U.S. General Accounting Office, U.S. Government Printing Office, January 7, 1977.

Sandall, H., Hawley, T. T., & Gordon, G. C. The St. Louis community homes program: Graduated support for long-term care. *American Journal of Psychiatry,* 1975, *132* (6), 617–622.

Santiestavan, H. *Out of their beds and into the streets.* Washington, D.C.: American Federation of State, County, and Municipal Employees, 1625 L Street, N.W., February 1975.

Senate Special Committee on Aging, Subcommittee on Long-Term Care. *The role of nursing homes in caring for discharged mental patients: And the birth of a for-profit boarding home industry* (Supporting Paper No. 7). Washington, D.C.: U.S. Government Printing Office, 1976.

Turner, J. C. Comprehensive community support systems for adults with chronically disabling mental health problems: Definitions, components, and guiding principles. *Journal of Psychosocial Rehabilitation,* 1977, *1*(3), 39–47.

Wolfensberger, W. The principle of normalization and its implications to psychiatric services. *American Journal of Psychiatry,* 1970, *127*(3), 67–73.

Wolfensberger, W. *The principles of normalization in human services.* Toronto: National Institute of Mental Retardation, 1972.

IV

THE INVOLVEMENT OF PARAPROFESSIONALS IN COMMUNITY MENTAL HEALTH

Chapter 9

A NEEDS-BASED SERVICE DELIVERY MODEL FOR COMMUNITY MENTAL HEALTH CENTERS

Robert Cohen*
Melissa E. Devine†

The functions performed by mental health paraprofessionals vary from agency to agency, in relation not only to clients' needs but also to the models of service delivery to which the given agency subscribes. Often implicit rather than clearly articulated, these models reflect the value systems and mental health ideologies of parties responsible for the given agency's programs. The authors conceptualize six frequently occurring service delivery models, examine the roles of paraprofessionals in implementing each model, and recommend as optimal a "competence building-resource enabling" model. This latter model requires that paraprofessionals be involved extensively in responsible and innovative functions. Thus, the authors advocate the use of paraprofessionals not as a goal in itself but as a means for making possible the delivery of services needed by a community and its residents. This chapter should help staff members of mental health centers to identify the service delivery model(s) that guide(s) their operations, and to examine the fit between the use of paraprofessionals and the service delivery model(s).

This source book focuses on the effective use of paraprofessionals in community mental health centers. In order to examine this issue clearly, it is first necessary to establish the assumptions, goals, and models of service delivery

*Chairperson, Department of Psychology, LeMoyne College, Syracuse, New York.

†Department of Psychology, LeMoyne College, Syracuse, New York.

upon which these centers are based. The roles and functions a paraprofessional performs are largely dependent on the manner in which his or her agency perceives and implements its mission. It is futile to attempt to design meaningful roles for paraprofessionals if we do not first understand what the center is trying to accomplish. This chapter is based on the premise that knowledge of the service objectives and style of the agency makes it possible to identify the tasks to be performed and to assess how paraprofessionals may function effectively in these tasks.

Six different approaches for service delivery are examined in this chapter. The approach recommended as optimal (the "needs-based" model) for achieving the goals of a community mental health center requires the extensive use of paraprofessionals in a wide variety of roles.

The community mental health center movement evolved in response to the need for more effective comprehensive approaches to the mental health problems of the total community. When the original Community Mental Health Centers Act was enacted in 1963, the national climate was conducive to the development of socially innovative programs, particularly those addressing the needs of low income and minority persons. Progressive sounding ideas such as "continuity of care," "community-based services," and "preventive intervention" were appealing. The availability of funds for the construction and operation of community mental health centers was tempting.

This combination—a strong sense of social consciousness and a substantial allocation of new funds—facilitated the development of many new programs. But it was not enough to insure the solution of problems for which traditional mental health programs had been failures. In addition to the political and economic obstacles and the diminished public expression of social concern that arose during the next decade, a number of conceptual and operational problems also impeded the achievement of an enlightened community mental health movement. Paramount among these problems was and is the lack of a clearly defined operational model of community mental health. The community mental health legislation indeed spelled out some general goals and priorities (e.g., emphasis on a total community or catchment area) and abstractly described the type of services to be utilized in achieving these goals (e.g., inpatient, outpatient, emergency services, consultation and education). However, this legislation did not set any uniform standard of how the centers may genuinely improve the mental health of the community.

To be effective in this mission, a center needs to have a precise definition of what is meant by community mental health, an operational blueprint of the resources and services appropriate to this definition, and a plan of action that will enable the center to work efficiently toward the defined ideal of a mentally healthy community.

In the absence of this precise operational model, community mental health centers have moved in many different directions. While some have made great strides in enhancing the quality of life within their communities, other centers have done little more than perpetuate traditional practices—the same practices whose limited value had given impetus to the creation of the community mental health center program. Still other centers—probably the majority —engage in the thankless struggle of trying to meet the day-to-day crises through a loosely bound patchwork of services, impeded by the bureaucratic demands of the mental health system and unaided by any cohesive framework of ideology and practice.

We are not proposing that the answer to the community mental health dilemma resides solely in a cogent definition or conceptual model. However, the first step in the process of developing a viable approach is to analyze the various models of mental health, particularly with regard to their implications for a system of community mental health services. Once an optimal model has been selected, the needs of the system can be identified, the resources to meet these needs can be calculated, and a plan of action can be designed to implement the system.

In this chapter we will identify the major models of mental health service delivery. In addition to describing the basic assumptions and methods of each approach, we will also examine the implications for both the community mental health movement and for the utilization of paraprofessional workers. After presenting the basic approaches, we will propose an integrative, conceptual model that enables agencies to incorporate the positive features of the previously described approaches. We will then illustrate how paraprofessionals can contribute to the functioning of community mental health centers within the context of this needs-based model. The chapter will conclude with a discussion of the issues and problems involved in implementing a needs-based model for mental health services.

ALTERNATIVE CONCEPTIONS OF MENTAL HEALTH SERVICES

There is a variety of ways in which mental health may be perceived and described. Each view, in turn, leads to a series of possible strategies, actions, and programs. In examining the various conceptions of mental health it may be helpful to condense each model into its most basic form, describing its fundamental elements in simple, concrete terms. Toward this objective we pose the following question for each service delivery model: *Who does what to whom, toward what purpose, and for whose benefit?* A summary analysis of the various models of mental health service delivery, based on this question, is presented in the appendix located at the end of this chapter.

Social Control Model

Whether one liked it or not, mental health agencies have always been, and to some extent still are, viewed as protective agents for society. While the more blatant examples of back-ward "snake pits" no longer prevail, there are many ways in which mental health centers function as instruments of social control.

At one end of the continuum are the legal mechanisms of involuntary commit-ment, ostensibly designed to protect the community from those whose personal difficulties may cause them to harm others, or to prevent the disturbed individ-ual from behaving self-destructively. Less obvious, but equally within the realm of social control functions, is the notion that mental health services are designed to remove deviant persons from the mainstream of society. This segregation may be for the purpose of "custodial care" or to facilitate the extinction of deviant behavior. Even outpatient mental health services may be viewed as social regulators when, as is so often the case, the purpose of treatment is to encourage conformity to pre-existing social norms of behavior. As Silverstein (1968) observes:

> Once within the therapeutic context, the patient then exists in the very salient world of social management. In many ways the primary objective of treatment is often regarded as a special form of social processing en-abling the psycho-socially maladapted to possess the necessary tools for a "normal life." (p. 11)

While it would be foolish to deny the importance of protecting communi-ties from acts of violence and other forms of abuse, serious doubts may be raised as to whether this is an appropriate function for mental health agencies. These control functions would be better served if they were delegated to agencies that are clearly identified as regulators. Not only does the social control function constrain and stigmatize many clients in the mental health system because of the security measures taken for a few violent individuals, but, as Heller and Monahan (1977) note in their thoughtful analysis of commu-nity intervention, "it is the conflict between support and control functions that often blurs the clarity of mission of some agencies" (p. 373).

Medical Disease Model

In the medical model the client is seen as having an underlying disease which manifests itself in symptoms of unusual or maladaptive behavior. The client is served by a professional care giver who, working from an office or hospital setting, generally takes responsibility for the diagnosis, prescription, and treat-ment of the mental health client (or patient). Rappaport (1977) identifies two distinguishable components within the medical model: *the conceptual compo-nent and the style of delivery component.* Traditionally, criticism of the medical model has been directed at its conceptual base. Critics have claimed that people who seek help are experiencing "problems in living" rather than physi-cal disease (Szasz, 1960); that the medical conception reinforces attitudes of personal defectiveness and inadequacy among those who are experiencing difficulty (Levinson & Gallagher, 1964); and that adoption of the medical model yields a "limited scope" of possible approaches and interventions

(Cowen, Gardner, & Zax, 1967). On the other hand, certain features of the medical model, such as the public health aspects which deal with environmental causation and preventive intervention, have been perceived as compatible with an enlightened community mental health approach.

Rappaport believes that the second component—*the medical style of delivery*—has been overlooked. He characterizes this style as the *waiting-mode,* in which an "expert" or "authority" possessing an advanced academic degree passively waits for the clients to find him in his office. An alternative to the *waiting-mode* is the *seeking-mode,* which Rappaport (1977) describes in the following passage:

> A service offered in the seeking-mode generally takes place outside of the expert's office or hospital. It may be delivered directly by any number of persons, either professional or nonprofessional. The professional generally assumes the role of consultant, program innovator, and evaluator. . . . A neighborhood service center staffed by indigenous nonprofessionals is a good example of the seeking-mode. . . . Here the professional reaches out of his traditional setting into the community by training others to deliver service. The role of the non-professional is one of direct service agent to the target population (p. 73).

It is apparent from this description that the medical model is not generally compatible with this vision of service delivery. Yet, there is reason to believe that many of the formal underpinnings of the community mental health center programs are in support of a medical model. In his comprehensive overview study of the community mental health movement, Bloom (1977) notes that:

> A careful reading of the Community Mental Health Centers Act and regulations leads inevitably to the conclusion that the single most important professional involved in the provision of mental-health services is the physician and that one of the objectives of the act is to further the social policy of uniting mental-health with general-health services (p. 28).

As the reader will discover in the section on our proposed model, this strong emphasis on professional medical service is not consonant with a needs-based system.

Personal Education Model

In this system, the client's difficulties are attributed to deficient or unrealistic attitudes, perceptions, or behavioral skills. The role of the mental health center is to provide educational or other learning experiences to help the client gain adequate coping skills.

A wide assortment of educational approaches exists. These range from Gordon's (1970) Effectiveness Training programs and Simon's (1972) Values

Clarification approach, both of which are generally conducted by nonpsychiatric personnel to relatively well functioning individuals, to approaches such as Goldstein's (1975, 1976) Structured Learning Therapy, which utilizes mental health professionals and paraprofessionals to enable severely disabled individuals to learn basic coping skills.

In the context of a community mental health program, the personal education model offers the advantages of providing a broad and flexible array of services which build competence. The format gives the greatest potential for personal choice and minimizes side effects which stigmatize the client. The limitation of this model is that it places the major burden of change on the client without necessarily working toward fundamental reforms in the social systems of the community.

Community-Based Intervention and Support Model

Accompanying the development of community mental health centers was a concerted effort to decrease the number of persons institutionalized in large psychiatric hospitals. The rationale behind this policy of deinstitutionalization was that it would be both more humane and more effective to treat people within their own communities.

The practical difficulties of implementing the community-based intervention and support model are exemplified by the fact that the results of the long-term effort of this movement are mixed. Bloom (1977) points out that while the number of mental patients in residence decreased from 600,000 in 1955 to 216,000 in 1974, the number of admissions increased from 170,000 to more than 400,000 during approximately the same period (p. 24). In other words, while the absolute number of persons living in psychiatric institutions has been decreasing, the support systems of the community have not been able to maintain adequately these individuals in their natural settings.

Looking more closely at this issue, we find that approximately two-thirds of these admissions are readmissions (Lee, Note 1), and of those people who might be considered chronically disabled, up to 70% of them become rehospitalized during the 18-month period following their release (Fairweather, Sanders, & Tornatzky, 1974).

Why has the deinstitutionalization program not been more successful? The answer to this question is simple. As Sheets (Note 2) says, "to change the locus of a chronic disabled client from a state institution to a community environment is not enough" (p. 4). Sheets proposes the development of a community service system comprised of two essential elements. First, a support network, including social, vocational and residential supports, must be instituted within the community. Ironically, Sheets believes that the prototype for these supports may be found in the state hospital, which, despite its detrimental impact on many clients, often provides positive sources of security and refuge for the chronically disabled. The second, and more difficult, task is the development of replicable ways to enable chronically disabled persons to participate in the community in a manner that maximizes their own sense of value and self-satisfaction (Propst, 1974).

Many of the features of the Community Mental Health Centers Act and its amendments are derived from the community-based intervention and support model. The use of crisis intervention approaches, the development of outreach and day-care programs, and the provision of early identification and treatment services for children all represent efforts to maintain people who are experiencing psychological distress in their natural environments.

The community-based intervention and support model contributes several positive conceptual and practical features to the development of a comprehensive community mental health system. First, this model represents a significant change from those previously described. The role of the mental health worker is no longer primarily directed at changing the client; rather, the worker serves as a facilitator and provider of support, helping the client to find sources of stabilization, sustenance, and growth within his/her immediate community. This model seems to challenge the predominant American value system of putting the onus of change on the individual. The community-based model—which is essentially an *ecological approach*—argues that the development and provision of environmental supports may be as important to the achievement of mental health as the "bootstrap" approach which stresses the necessity of changing the identified client's behavior.

In a practical sense, this community support model is quite compatible with the paraprofessional concept. The role of mental health personnel is to help the client negotiate the obstacles and complexities faced in daily life. This assistance involves the functions of advocacy and support, and a general ability to make use of community resources. As Reiff and Riessman (1965) point out in their classical treatise on the indigenous nonprofessional and community mental health programs, these are the kinds of skills paraprofessionals are likely to possess by virtue of their social position, know-how, motivation, and life-styles. In fact, it might be argued that the cerebral, introspective style of many middle-class professionals would be detrimental to the performance of these tasks.

Prevention Model

In his essay on community psychiatry, Dumont (1971) suggests that, rather than focusing our attention on the individual as the target for our psychiatric ministration, we should consider the city to be our patient and channel our energies into creating social and structural changes that will enhance the mental health of this ailing organism.

Dumont's position (in spite of his medical analogy) represents the radical extreme on the prevention continuum. In Caplan's (1964) model, this would be considered *primary prevention*, the goal of which is "to ensure the adequate provision of supplies to members of a population and to help them deal constructively with their developmental and accidental crises [through] . . . social action and interpersonal action" (p. 56).

Primary prevention strategies are focused on population rather than on individuals; their aim is to reduce the rate of initial incidence of mental health problems in the community. A major primary prevention strategy involved helping individuals to turn potentially damaging life crises (e.g., starting one's first job) into springboards for change and growth. Caplan also speaks of *secondary prevention* (early detection and treatment) and *tertiary prevention* (reducing the rate of residual defect after the mental disorder has run its course), but as Bloom (1977) suggests, it might be more accurate and less confusing to refer to these interventions as *treatment* and *rehabilitation,* respectively.

Those who have attempted to implement the primary prevention model within a community mental health setting are painfully aware of the obstacles impeding these efforts. Not only do the pressing demands for crisis-oriented treatment and rehabilitation services absorb the lion's share of staff resources, but there is a reluctance to deviate from traditional clinical roles. These factors combined with the conservative attitude of the 1970s toward social action and institutional change make it next to impossible to mount an effective primary prevention program.

This does not mean that the primary prevention approach is not worthwhile, only that it is difficult to achieve. In fact, in the long-term perspective of the future, the primary prevention model holds the greatest promise for enhancing the mental health of our communities.

Many variations exist for implementing the prevention model. Within the framework of the community mental health centers' mandate, consultation and education services (indirect services) comprise the most popular vehicles for prevention. Staff members (professional and paraprofessional) may work with those individuals and entities that have a significant impact on the development and mental health of the community's citizens. The focus of their work is typically to enhance the individual's or organization's ability to understand and relate positively to people they serve, as well as to increase the consultee's awareness of other helpful resources. The Community Mental Health Centers Amendments of 1975 specify that centers wishing to receive funding need to provide consultation and education services to the following: health professionals, schools, courts, state and local law enforcement and correctional agencies, members of the clergy, public welfare agencies, health service delivery agencies, and other appropriate entities, New Section 201 (b) (1).

Activities that might be considered preventive efforts include: the development and support of special enrichment programs for children and other at-risk groups; community organization and other forms of direct community involvement directed at improving the quality of life; and attempts to develop alternative social institutions, such as alternative schools (Heller & Monahan,

1977).[1] Specific preventive programs might include: meaningful work experiences for adolescents; procedures for involving factory employees in the design of more rewarding work functions; and seminars on the use of leisure time for working adults who will soon retire.

THE COMPETENCE BUILDING-RESOURCE ENABLING MODEL: AN INTEGRATED NEEDS-BASED ECOLOGICAL APPROACH

The Rationale

A careful examination of the various models of mental health yields a simple, but critical, insight: *The definition of mental health and the accompanying model of service delivery one chooses is dependent on one's personal value system and set of vested interests.* Thus, an individual or group that believes in a strong hierarchy of authority and that stands to gain from maintaining the status quo would obviously prefer the social control model; while the party concerned about equalizing the distribution of power and resources would probably favor the primary prevention model, as espoused by Dumont (1971).

Having arrived at this conclusion, we can lay aside any illusions we may have had about the existence of a "true" definition of mental health or a "right" or "wrong" model of service delivery. The choice we make will be based on our personal belief system. Only the structural and mechanical elements of implementation and some of the outcomes for the individual and the community can be subject to empirical verification.

Our choice of the competence building-resource enabling model is based on six premises.[2]

1. A system that enables individuals to increase their intellectual, emotional, and behavioral options will ultimately benefit both the individual and the community.
2. A model based on the notion that the quality of the physical and interpersonal environment has a significant impact on the individual should provide channels and methods for upgrading the quality and accessibility of those environments.
3. In contrast to the traditional mental health system's obsession with deviance and pathology, an effective model should emphasize bolstering existing strengths and building competencies in individuals and groups.
4. Ultimately, it is not possible to resolve the issue of whether the individual or the social system should be exclusively attended to since they are inextricably intertwined and there are too many distressed individuals and impoverished social systems. Therefore, the model of choice should be comprehensive and flexible enough to provide attention to both individu-

als and social systems, with particular emphasis on their interactions and compatibilities.

5. Because human service agencies are so vulnerable to social and political influences, an adequate model should utilize concepts and ideas that address the basic personal and environmental sources involved in the fulfillment and curtailment of human potential. The language of the model should be fundamental and functional so as to minimize arbitrary alteration of the resultant service system. For example, the basic supplies and skills required for positive self-esteem and functioning need to be identified and described. A great deal of human and financial resources is wasted when governmental agencies switch their emphasis from one popular concern (e.g., narcotics addictions) to another symptomatic problem that has captured the public's interest (e.g., alcoholism). Vast organizational and programmatic changes are made to accommodate to the new "crisis," even though the root causes, fundamental needs, and essential resolutions may actually be the same for both problems.

6. The ecological perspective takes into account the complex interactions and influences that affect both individuals and their communities. According to the ecological approach, one cannot understand and assist an individual apart from the many environmental forces that have an impact on that person. In subscribing to this approach, it is necessary to select concepts that are capable of generating a comprehensive array of interventions and supports. The concepts that most adequately meet these criteria are: (a) identification and assessment of needs; (b) identification, procurement, and development of appropriate resources; (c) enhancement and development of competencies; and (d) creation and utilization of social and service networks, both for consumers and the agencies serving them.

Basic Conceptual Elements

In its simple form, the *competence building–resource enabling model* may be conceptualized in the following manner.

1. People grow and develop positively when their basic needs are being met. The fulfillment of these needs—which include biological, psychological, spiritual, and social needs—requires a variety of supplies and resources (physical and nonphysical).

2. This fulfillment of needs is dependent on two conditions: the availability and accessibility of resources, and the ability to acquire and utilize these resources. Positive mental health may be defined as the favorable existence of both these conditions. A mentally healthy community would be one that provided the necessary resources for all of its citizens and enabled the members of the community to develop the skills needed to utilize these resources.

3. Persons whose needs are not met are likely to experience frustrations, distress, and an inability to cope well with the demands of their environment. The consequences of this lack of need fulfillment are a loss of functional ability, a diminished sense of self-esteem, and an attitude of demoralization and helplessness. These three conditions have an interactive effect on each other. When one attribute is strengthened, the other two are also likely to be affected positively, and vice versa. For example, if a person learns a new social skill, the use of that skill will satisfy a social need. At the same time, the successful application of this skill will probably bolster the individual's self-esteem and sense of personal power. This increase in confidence will, in turn, make it easier for the person to confront new social situations. This snowball effect may work in reverse if social needs cannot be met due to a lack of ability or opportunity.

4. Within this needs-based framework, the job of the community mental health system is to (a) assess the degree to which needs are being met on an individual and community-wide basis; (b) identify and develop resources (including supplies, settings, supports, and outlets) appropriate to the unmet needs, and work to increase the accessibility of these resources to those who do not have access to them; (c) assist and support those individuals who do not have the skills necessary to successfully pursue these resources; and (d) work to increase the level of tolerance and acceptance of the community toward those who have already suffered because of the long-standing inaccessibility of resources to them.

Implications of This Model for a Community Mental Health Service System

How do we operationalize the four functions of the competence building model listed above? What are the implications of this approach for community mental health centers or for other agencies that might adopt this model? Let us answer these questions by briefly examining these four functions (indicated by the four subheadings that follow).

Assessing the Degree to Which Needs Are Being Met on an Individual or Community Basis. The first task is to establish what the needs are and to devise appropriate methods to measure where these needs are being fulfilled.

In his recent book on the biosocial approach to persons in distress, Hansell (1975) presents an interesting variation on the needs-resources issue. He describes seven essential attachments necessary for the survival of an individual. These attachments provide a useful framework for those wishing to identify the elements required to maintain a basic level of functioning.

1. Food, oxygen, and information of requisite variety; biochemical and informational supplies.

2. A clear concept of a self-identity, held with conviction.
3. Persons, at least one, in persisting, interdependent contact, occasionally approaching intimacy.
4. Groups, at least one, comprised of individuals who regard this person as a member.
5. Roles, at least one, which offer a context for achieving dignity and self-esteem through performance.
6. Money or purchasing power to participate in an exchange of goods and services in a society specialized for such exchanges.
7. A comprehensive system of meaning, a satisfying set of notions which clarify experience and define ambiguous events (p. 33).

Maslow (1970) spoke of a hierarchy of needs, with the basic biological needs requiring adequate attention before a person is able to strive toward higher level, self-actualization needs. Put in this context, it is easy to understand why severely distressed individuals have found little solace or assistance in the more abstract forms of psychological therapy. The needs-based model, taking into consideration these fundamental human requirements, obviously seeks a revision of traditional mental health assessment approaches. First, the esoteric pathology-seeking diagnostic instruments would be discarded in favor of more functional indices measuring competence and the availability of support systems. Second, the exclusive focus on assessing the individual in a clinical setting would be replaced by an emphasis on studying behavior in natural settings and assessing needs and resources on a community-wide basis.

For example, the observation that a group of school children was experiencing problems, such as social isolation or academic failure, might lead to an assessment of community resources which could provide help to enhance the children's self-esteem, social interactions, and academic achievement. Finally, implementation of this system of assessment would not be limited to a small group of highly trained professionals. Instead, it would make use of people who were familiar with the workings of the community and the functioning of its residents—an ideal task for the indigenous paraprofessional (Reiff & Riessman, 1965).

Identifying and Developing Appropriate Resources and Working to Increase the Accessibility of These Resources to Those Who Do Not Have Access to Them. A decade ago, proponents of upgrading mental health services began most discussions with a plea for spending more money. However, recent experiences with economic decline and energy crises have heightened our awareness of the problem of limited resources. Today, although the need for additional funding is still recognized, pleas for improvement and reform are generally couched in terms of making better use of *existing resources*. Within the framework of the proposed model, improved utilization of current resources may take several forms.

First, good working relationships must be developed between the mental health center and the agencies and groups which are able to provide basic resources related to biological, social, vocational, educational, residential, and other self-care needs. It would be presumptuous and inefficient for a mental health center to attempt to provide all these services. However, a holistic approach recognizes that it is neither desirable nor effective to view these needs as separate and unrelated. An effective *human services* program—and that is really what is being proposed—requires coordination and integration of all services on a practical level. Some examples of resource identification are: (a) identifying supportive, nonstigmatizing sources of shelter for those who do not have access to existing home environments; (b) finding suitable sources of preparation and employment for those who need purposeful activity which will provide social and economic reinforcement, as well as a sense of personal accomplishment and esteem; (c) creating or helping to create alternative settings to provide for unmet needs (e.g., neighborhood centers, social clubs, group homes, child care centers); (d) assisting established settings to provide better psychological nurturance and support (e.g., school consultation); (e) engaging in the collection and dissemination of information on where and how basic goods and services can be found, on the assumption that knowledge is an important component of personal power—possession of this information should help community residents to feel that they can control their own lives; (f) identifying and collaborating with people who serve either formally or informally as community leaders for the purpose of finding additional sources of physical and social support; and (g) identifying and using, in a creative way, the resources of community members who wish to become engaged in supportive interpersonal relationships; foster grandparents, big brothers and sisters, and paraprofessional advocates represent but a few examples in this area.

Paraprofessionals familiar with the community are well suited for creating good working relationships between the mental health center and individual community agencies, groups, and leaders. For example, consultation and education service paraprofessionals can conduct a survey to create a service referral directory for use by mental health center personnel from all of the 12 service areas now required of community mental health centers by 1975 federal legislation (Public Law 94–63). While conducting the survey, the paraprofessionals can describe the mental health center to the community professionals and nonprofessionals with whom they come into contact. Through a similar process, consultation and education paraprofessionals can also gather together a list of names of community people who are willing to help create new services (e.g., cooperative housing for discharged state hospital patients) that can fill unmet community needs.[3]

Second, a service delivery system must be developed which emphasizes the full use and development of all available community resources as well as the traditional clinical contact. Most people in the mental health field have acknowledged that no single agency has the capability of providing directly for all client needs. To put this concept into practice requires a major revamping of the mental health delivery system. Mental health personnel need to become active seekers of resources and developers of social networks. While the mental health centers would continue to provide certain specialized services and resources (e.g., crisis support, social skills training), the staff would devote much of its energy to expediting and advocating attention and collaboration with other agencies on behalf of mental health consumers. A notable example of this service mode is the Bridge Program in Syracuse, New York, which utilizes family advocates to help families with troubled children make use of appropriate resources and supports (Apter, in press).

A further example is provided by paraprofessionals from the consultation and education program at the Dr. Solomon Carter Fuller Community Mental Health Center in Boston, Massachusetts (Alley, Blanton, Feldman, Hunter, & Rolfson, 1979). Paraprofessionals and professional staff members from the program serve on the boards of health agencies that serve the catchment area. These affiliations have enabled the staff members to organize a health task force for non-English-speaking minorities. Its membership includes both health care providers and the non-English-speaking consumers of health services.

Third, in conjunction with the professional staff members, personnel who are capable and willing to serve as active problem solvers must be employed. There is a strong need for workers who directly assist clients in planning and organizing daily activities such as household budgeting and job seeking. Using this type of worker will significantly increase the scope of the agency, both in terms of the amount of resources provided and the number of consumers served. Recent overview studies have reported that many paraprofessionals are particularly suited for this active problem-solving role (Cohen, 1976; Gartner, 1971; Social and Rehabilitation Service, 1974).

Paraprofessionals serve as active problem solvers in the Hillsborough Community Mental Health Center aging program in Tampa, Florida (Alley et al., 1979). The paraprofessionals make the initial evaluations of the clients' needs. Then they assist the clients in taking care of these needs so that the clients can become autonomous. The assistance from the paraprofessionals can involve physical touching, such as hand-holding or hugging, and is a way of relating that is uncommon between professionals and clients. The paraprofessionals make home and community visits to help clients learn skills such as those involved in balancing checkbooks, making shopping lists, writing letters, buying eyeglasses, securing food stamps, or establishing proper nutritional habits. The paraprofessionals supplement these direct services to individual clients by leading or coleading insight therapy, support, and activity groups. Furthermore, through consultation and education activities, the paraprofessionals teach their clinical and social intervention skills to the staff members of nursing homes, retirement centers, and hospitals.

Assisting and Supporting Those Individuals Who Do Not Have the Skills to Pursue These Resources Successfully.   While the primary thrust of the competence building-resource enabling model is to restructure the environment in order to enhance the availability of resources, we need to acknowledge that some of these changes will take considerable time. Besides, there are some people whose competence level is so low as to make it difficult for them to meet even their basic needs (e.g., nutrition, shelter). For these reasons, it is necessary for a community mental health center to facilitate the direct provision of competence building services to individual consumers.

The manner in which these services are delivered is critical. If the client is seen as a deviant individual *who must learn to adjust,* we have returned to the social control position of "blaming the victim" (Ryan, 1971), carrying with it the implied notion of "changing the victim." On the other hand, it is possible to offer consumers of mental health services the opportunity to increase their affective and behavioral alternatives without infringing upon their personal rights.

To assure appropriate and effective provision of mental health services to those in need, it is first necessary to develop an adequate system of delivery (National Institute of Mental Health, 1976). One of the systems that seems well suited for this purpose is the Balanced Service System[4] (Gerhard & Dorgan, 1976; Miles & Gerhard, 1972) originally developed within the New York State Department of Mental Hygiene. The Balanced Service System (which the Joint Commission on Accreditation of Hospitals used as its basic source for generating the principles, indicators, and standards for the accreditation of community mental health centers [Joint Commission on Accreditation of Hospitals, 1976]) is a comprehensive functional approach that relies on a case management process to provide continuity of services. Under this system, case managers work to link mental health consumers with a service system offering services in such areas as crisis stabilization, growth, and sustenance. The case manager—who might well be a paraprofessional—facilitates the relationship between the consumer and other significant entities, including all internal and external services, as well as the consumer's folk-support system. The case manager has "the primary responsibility for assuring the assessment, planning, linking, monitoring of, and advocacy for, consumers in response to their changing needs" (Gerhard & Dorgan, 1976, pp. 21–22).

Beyond providing a systematic method for organizing and coordinating services and a responsive mechanism for guiding clients through this system, a community mental health center needs to make available functional resources to enable clients to develop critical skills. It is in the area of competence-building that the utility of the *personal education* and *community intervention and support* models becomes apparent. Whether through the use of behavioral procedures (Nietzel, Winett, MacDonald, & Davidson, 1977), humanistic approaches (Rogers, 1977), or formal social support systems (e.g., Fountain House in New York, New York), it is crucial for mental health consumers to be given an opportunity to participate in experiences that will enhance their personal, social, and vocational skills.

Paraprofessionals act as case managers in the Cambridge-Somerville

Mental Health and Retardation Center aftercare program in Cambridge, Massachusetts (Alley et al., 1979). In that program paraprofessionals remain as primary care givers with clients as long as the clients need assistance. Prior to their discharge from the state hospitals, patients are helped by their paraprofessional case manager to assess their own needs. In addition, before clients leave the hospital, the paraprofessionals take them on community visits for familiarization with grocery shopping, choice of housing, and other matters important in community transition. After clients are discharged, the paraprofessionals help them in many matters, including disputes with welfare or landlords, arrangement for placement in a vocational rehabilitation program, and consultation with personnel of a community day-care facility attended by the client. In several instances, the paraprofessionals have created new programs (e.g., a loan fund for discharged patients) to fill needs otherwise unmet by existing resources.

Working to Increase the Level of Tolerance and Acceptance by the Community. One further task remains for community mental health centers. It is fine to restructure resource systems and enhance individual competence. However, if we are concerned with developing mentally healthy communities, and if we wish to integrate people who have long-standing histories of inaccessibility to critical resources into the mainstream of community life, then we must make a concerted effort to increase the tolerance and acceptance of the many citizens and institutions who resist this movement. Only through a program of education, exposure, and—it is hoped—productive involvement with people who have special needs, will the fear and misunderstanding of the established community be diminished.

In the Rutgers, New Jersey, day-care-transitional-aftercare program (Alley et al., 1979), paraprofessionals have helped to increase acceptance by the business community of discharged state hospital patients. The potential employer trains a paraprofessional to do the job. Subsequently, the paraprofessional takes responsibility for training all future discharged patients who occupy the position. Job coverage is guaranteed, for the paraprofessional will fill in whenever a discharged patient is unable to work.

Paraprofessionals and the Competence Building–Resource Enabling Model

While the other chapters in this source book provide numerous examples and considerable evidence of the functional contributions paraprofessionals have been making in the delivery of community mental health services, there is a need to place the role of paraprofessionals in an appropriate context.

The changing concepts of mental health and mental health services have resulted in several modifications of the traditional perception of the problems of mental health. First, there is an increasing tendency to view mental health as a complex social issue, subject to the influence of political and cultural values, rather than one of precise medical determination or intrapsychic adequacy. This change has served to remove the problem of mental health from the realm of absolute truth and bring it into the arena of social judgment based on relative values and standards of human behavior. In turn, the focus of attention has moved toward an assessment of social conditions that affect behavior and the compatibility of the individual with a particular environment, since we can no longer be assured that the problem rests with the individual whose behavior is in question.

In accordance with these altered perceptions, new models of mental health service delivery have evolved along with modified roles for mental health workers. If one does a brief task analysis of the model being proposed in this chapter (Wiley & Fine, 1969), it soon becomes evident that the functions required to implement this model are, in many ways, different from those of traditional mental health models. A good working knowledge of the community and its resources is essential. An ability to negotiate actively with the institutions and social networks that affect the consumer is critical. Effective linkages need to be established among the mental health center, the consumers of service, and various other human service agencies. An active, practical, problem-solving orientation must prevail. And, finally, good rapport must be established with consumers in order to ensure an ongoing relationship of mutual trust and respect.

To describe these attributes as being compatible with the working style of the paraprofessional would be to underestimate the significance of this relationship. These attributes represent the basic qualities that formed the rationale for *creating* the paraprofessional program. They constitute the essential assets that well prepared paraprofessionals bring to the job.

Thus, it may be said that the competence building–resource enabling system of mental health service not only would benefit from the utilization of paraprofessionals, but that the *foundation of this approach is based on the notion of employing paraprofessional workers, and its success is dependent upon their effective participation.*

Additional Issues and Problems

Having described the rationale, theory, and methods of the competence building–resource enabling model, there remains the task of identifying the major issues and problems related to putting this system into practice.[5] Space limitations do not permit an extensive analysis. However, a brief listing of the basic factors and forces that need to be considered will be presented.

1. Any effort to move toward a functional needs-based system of mental health services must take into account the intense resistance that may come from those who have a strong, vested interest in the traditional

model of service. The issue is broader than simply introducing a new type of worker (i.e., paraprofessional) into the system; it also involves making fundamental, substantive changes in the way mental health services are conceptualized and delivered.

2. The development of a client-responsive system is difficult. It not only requires a sophisticated understanding of community needs and resources but also demands a great deal of flexibility and cooperation among the staff, as well as an agency operation that is well planned and efficiently organized.

3. By definition, the proposed needs-based model requires community mental health centers to establish numerous linkages and networks with formal and informal groups and sectors of the community. The barriers impeding coordination of human services are formidable, and the skills needed to overcome these barriers are complex and not easily acquired (Aiken, Dewar, DiTomaso, Hage, & Zeitz, 1975).

4. The problems of establishing an effective system are not made any easier by the fact that in any one community a myriad of private, city, county, state, and federal agencies may be involved in the delivery of mental health and other human services. Issues of territoriality and jurisdiction, with their accompanying problems of funding competition and bureaucratic bickering, drain off valuable time and energy that could be better spent on the delivery of service.

5. Related to the issue of jurisdiction is the problem of governance and accountability. With its emphasis on citizen participation, the community mental health program needs to develop effective ways to obtain meaningful community input. This requires not only reasonable mechanisms for representative governance, but also an intensive program of citizen education to ensure enlightened participation and decision making.

6. Finally, there are the inevitable, non-service-related obstacles that play such an important role in the formation and maintenance of a human service program. We should not underestimate the impact of factors such as the state of the economy, the prevailing political orientation (both locally and nationally), the existing social climate, and the willingness of the community to accept a mental health system that no longer serves as a vehicle for removing "deviant" persons from the community, but insists on providing community-based services.

CONCLUSION

The competence building–resource enabling model is ambitious in intent, complex in design, and radical in its departure from traditional modes of mental health service delivery. The notion of a needs-based approach that places responsibility for adaptation and change on the structures and systems of the community, rather than on the individual client, represents a major revision in orientation. Effective implementation of this model will require appropriately trained paraprofessionals, but effective implementation of this approach will not come easily. There are formidable obstacles, both of a technical and human nature.

But the potential payoff is considerable. This approach holds the promise of enhancing personal and community competencies as well as diminishing suffering, distress, and the sense of helplessness. The needs-based system facilitates the return and integration of people with special needs into the natural environment of their home community. It may help to reduce the deep-rooted stigma that has been attached to mental health problems. The model is comprehensive enough to encompass all of the basic needs and skills involved in effective functioning as well as broad enough to incorporate the positive features of the other mental health approaches described in the beginning of this chapter.

And, finally, the competence building–resource enabling model provides an appropriate vehicle for transforming the community mental health center from a quasi-traditional agency, providing a limited range of mental health services to individuals *in the community,* to an authentic human service system concerned about and involved in enhancing the mental health *of the community.*

NOTES

[1] Interestingly, Heller and Monahan also consider the New Careers program to be an alternative to existing institutional arrangements (1977, p. 306).

[2] The ideas and concepts listed come from many sources, including personal experience. Some of the most influential scholarly sources have been Bloom (1977), Caplan (1964), Cowen, Gardner, and Zax (1967), Dumont (1971), Gerhard and Dorgan (1976), Heller and Monahan (1977), Pearl and Riessman (1965), Rappaport (1977), Reiff and Riessman (1965), Sarason (1974, 1976), Sarason, Levine, Goldenberg, Cherlin, and Bennett (1966), and Sheets (Note 2).

[3] Karen Signell describes the use of volunteers in community mental health centers in Chapter 13.

[4] Richard Dorgan and Ronald Gerhard describe relevant ideas in detail in Chapter 5.

[5] Louis Tornatzky describes the role of the indigenous change agent in Chapter 7.

REFERENCE NOTES

1. M. Lee, *Readmission and the community mental health center.* Unpublished report, Research Department of the Hutchings Psychiatric Center, Syracuse, N.Y., 1973.
2. J. Sheets, *The fourth revolution in psychiatry: Community chronic care.* Unpublished master's thesis, University of North Carolina, 1977.

REFERENCES

Aiken, M., Dewar, R., DiTomaso, N., Hage, J., & Zeitz, G. *Coordinating human services.* San Francisco: Jossey-Bass Publishers, 1975.

Alley, S. R., Blanton, J., Feldman, R. E., Hunter, G. D., & Rolfson, M. *Case studies of mental health paraprofessionals: Twelve effective programs.* New York: Human Sciences Press, 1979.

Apter, D. Getting it together at camp and beyond. *Innovations.* Palo Alto, Calif.: American Institutes for Research, in press.

Bloom, B. L. *Community mental health: A general introduction.* Monterey, Calif.: Brooks/Cole, 1977.

Caplan, G. *Principles of preventive psychiatry.* New York: Basic Books, 1964.

Cohen, R. *"New Careers" grows older: A perspective on the paraprofessional experience, 1965–1975.* Baltimore: The Johns Hopkins University Press, 1976.

Cowen, E. L., Gardner, E. A., & Zax, M. *Emergent approaches to mental health problems.* New York: Appleton-Century-Crofts, 1967.

Dumont, M. P. *The absurd healer.* New York: Viking Press, 1971.

Fairweather, G. W., Sanders, D. H., & Tornatzky, L. G. *Creating change in mental health organizations.* New York: Pergamon Press, 1974.

Gartner, A. *Paraprofessionals and their performance: A survey of education, health and social service programs.* New York: Praeger, 1971.

Gerhard, R., & Dorgan, R. E. *The balanced service system.* Albany, N.Y.: New York State Department of Mental Hygiene, 1976.

Goldstein, A. P. *Structured learning therapy: Toward a psychotherapy for the poor.* New York: Academic Press, 1975.

Goldstein, A. P., Sprafkin, R. P., & Gershaw, N. J. *Still training for community living: Applying structured learning therapy.* New York: Pergamon Press, 1976.

Gordon, T. *Parent effectiveness training: The no-lose system for raising responsible children.* New York: Peter Wyden, 1970.

Hansell, N. *The person-in-distress: On the biosocial dynamics of adaptation.* New York: Human Sciences Press, 1975.

Heller, K., & Monahan, J. *Psychology and community change.* Homewood, Ill.: Dorsey Press, 1977.

Joint Commission on Accreditation of Hospitals, Accreditation Council for Psychiatric Facilities. *Principles for accreditation of community mental health service programs.* Chicago, 1976.

Levinson, D. J., & Gallagher, E. B. *Patienthood in the hospital: An analysis of role, personality and social structure.* Boston: Houghton Mifflin Company, 1964.

Maslow, A. H. *Motivation and personality* (2nd ed.). New York: Harper and Row, 1970.

Miles, D., & Gerhard, R. *The balanced service system.* Albany, N.Y.: New York State Department of Mental Hygiene, 1972.

National Institute of Mental Health. *A client-oriented system of mental health service delivery and program management: A workbook and guide.* Washington, D.C.: Department of Health, Education, and Welfare, 1976.

Nietzel, M. T., Winett, R. A., MacDonald, M. L., & Davidson, W. S. *Behavioral approaches to community psychology.* New York: Pergamon Press, 1977.

Pearl, A., & Riessman, F. *New careers for the poor: The nonprofessional in human service.* New York: The Free Press, 1965.

Propst, R. N. Creating alternatives for optimal residential care in the community. In *Creating the community alternative: Opinions and innovations: Proceedings of Horizon House state-wide conference.* Hershey, Pa.: Horizon House, 1974.

Rappaport, J. *Community psychology: Values, research and action.* New York: Holt, Rinehart and Winston, 1977.

Reiff, R., & Riessman, F. The indigenous nonprofessional: A strategy of change in community action and community mental health programs. *Community Mental Health Journal Monograph,* 1965, No. 1, 3032.

Rogers, C. *Carl Rogers on personal power.* New York: Delacorte Press, 1977.

Ryan, W. *Blaming the victim.* New York: Random House, 1971.

Sarason, S. B. *The psychological sense of community: Prospects for a community psychology.* San Francisco: Jossey-Bass, 1974.

Sarason, S. B. Community psychology, networks and Mr. Everyman. *American Psychologist,* 1976, *31,* 317–328.

Sarason, S. B., Levine, M., Goldenberg, I. I., Cherlin, D. L., & Bennett, E. M. *Psychology in community settings: Clinical, educational, vocational, social aspects.* New York: John Wiley and sons, 1966.

Silverstein, H. (Ed.). *The social control of mental illness.* New York: Thomas Y. Crowell Company, 1968.

Simon, S. B., Howe, L. W., & Kirschenbaum, H. *Values clarification: A handbook of practical strategies for teachers and students.* New York: Hart Publishing, 1972.

Social and Rehabilitation Service. *National study of social welfare and rehabilitation workers, work and organizational context: Overview study of employment of paraprofessionals (Research Project No. 3).* Washington, D.C.: Department of Health, Education, and Welfare, 1974.

Szasz, T. S. The myth of mental illness. *American Psychologist,* 1960, *15,* 113–118.

Wiley, W. W., & Fine, S. A. *A systems approach to new careers: Two papers.* Kalamazoo, Mich.: W. E. Upjohn Institute for Employment Research, 1969.

Appendix   Analysis of Mental Health Service Delivery Models

Models	Who delivers	What services/where offered
Social control	Mental health workers—professional and paraprofessional, often in conjunction with representatives of judicial system	Removal from natural community (partially or totally); segregation; intense observation and supervision; constraint; modification of "deviant" behavior to acceptable standards; social regulation; generally delivered in a total institution or highly regulated setting
Medical disease	Professional mental health workers—frequently with medical orientation—with paraprofessionals sometimes assisting in a "handmaiden" fashion	Treatment of disease through some form of psychotherapy or chemotherapy; generally provided in an institutional setting
Personal education	Mental health worker as educator; other significant individuals who have been trained (e.g. clergy, parents, teachers)	Educational experience dealing with behavior, feelings and/or attitudes; may be delivered in a variety of settings, including mental health centers, schools, homes, churches, etc.
Community-based intervention and support	Mental health workers as facilitators and providers of support, reliance on paraprofessionals	Guidance, advocacy, support and assistance in finding sources of stabilization, sustenance and growth; provision of environmental supports; some service delivered at mental health center, but most provided in community settings
Prevention	Mental health professionals and paraprofessionals, as well as many not directly associated with mental health (e.g. parents, educators, politicians)	Alteration of the style and substance of social systems that have a significant impact on people; provided through the community

Competence building—resource enabling model: see pp. 226–227.

To whom	Toward what purpose	For whose benefit
Identified clients who exhibit bizarre or "deviant" behavior; people displaying disruptive or violent behavior, as well as those seen as inclined in this direction; people viewed as not able to take care of themselves or capable of harming themselves	Reduce the frequency of "deviant" behavior within natural community; change behavior of maladjusted individuals	Protect those who might be threatened by the behavior of the client; protect the community, supposedly on behalf of the client, but not usually with client's consent
Individual clients (or patients) who report or display distress or dysfunction	Relieve symptoms and distress; alleviate inner conflicts and stresses	The identified client or significant other making referral (e.g. child's parent); the medical establishment
Consumers, clients and individuals who voluntarily initiate contact with educational services	To increase the number of intellectual, emotional and behavioral options available to the individuals	Primarily for the consumer; indirectly for the community and society
Individuals and families in crisis; chronically disabled persons, including those who have been institutionalized for lengthy periods	To maintain people with special needs in their natural environment or in community settings that closely approximate these environments (e.g. group homes); "normalization"; develop coping skills; to provide self-esteem, bolstering experiences	People with special needs; those persons who benefit from associating with people with special needs
Formal and informal social entities, structures and systems, and the individuals responsible for their functioning (e.g. schools, work place, families, social groups)	To increase the availability of social, psychological, educational and economic resources to *all* people of the community	Individuals living in the community; the community-at-large due to enhanced quality of life and reduced number of problems and disabilities putting a strain on community's limited resources

Models	Who delivers	What services/where offered
Competence building–resource enabling	Mental health professionals, and paraprofessionals; other human service workers; interested citizens	Assess the degree to which needs are being met on an individual and community-wide basis; identify and develop resources appropriate to the unmet needs, and work to increase the accessibility; assist and support those individuals who do not have the skills necessary successfully to pursue these resources; work to increase the level of tolerance and acceptance by the community toward those who lacked accessibility to resources; borrow and integrate the positive aspects and services from other models provided in all sectors and settings of the community where significant resources are available

To whom	Toward what purpose	For whose benefit
Formal and informal social networks and systems; people with special needs; other citizens of the community	To fulfill individual and community needs and improve the quality of life by increasing the availability and accessibility of resources, as well as enhancing the competence and ability of people to acquire and utilize these resources	The community; groups and systems within the community; mental health consumers and citizens whose access to resources has been enhanced

THE COMMUNITY MENTAL HEALTH WORKER: THE ROLE AND FUNCTION OF INDIGENOUS PARAPROFESSIONALS IN A COMPREHENSIVE COMMUNITY MENTAL HEALTH CENTER

Mark Tarail, DSW*

This chapter describes a comprehensive community mental health center in which paraprofessionals play a broad set of key roles and make it possible for the center to offer services consistent with its guiding principles. The particular center, the Maimonides Community Mental Health Center, is located in New York City and serves an ethnically heterogeneous population.

All paraprofessionals and nonprofessionals at Maimonides are indigenous to and must be recruited from the catchment area population and, thus, can serve as representatives of the clients and the community. In addition, these staff members participate in a diverse set of activities including: outreach work, community organization, primary prevention, and clinical intervention. A career development program includes many safeguards against the confining of paraprofessionals at the bottom of the career ladder. The chapter includes sections on funding issues and on the special problems that arise when a mental health center employs indigenous paraprofessionals in positions of considerable responsibility.

*Dr. Tarail is Director of Maimonides Community Mental Health Center of Brooklyn, Director of the Department of Community Medicine and Community Health Services at the Maimonides Medical Center, Professor of Community Mental Health Practice at New York University, and Clinical Associate Professor of Psychiatry at Downstate Medical Center, State University of New York.

places an emphasis on the provision of a full spectrum of services and programs aimed at the maintenance of mental health and the prevention of illness. Such programs as community mental health education, rehabilitation and social restoration services are offered to all individuals and families and to other larger social agencies in the service area.

3. The community mental health center provides services at the places in the community where the need for those services arises. The experience of many mental health centers has demonstrated that the fundamental arena of services and care for the mentally ill is frequently not the therapist's office or the hospital, but rather the community itself. The given problem may originate in the community, the home, the social organization, the public and parochial school, or the church. Problems may be found in the trade union hall, the neighborhood, or even in the street. The staff members of a community mental health center do not wait for the problem to come to them; rather they go to the people needing services by providing help directly on their own turf. It is also important that programs involving preventive, educational, community training and consultation services, as well as those involving the maintenance of mental health, frequently take place out of the center building and its offices, and are provided within the community, in its homes and in its institutions. Even the direct, clinical diagnostic and treatment services are often more effective and more accessible when they are decentralized, at least in part, and through satellite clinics, housed in neighborhood storefronts or other nontraditional settings in different parts of the catchment area.

4. Services in a community mental health center should be designed to meet the specific needs and priorities of the clients and the community served. All service programs, the modalities of care and treatment, and the organizational modes and forms should reflect the unique needs of these particular patients and clients, as well as the priorities and needs of the community within the catchment area. In traditional health facilities, especially in psychiatry and mental health, patients and programs often are squeezed into limited, preconceived and prestructured settings and modalities which have been determined by the needs of the organization rather than by the primary needs of the patient and client population.

5. It is also the common experience that almost every catchment area contains a number of different, specialized subcultures. The local heterogeneous population often has within it different racial, national, religious, and class groups, as well as the usual grouping by age and sex. The community mental health center model is characterized by its efforts to serve the differing mental health needs of these various subgroups, especially those of the minority, racial, ethnic, and class groups, and to serve them in ways which are indigenous to these groups and reflect their different characteristics.

6. The people who are served have the right to determine the nature and priorities of the services offered by the community mental health center,

The comprehensive community mental health center, probably more signifi
cantly than any other type of psychiatric or mental health facility, has provide
a setting which demonstrates the effectiveness of using substantial numbers o
paraprofessionals in the direct provision of mental health care. The principle
and concepts fundamental to the development of a community mental health
center have made possible this extensive use of indigenous paraprofessionals
in a wide variety of roles and functions. This chapter will present some of these
basic principles and discuss some of the problems, solutions, and strategies
involved in the use of this indigenous group of mental health workers.

These special concerns include the recruitment and selection, roles and
functions, and the career development of the paraprofessionals themselves.
Other concerns are the funding problem and those issues, both internal and
external, inherent in the field, which affect a center's ability to use and train
the indigenous paraprofessional workers.

The content of this presentation is, in the main, based on the rich experience of the Maimonides Community Mental Health Center of Brooklyn during
its eleven years of existence, as well as the author's observation and knowledge
of the experiences of a number of other mental health centers.

Some Working Principles Underlying the Operation of Programs at the Maimonides Community Mental Health Center

The Maimonides Community Mental Health Center, in its organization, development and operation, reflects a philosophy and an innovative service system
based on a number of fundamental principles. Some of these principles are
fundamental to a policy which has resulted in the effective use of paraprofessionals in a wide range of mental health programs.

1. Services must be available and accessible to all who need them. The
   community mental health center model represents the first incidence in the
   history of health services in this country in which mental health services
   are provided to all individuals and families as a *right* and not as a privilege.
   This principle is safeguarded by federal law. Thus, the mental health
   center must make its services accessible to all individuals and to all families residing in a given catchment area regardless of their ability to pay,
   their age, sex, race, religion, ethnicity or national origin, their diagnostic
   category, or the severity of their illness.
2. Maintenance of good mental health and the prevention of illness are part
   of the responsibility of the community mental health center. Most so-
   called mental "health" facilities are really illness agencies; they are preoc-
   cupied almost exclusively with diagnostic and treatment services for the
   mentally ill. The community mental health center, on the other hand,
   while providing diagnostic and treatment services to those who are ill, also

and the center must recognize the participation of the community as essential to the achievement of its objectives. The development of formal channels for this kind of active involvement of service consumers and community leaders in the center has been an important contribution to the field. Indigenous community involvement is relatively new in this country in the health field, and particularly in mental health. The concept and the practice tend to be threatening to administrators and to professional workers in traditional facilities. There are many models for community participation, from the token advisory board to the direct governing board structure. This principle of community and consumer involvement in policy decision making, budgeting, evaluation, political action on behalf of the center, funding, etc. through formal channels of participation and authority currently is built into the present federal law which mandates and funds community mental health centers, namely, P.L. 94–63. For a detailed description of the various models, objectives and methods of community participation, the reader is referred to Tarail, 1972 (Note 1).

A concomitant principle is that every mental health center needs the support and advocacy of its local community in order to survive and develop. The experience of the Maimonides Mental Health Center, and other similar facilities, demonstrates that this support will be granted to the center by the community only if the center's administration and its staff can present themselves as advocates of the people's needs, and demonstrate this position not only in words, but in deeds. Thus, in most effective centers a system of mutual advocacy has developed between the community, the consumers, and the service providers.

7. Experience in many mental health centers has demonstrated that most persons seeking help and treatment have social and biomedical, as well as emotional and psychological problems. This situation is especially true of poor, working class and lower middle class populations. Since the mental health problems of individuals and families are influenced by and related to biopsychosocial factors, therapeutic service should provide comprehensive biopsychosocial models of intervention. This holistic approach, treating the whole human being, is a principle which underlies the diagnostic and treatment services in a mental health center.

Additional principles and concepts underlie the goals, development and operation of a mental health center. For a more detailed description of these concepts, the reader is referred to Tarail (1977).

ROLES AND FUNCTIONS OF INDIGENOUS PARAPROFESSIONALS

These principles which have guided the development and organization of the programs undertaken at Maimonides Community Mental Health Center may also be seen as the foundation of the very effective and widespread use of paraprofessionals in the Center's operation. The roles they maintain and their function as part of the mental health field are varied and extensive.

In a number of mental health centers, including the Maimonides Center, substantial groups of indigenous paraprofessionals work with and beside trained mental health professionals; such as, psychiatrists, social workers, psychologists, nurses, and special educators. In the Maimonides Community Mental Health Center over 40% of the total salaried staff are paraprofessionals and nonprofessionals.[1] As a matter of administrative policy, all paraprofessionals and nonprofessionals are indigenous to and must be recruited from the local catchment area population.

The paraprofessionals, classified as community mental health workers at Maimonides, are essential to the mental health center's ability to implement its objectives and mandates. They perform vital roles and functions which are different from and supplementary to the work and tasks of the trained professionals. These roles include the following.

Representatives of the Clients and the Community

The indigenous paraprofessionals not only enhance the immediacy, the identification and the effectiveness of the services offered to the local client, but also are valuable assets to the nonindigenous professional. They bring knowledge and insight about the needs of the local community, and the special needs of subcultural groups to the professionals on the staff. They act as educators to the staff, administration, and policy-making groups in the center by giving a realistic assessment of the nature of the local community and its need priorities. They provide a channel for interpretation and education to the local organizations and residents in the community about the nature of the services in the mental health center, about how to use them effectively, and about the various funding and organizational problems of the center.

Because of this special insight the indigenous paraprofessionals, through their various roles and functions, can truly provide an important and essential influence in the center. If the professional administration and staff are willing to accept this nontraditional, but invaluable source of accurate information about the clients they wish to serve, a great many policies, services, and decisions may evolve in a way that will produce the most appropriate and effective results in the community. The proper use of this information can lead to the paraprofessionals' influencing the nature and methods of the service system, providing educational interpretation and therapeutic liaison between the providers and consumers, and bring knowledge about the indigenous needs of catchment area residents and their subcultural groups to the attention of the professional staff. These functions serve to maximize the ability of the mental health center to provide the most effective, high quality mental health services, and to relate the programs directly to the mental health needs of the local population and local institutions and agencies.

Generalists and Advocates in Outreach Work

The majority of the paraprofessionals at Maimonides work in the neighborhood-based satellite clinics. They are the chief providers of services in outreach programs, particularly those offered at neighborhood storefront centers, where local individuals and families may go to get help with the many kinds of personal problems which can affect their mental health. As generalists, these paraprofessionals have been trained to be involved effectively in the total biopsychosocial needs of the individuals and families who come to the outreach centers for service. The clients may have problems which can be characterized as social, economic or educational; they may be experiencing difficulties with housing or with their marriages. The paraprofessionals frequently act as advocates, or as ombudspersons, in relation to the services of the mental health center, or to those of the hospital, the local public welfare agency, the schools, the correctional system, or other community services. They work under the supervision of trained clinical professionals and community organizers. The varied skills of paraprofessionals, thus, are used at Maimonides in all service areas in ways which will most benefit the client. In contrast, at some community mental health centers the activities of paraprofessionals are confined to particular service areas (e.g., inpatient or aftercare) where paraprofessionals traditionally play roles.

Community Organization Workers

Paraprofessionals also assume an important role as neighborhood community organizers, organizing projects and activities in response to mental health needs and problems. They help to train community leaders who are involved in developing programs in parent associations, in trade unions, in women's groups, in church groups, in neighborhood associations, and in other local community organizations. Paraprofessionals, as neighborhood organizers, are especially helpful in working with gang groups on the streets and other youth groups historically unable to be reached by traditional psychiatric facilities and professional workers.

Advocates for Citizens Dealing with Public Agencies

The paraprofessionals provide an important source of knowledge and expertise in helping clients and patients to maneuver through the various service bureaucracies in the local community and in the city. At the Maimonides Community Mental Health Center they often supplement the formal liaison arrangements for mutual referral and relationships by establishing a personal relationship between the mental health center and the other service providers. They also perform advocate roles on behalf of clients and patients who reside in the local community and who find it difficult to get the help they need from the other agencies and institutions. This role includes breaking through bureaucratic resistance in the mental health center itself on behalf of the people in the community who need help.

Workers in Primary Prevention Programs

Paraprofessionals at Maimonides Community Mental Health Center are involved in many primary prevention programs. In this work they often are instrumental in organizing self-help groups in the client population. The activities of many of these groups are designed to make an impact on the pathogenic social conditions which influence the development of mental illness and mental health.

Three examples from Maimonides illustrate the variety of primary prevention efforts that paraprofessionals can spearhead: (a) Paraprofessionals organized a self-help group of normal mothers to discuss the mothers' daily living problems; the ensuing discussions resulted in the mothers carrying out a successful fight for a new day-care center in their community. (b) Paraprofessionals organized gangs and other youths into a self-advocacy group that succeeded in persuading the city government to renovate a local swimming pool and park; as a result, the youths were able to use the facilities for recreation during the summer. The youth groups benefited also by substituting constructive civic action for previous antisocial delinquent activities. (c) Paraprofessionals organized a tenants group that forced apartment and tenement house landlords to remove paint that causes lead poisoning.

Mental Health Education Workers

The paraprofessionals play a vital and primary role in the organization of community mental health education programs at Maimonides. For instance, paraprofessionals have organized committees of presidents and education officers of the various parents associations in the public schools and parochial schools. These community members, in turn, have organized groups and workshops concerned with such subjects as "Normal Child Development" or "How To Be A More Effective Parent." The principle involved in these programs is that it is the most effective practice to motivate local residents themselves to organize local mental health education programs in relation to their interests and needs. The professionals provide the teaching and expertise for the various education groups. It has been found at this particular center that the role of the indigenous paraprofessional is the key to the breadth, motivation, and ability to reach large numbers of people in such programs.

Workers in Secondary Prevention and Case Identification

In equally important roles, paraprofessionals are involved in secondary prevention functions and in early case finding. Since they are indigenous to various community organizations in the local catchment area, such as parents associations, church organizations, public and parochial schools, gang groups, fraternal organizations and trade unions, they often are able to identify individuals and families who need help in the critical, early stages of the mental health problem. Thus, they are often able to bring these people and the services of the center together at an earlier phase of impending mental health crisis than would have been possible without their help. They also are active in developing formal as well as informal liaisons with local indigenous organizations through which easy and confidential channels are established for referrals. In another important aspect of this work, paraprofessionals work on duty schedules which make them easily accessible to local residents who need help during hours and periods of time, such as nights and weekends, when a fewer number of professionals are at work in the mental health center. It follows that accessibility to the center at Maimonides is eased for the local residents who will often find it more comfortable to enter the mental health service system by talking first to the paraprofessional, whom they know as a neighbor or a friend and as a member of their own subcultural group.

Agents for Reducing Stigma

Another especially important function undertaken by the paraprofessionals in this area is that of helping many families and children to overcome the profound sense of social stigma connected with mental illness or helping them to cope with mental health problems of the children. Such families too often initially tend to resist coming to the clinical services of the mental health center for help.

Workers for Patient Re-entry

As all mental health workers know, one of the difficult problems in the treatment of mental health patients comes to the fore when the patient is ready to re-enter normal family, community, and worklife after treatment, or at particular stages of treatment, in the mental health facility. It is at this time that community mental health workers provide a vital function, not only in staffing re-entry programs, but also in helping the patient make contact with local groups and organizations in the neighborhood. The paraprofessional can help the re-entering patient to bridge the gap between families', neighbors', and friends' perceptions of the patient as mentally ill and the fact that the patient has recovered or is in the process of recovering.

Liaison Personnel between Professional and Community

Many of the professional workers in the mental health center are not indigenous to the local catchment area. They often are not of the same racial, ethnic,
or class background of the people they serve, and frequently do not live in the
local community. The professional, therefore, often finds it difficult to connect
with patients and clients, or prospective clients, who are part of local community groups. He or she may not have the ability to immediately assess the needs
of these clients at the time that they need help, or the cultural empathy to
understand the clients' perceptions of the kind of help they do need, when they
need it, and how they wish that need to be filled. On the other hand, the
paraprofessionals, being indigenous to the local populations, usually have easy
connections with their own subgroups and neighborhoods and can act frequently as effective liaisons between the professional providers and the potential users of the center's services.

Participants in the Delivery of Clinical Intervention Services

Paraprofessionals in the center are also involved in therapeutic intervention
and mental health counseling roles with individuals and families under the
supervision of clinical professionals. They provide such services under a wide
range of circumstances: in the 24-hour inpatient psychiatric unit, in the day
hospital and the day treatment center, in outpatient clinics, in emergency
services, in work with selected families, in programs for the elderly, and in
prevention, treatment and rehabilitation programs with patients and clients
involved in alcohol and drug abuse. They also work as members of interdisciplinary and interclassification teams with patient and client service units. In
these units, clients are assigned to individual staff members or to teams of staff
members on the basis of a match between the clients' needs and the competencies of the staff member(s). In contrast, in many psychiatric facilities, the staff
members pick and choose the patients with whom they would most like to
work. At Maimonides, this process has been built into the institutional system
as a standard operating procedure. Thus, the process will survive changes in
the composition of the administrative and treatment staff.

Experience at the Maimonides Community Mental Health Center, and at
other mental health centers, has demonstrated that, while some problems are
associated with the effective functioning of indigenous community mental
health workers, the achievement of the objectives of the center have been
considerably enhanced by their presence and their work. Without substantial
groups of indigenous paraprofessionals performing in the roles that have been
described, the mental health center tends to revert and regress to a more
traditional form of psychiatric facility, and the staff finds that it is difficult to
carry out the concepts, principles and objectives which are the foundation of

the philosophy on which the services of the mental health center have been developed.

Career Development for the Paraprofessional

In many communities, the mental health center represents one of the largest employers of local people in the catchment area. Local residents are happy to have an opportunity to have jobs and be involved in productive work at the center, especially in these times of large scale unemployment.

However, within a year or so after being hired, many of these new workers tend to develop roots and aspirations within the hierarchical professional value system of psychiatry and mental health. They become interested in advancing from their original position to one of more responsibility and higher status; they seek opportunities for career development, professional advancement, promotions and increases in salaries. As an important principle of good personnel practice, the mental health center should take responsibility for helping to provide professional and career advancement opportunities for these aspiring paraprofessionals. This responsibility is especially significant in light of the historic inhibitions to advancement in any field that have been the lot of society's minority poor, and in particular the black and Puerto Rican people. The community mental health center must recognize the fact that this population has long been denied their human right to both career advancement and higher education.

The Maimonides Community Mental Health Center has developed a number of different interrelating approaches to the upgrading of skills and the career development of paraprofessional mental health workers. These approaches include the following:

1. Measures to prevent the exploitation of the paraprofessional worker as well as opportunities for mobility upward within the mental health center have been established as policy at the center. The classification system for paraprofessionals, built into union contracts, provides for a five year salary scale with five steps between a minimum and a maximum earning figure. This system also provides opportunities for promotion to Senior Community Mental Health Worker, or Team Leader, with a higher level of salary and salary scale.

    In addition, salaries of mental health workers and other mental health paraprofessionals are higher in the mental health center than the salary levels of nursing aides and other paraprofessionals in the general hospital. This differential is based on the requirements for a higher level of work and training built into the official job descriptions for positions in the mental health field.

2. All paraprofessionals are provided with intensive in-service training pro-
    grams designed to: (a) familiarize them with mental health problems and
    concepts; (b) develop counseling and other therapeutic skills for use in
    patient and family interviewing and referral; (c) develop skills in commu-
    nity organization, education and preventive programs; (d) communicate
    knowledge of human behavior and the ideology and characteristics of
    various mental illnesses; and (e) teach the skills and methods needed for
    working with families and groups.
3. In addition, paraprofessionals participate in the extensive and intensive
    interdisciplinary in-service training programs provided by the center for
    its entire staff within each element of service.
4. Group and individual supervisory conferences are held on a regular
    weekly basis as part of the training and education of the paraprofessional.
    These conferences are conducted by senior professionals who are particu-
    larly selected and trained to work with the community mental health
    workers.
5. Paraprofessionals who have completed a number of seminars are provided
    with a certificate, indicating successful completion of a cluster of educa-
    tional training programs. These certificates not only provide the para-
    professional with a concrete symbol of achievement; they may also be
    used by the paraprofessional who can offer them as evidence in applica-
    tion for life-experience credit when enrolling in an academic institution.
6. Special training programs are provided for paraprofessionals who are
    assigned to work in specific areas of service. These programs are geared
    to the development of knowledge and skills relevant to their assigned
    tasks, such as: the 24-hour Hospitalization Services in relation to work
    with psychotic and other profoundly ill patients; work with the elderly,
    work with children with mental health problems; home visiting services;
    follow-up and after care services; activity therapies; and neighborhood
    mental health organizations.
7. Work-study programs have been arranged with local community colleges
    and universities, so that the paraprofessionals can matriculate in pro-
    grams providing Associate Degrees, Bachelor Degrees, and Masters De-
    grees in Psychology, Social Work, Special Education, Mental Health, and
    other health related fields. The mental health center arranges on-duty
    work schedules and assignments for each worker, taking into consider-
    ation working hours and attendance at school, so that he or she can
    continue to earn a salary while going to school. Since the center is open
    24 hours a day, 7 days a week, it is possible to arrange such assignments
    in a way that will facilitate college attendance for the working paraprofes-
    sional.
8. The Maimonides Community Mental Health Center has made arrange-
    ments with the local institutions of higher education to provide academic
    credit for life experience, work experience and in-service training pro-

grams for the paraprofessional mental health worker. Because of this agreement, the educational programs in the colleges can provide accelerated courses, geared to the special needs of the paraprofessionals, who often begin their formal studies with as much as two years of academic credits granted for their experience in the center. These agreements are usually made through a letter written by the center director to the dean describing the experiences of the specific paraprofessionals. Since Maimonides serves as a training locale for many colleges, there is a mutual foundation of confidence which makes possible such arrangements.

9. Full-time college attendance is also an option for some mental health workers at the Maimonides Mental Health Center. Several years ago by arrangement with the New York City Department of Mental Health and Mental Retardation Services, and with the use of federal, state, and city funds, the Center was able to organize official professional career ladder training and education in collaboration with several colleges and universities in the city. In this program the worker went to school full time, received a stipend from the special program, and continued to work part-time in the center. Academic field work and practice credit was provided by the college of the student's choice. Unfortunately, the federal funds stopped and the current financial crisis in New York State and New York City prevented further funding of this successful and impressive program from which 15 paraprofessionals in the Maimonides Center graduated. However, continuation of the program after termination of funding was provided by the individual work-study arrangements between the mental health center and local colleges.

It is essential to emphasize again that such arrangements as enumerated above are essential for the constructive use and enhancement of the contribution of paraprofessionals in a mental health center. The benefits accrue not only in terms of the paraprofessional career aspirations of the workers, but also in their increased effectiveness in providing clinical and non-clinical services to the local community. Experience at the Maimonides Center reveals that paraprofessionals who have participated in and completed the total training tracks—or any part of them—develop into some of the most effective, skilled. sensitive, and committed professionals available to the field. Examinations of their performance have consistently found that they make high level contributions to the patients, the clients and to the organization.

FUNDING

There can be general agreement, based upon experience, that indigenous paraprofessional mental health workers are essential to the provision of mental health services to the community, and that they make an important contribution to the operation and survival of the comprehensive community mental health service facility. There also can be general agreement that for paraprofessionals to perform the important roles and functions described, they need intensive and extensive training as well as the opportunity for career advancement in an organized formal manner. However, the staff and administration of many mental health centers who wish to move in this direction have been unable to do so because of the lack of funds.

Thus, a contradiction exists in the field. On the one hand, paraprofessionals with training, experience, and the provision of a career ladder are essential to the operation of a community mental health center; on the other hand, most mental health centers are not able to provide the opportunities for training or the career ladder needed to assure full and effective use of paraprofessional workers. The reasons for this difficulty include the following:

1. Community mental health facilities are barely able to survive as it is, and are having difficulty providing even the minimum service needed due to lack of city, county, and state tax levy funding support. In a fiscal containment period, therefore, the assignment of local budget funds to subsidize the training of paraprofessionals does not have a high priority.

2. While a great deal of money has been spent by the federal government in the last five years for paraprofessional training programs, the grants have, in the main, been given to educational institutions, particularly community and four-year colleges, rather than to service facilities and centers.

3. Many mental health centers are located in areas where it is not possible to find an accessible college willing and able to establish an educational career ladder program on a work-study basis; and most paraprofessionals cannot afford to go to school and pay tuition without working for an income.

4. Even when federal funds were available, the federal government distributed them, for the most part, under a destructive and irrational grant policy which was impossible to implement. The requirement for local matching and policy of time limited grants with gradually decreasing federal support has resulted in the termination of excellent programs within several years of their initiation. This policy also has inhibited agencies and communities from applying for federal funds and from starting programs, for fear that their termination will have antagonistic consequences in the community and because it does not seem just to raise the expectations of paraprofessionals, and their communities, only to frustrate them when time and funds run out.

5. With all the pressures on local counties and states for cost containment in the fields of health and mental health, and in the light of other mandates to spend tax funds on such things as welfare, education, police and

sanitation, local funds are just not available for paraprofessional training programs.

Four major funding policy changes are essential to the growth and establishment of effective training programs:

1. Federal funds are needed to support such programs.
2. Federal funds should be granted on a permanent basis, without time limit, without requiring local matching funds, and on a program cost basis without gradual decrease in the amount.
3. Federal training grants should be given to provider agencies and community mental health facilities as well as to colleges, or to consortiums of service providers and educational institutions.[2] Experience has demonstrated that paraprofessional training programs are more effectively organized, and jobs more easily provided to the graduates when the service facility has the responsibility for administration and organization of the program. In addition, in such instances, the program tends to build in its own pressure for continuation from the local community which has a stake in its existence.
4. A special federal grant program should be created to support specific professional and semi-professional career ladder training programs for indigenous paraprofessionals.

These approaches and the use of federal funds will go a long way toward the development and institutionalization of paraprofessional training and career advancement programs.

SPECIAL PROBLEMS

Extensive use of paraprofessionals, especially in mental health centers and other facilities with the most effective paraprofessional programs, has demonstrated the existence of a number of real problems which are not easy to solve. Identification of these problems and implementation of programs aimed at their solution are tasks important to the attainment of maximum effectiveness in the use of paraprofessionals in community mental health services. These problems include the following:

1. Special funding for training programs is essential. This matter has been discussed above.
2. The training of paraprofessionals by professionals can result in the transfer of pseudo-professional attitudes and characteristics to paraprofessionals which can inhibit rather than enhance paraprofessional effectiveness.

Professionals tend to train paraprofessionals in their own image. Sometimes some of the more dysfunctional elements of the professional image are produced. A not all-inclusive list might include: preoccupation with hierarchical status; competition with other mental health disciplines; concentration on the use of psychotherapy as the main modality of treatment; inability to provide holistic services reflecting the biopsychosocial needs of the patient or client; preoccupation with matters of certification and licensing; emphasis on the development of polysyllabic language and communication often as a substitute for substance and knowledge; tendency toward alienation from the people who are served; and a push toward the development of their own discipline through a separate, professional organization with a consequent move away from interdisciplinary and interclassification participation in the provision of services. The Maimonides Community Mental Health Center employs knowledgeable professionals who because of their community mental health orientation value and are able to implement community-based, non-elitist approaches to service delivery. After receiving some specialized appropriate training, such professionals are most effective in training paraprofessionals.

3. Some mental health professionals, especially those from the disciplines of psychology, social work, and nursing, are threatened by the development of trained paraprofessionals and their use in the mental health facility. Such professionals tend to "put down" the paraprofessionals and resist the development of paraprofessional training programs or the use of such workers in roles involving therapeutic intervention. These attitudes tend to intensify conflict and competition between the two groups.

4. There is a danger that the administrations of some facilities, pressed for funds, may resort to substituting the lower paid, trained paraprofessionals for the more expensive professional workers, disregarding the needs of patients and clients. Such a policy of exploitation of the paraprofessional hurts not only these workers, but also the health facility itself, by minimizing its ability to achieve service objectives.

In fact, special problems have been created by the tendency in some facilities to use paraprofesionals almost exclusively as substitutes for professionals in providing outreach services and ambulatory programs to poor, working class, and minority group communities. This practice prevails, especially where professional personnel resist going out into communities, preferring to restrict their rendering of services to their offices and therapeutic service units housed in the facility. There also have been a number of instances in which clients or patients in poor and minority communities have indicated their distress at being served by paraprofessionals while more well-to-do populations are served by "Doctors and PhD's." It must be emphasized that the community mental health philosophy rejects the establishment of a two-class system for its patients and clients as well as for its professional and paraprofessional workers. The use of paraprofessionals is intended, not to downgrade the poor and the minorities, but to expand and enrich the capabilities of the mental health working force so as to provide high quality services to all in accordance with their needs through interdisciplinary and interclassification teams.

5. Sometimes the recruitment of paraprofessionals is influenced by political considerations on the part of community boards and administrators. An employment process based on political pressure will come into conflict with the essential principle of ethnic and racial representation in the salaried staff, and will diminish the ability of the mental health facility to employ mental health workers who reflect the subcultures indigenous to the local population. This problem occurs most often in those facilities where the majority of the professional staff members do not reside in the local community and do not share the ethnic, religious, class, national, or racial origins of the people they serve. The impact of such an employment process is a serious problem in communities which have substantial minority group populations. These are the communities in which the residents historically have had the greatest difficulty in finding jobs and opportunities for career advancement and higher education.

These political pressures usually follow three patterns, either individually or in some combination. First, local community leaders may try to use employment in the local mental health center as a vehicle for giving favors to political supporters or to relatives. Secondly, members of the dominant ethnic group, especially if the majority is white and non-Hispanic, may attempt to have all the jobs allocated to members of that group. Finally, the members of the middle class may attempt to have jobs given to members of their social class.

The community, administration, and staff members at Maimonides Community Mental Health Center have developed three strategies for counteracting these pressures. The most basic strategy is to involve members from two committees jointly in writing detailed job descriptions and outlines of required experience and educational qualifications for the new employee. One committee is comprised of professional providers of services from the mental health center; the other committee consists of community board members who act as representatives for consumers of mental health services. This strategy causes both provider and consumer groups to become invested in the objective choice of the new employee. The second strategy is the requirement that both committees agree on a candidate before an applicant is hired. In cases of unresolvable conflict, the director of the center makes a decision, usually in favor of the recommendation of the community committee. The third strategy provides for a probationary period for each new employee. At the end of this period, the employee's performance is evaluated internally by mental health center staff members and the consumer personnel committee; subsequently a decision is made to retain or to dismiss the new employee.

6. Civil service and trade union position classification systems frequently do not contain job descriptions and salary levels necessary to match the career ladder and training programs for the paraprofessionals. Administrators have found it almost impossible to get increases in salaries for community mental health workers commensurate with the different levels of advanced training and experience built into the program.

Trying to change these existing classifications is a less effective way of solving the problem than negotiating new promotive classifications and higher salary levels, based on the creating of new job definitions and new job titles. These new titles and definitions will then become part of the civil service or trade union classification system. Every program of advanced training should include guaranteed opportunities for jobs and for the upgrading of task assignments and salaries.

At the Maimonides Community Mental Health Center, the career ladders and associated salary levels are the product of a careful and prolonged negotiation process. The process involved the director of the mental health center, representatives from the Maimonides Hospital personnel department, the union representing paraprofessionals and nonprofessionals at the hospital, and, where appropriate, the New York State Civil Service Commission. The strategy of providing a higher salary in the community mental health center for the same job classification positions and work assignments as in the hospital was not feasible, for the mental health center then would have been an exception to the policy of parent hospital. Pressures then would have been exerted on both the hospital management and union by the employees of other sections of the hospital for the same higher levels of pay. Accordingly, the mental health center paraprofessionals and nonprofessionals were given new and additional tasks as well as new titles. Furthermore, funds were set aside in the regular budget to compensate workers who have achieved the requirements for advancement within the career ladder. The possibility of advancement for eligible current staff members is assured by giving trained workers fiscal advancement and promotional priority over the hiring of new employees.

7. Many colleges which have received federal and local funds to provide career ladder training programs for paraprofessionals have not built into their vocational programs commitments to obtain jobs for the students upon completion of their training. This situation is especially true of the two-year community college programs for the training of community mental health workers. As a result, hundreds of such paraprofessionals with associate degrees and other diplomas have found it necessary to take jobs requiring lower skills and offering lower pay, often jobs similar to the ones they held before they went to school. This lack of job opportunity undercuts and subverts an aspirant's motivation to enter the career program while frustrating and disappointing the newly created hopes of the

paraprofessionals. All grants and funds provided for career ladder programs should mandate not only effective training programs but also prearranged collaboration with the provider agencies to secure jobs for the trainee after completion of the training.

8. Programs for paraprofessionals, such as described above, have raised the controversial question of confidentiality in mental health facilities. An examination of this problem at the Maimonides Community Mental Health Center resulted in the following conclusions:

A. The problem of confidentiality is raised almost exclusively by professionals, and not by patients or their families or by the paraprofessionals.

B. Most patients interviewed concerning this matter are more concerned with obtaining service and getting well than with confidentiality.

C. Paraprofessionals in general have tended to be more sensitive to the need to keep patient matters confidential than the professionals. Professional workers have been heard discussing patients and their problems by name publicly in the staff-patient cafeterias and in hallways more often than paraprofessionals have been heard to do so.

D. In general, confidentiality has frequently been used as a smoke screen behind which health and mental health professionals hide the strong desire to avoid being publicly accountable for their competence.

E. This problem is in the main nonexistent in facilities which function on the basis of a profound commitment to serving the needs of their patients and clients.

9. Racism and sexism are problems in the broader community that unavoidably impinge to some extent on the relationships among staff members at the mental health center. These problems have been successfully minimized at the center, however. In fact, the mental health center is one of the few places in the community where different ethnic and religious groups will meet together after confrontation and conflict have occurred. Members of the center's administrative staff view racism and sexism as causes and pathogenic factors influencing mental health problems, and support strategies aimed at reducing these problems in the community and within the center. Thus, the administration and rank-and-file staff members have struggled together to achieve integration and equality within the staff at the center. Furthermore, both groups have consistently fought for career ladders that will provide all staff members with equitable opportunities for upward mobility regardless of ethnicity, race, or sex.

Some of the problems associated with the use of paraprofessionals are difficult to resolve in some settings and in the mental health field in general because the field has not totally committed itself, as yet, to a community mental health orientation. The most prevalent approach is still to provide services through more traditional psychiatric programs and facilities. Experience, nevertheless, has demonstrated that none of these problems are incapable of solution. There are no insurmountable obstacles which can prevent the development of effective programs involving the high level use of paraprofessionals in the provision of service, or their exposure to the high quality of training essential to the paraprofessionals' effective integration into the field.

CONCLUSION

As the field of mental health moves further toward the establishment of community mental health centers and other comprehensive service systems, the need increases for the employment of substantial numbers of trained indigenous paraprofessionals within the community mental health facility. The provision of important roles and functions for paraprofessionals, such as those described in this paper, not only reflects the principles and goals of a community mental health center, but also enhances the ability of the center to implement these principles and effectively achieve its mandated objectives. A community mental health approach to the provision of services represents a profound social commitment to serving the mental health needs of the population through the provision of prevention, mental health maintenance, community mental health education, diagnostic and treatment services, rehabilitation and social restoration programs. The professional workers in large measure are helped in fulfilling this commitment by the supplementary and complementary functions of indigenous trained paraprofessionals.

NOTES

[1] The term "non-professional" is characteristically applied to clerical workers, food service workers, and other persons who do not specialize in mental health services. At Maimonides, however, this distinction is not made, for these "non-professionals" can have an impact on the mental health of the clients with whom they come into contact.

[2] The faculty members at colleges may not revise their courses to keep abreast of changing patterns of practice. This tendency is especially pronounced in times of rapid change.

REFERENCE NOTE

1. M. Tarail, *Community participation: Issues and implications for administrators.* Unpublished manuscript, 1972. (Available from the author at the Maimonides Community Mental Health Center in New York, New York.)

REFERENCE

Tarail, M. New trends in mental health services—What are we evaluating? In W. Neighes, R. J. Hammer, & G. Landsberg (Eds.), *Emerging developments in mental health program evaluation.* New York: Argold Press, 1977.

Chapter 11

A SYSTEM-WIDE PROGRAM FOR MENTAL HEALTH WORKER UTILIZATION

E. Mansell Pattison, MD*
Ernest Kuncel, MS†
Frank R. Murillo, MSW‡
Razmig Madenlian, MA§

This chapter describes a comprehensive community mental health center in which paraprofessionals play an integral, system-wide role in the delivery of services. The particular center, the Orange County Department of Health, is located in a suburban region of Southern California and serves a primarily lower- to middle-income population.

The chapter presents the relevant goals and organizational features of the Orange County mental health system, provides data indicating that paraprofessionals comprise a valuable component of the local system, and describes both the advantages and disadvantages of using paraprofessionals. Mental health workers are defined as professionals engaged in a professional career in mental health service; their identity is based more on their new function and professional norms of universal responsibility than on their community of origin or past life. The chapter and appendices provide guidelines for the selection of such mental health workers, and present detailed information on an in-service training program/career ladder sequence.

*Professor of Psychiatry and Human Behavior, Social Science and Social Ecology Vice-Chairman, Department of Psychiatry and Human Behavior, University of California, Irvine; and Deputy Director, Training, Consultation and Education Division, Orange County Department of Mental Health, California.

†Research Assistant, Training, Consultation and Education Division, Orange County Department of Mental Health, California.

‡Outpatient Service Director, East Central Regional Services, Orange County Department of Mental Health, California.

§Director of Regional Programs, Training, Consultation and Education Division, Orange County Department of Mental Health, California.

This chapter will focus on the use of mental health paraprofessionals as integral components of a total mental health delivery system in Orange County, California.[1] The passage of the State of California Community Mental Health Act (the Lanterman-Petris-Short Act) in 1968 mandated the development of local county community mental health programs to provide a comprehensive program similar to federal guidelines. In 1968 no formal community mental health services existed in Orange County, which had a population of 1.8 million. Therefore, the opportunity to construct an innovative system-wide program was presented to us in 1969 when the Orange County Department of Mental Health (OCDMH) was formed.

Concepts of comprehensive community mental health services, community involvement, multidisciplinary staff roles and tasks, and innovative manpower deployment were critical factors in the construction of the program. A system-wide use of paraprofessional mental health workers was built into the fabric of the delivery system at the inception. The OCDMH has grown to a large county-wide enterprise encompassing six regional catchment areas, a budget of over $27 million, and a full-time staff of over 600. The development of mental health worker personnel within the organization was undertaken at the beginning by the Training, Consultation and Education Division with grant assistance from the National Institute of Mental Health. In this chapter we will, therefore, present our experience in the system-wide utilization of mental health workers, based upon institutionalized program processes.

A WORKING PHILOSOPHY OF THE MENTAL HEALTH WORKER

The community mental health movement is a major innovation as a delivery system of mental health care. Mental health manpower issues are interwoven with the entire philosophy of a community mental health delivery system. In fact, the development of new mental health manpower is both a cause and consequence of the community revolution in mental health delivery (Fisher, Mehr, & Truckenbrod, 1974; Kalafant & Borato, 1977). Reviews of the mental health staff deployment literature point out that this new pattern of service delivery requires a different staff deployment pattern; at the same time, the increased personnel changes the nature of the delivery system itself (Cowne, 1969; Pattison & Elpers, 1972).

There are six major considerations in the development of new personnel:

1. National surveys of mental health service staff production have shown that there is a growing gap between population growth with attendant mental health needs and the production of highly trained professionals. In fact, since the federal support of community mental health programs has spawned widespread development of local mental health services,

there has been an increased national shortage of professional staff members (Albee, 1959).

2. National studies of staff member education costs have shown that it is prohibitive to meet personnel requirements solely through extended professional training programs and then to staff these programs with high-cost professionals; thus, less costly trained and less costly employed paraprofessionals are needed (Arnhoff, Rubenstein, & Speisman, 1969).

3. Traditional mental health professionals generally come from the upper social classes and display consistent social class biases toward the lower social classes. This has resulted in skewed and ineffective services for the lower social classes who are major consumers of community mental health services (Jones, 1974; Lorian, 1973).

4. The need for mental health personnel who understand local community populations and who have similar social class and ethnic identity as well as similar life experiences has been underscored. Thus, stress has been put on indigenous community recruitment to answer the need for mental health manpower (Pearl & Riessman, 1965).

5. Community mental health stresses the importance of community outreach, primary preventive activities in the community, and the extension of mental health services into community life. Such new patterns of services are not typically defined within the repertoire of traditional mental health professionals (Grosser, Henry, & Kelly, 1969; Reiff & Riessman, 1965).

6. Community mental health further stresses the value of continuity of care with the linkage of clients in the treatment system with their community systems and resources. This type of service is not typically provided by traditional mental health professionals (Guerney, 1969; Hesse, 1976).

To conclude, the development of cost-effective mental health services is required to serve neglected populations that include the lower social classes and ethnic minorities and to emphasize community-linked services. The new mental health worker is seen as a relatively less expensive classification of employee to train and employ, one which would be more representative of the clientele to be served and more able to provide new extensions of mental health service directly linked to ongoing community life. In addition, in the last 10 years, program studies have reported that mental health workers can be successfully recruited and trained to perform many of the mental health tasks conducted by professionals (Alley & Blanton, 1976; Baker, 1973; Gartner, 1971; Young, True, & Packard, 1976). In fact, mental health workers have moved into innovative roles and tasks representative of the outreach thrust of community mental health (Egan, 1975; Matarazzo, 1971; Sobey, 1970).

Thus, the philosophy of the mental health worker as a new labor resource has been shown to be viable. Mental health workers can be recruited, trained, employed, and deployed to meet the labor needs of the community mental health delivery system. The theory and practice work in experimental programs within individual service areas; however, a new group of issues must be addressed and evaluated in the case of an institutionalized (ongoing) program implemented on a system-wide basis.

System-Wide Issues

We cannot easily dissect personnel issues from other critical issues in the construction of a community mental health delivery system, but we can identify certain issues that directly involve the mental health worker. We shall identify each issue and then offer our program solution.

1.   What are the treatment goals of a community mental health service? Traditional mental health services have emphasized long-term, intensive psychotherapies aimed at producing characterological change with patients who were essentially functional in society but suffering internal distress. The "worried well" with existential conflicts in life have been over-represented in the theory and practice of psychotherapy. The pursuit of personal satisfaction, however, is personal privilege and *not* a right. Note that the preamble to the American Constitution guarantees the right to life, liberty, and the *pursuit* of happiness. Personal happiness is not guaranteed!

In contrast, community mental health programs, which are primarily public-funded services, seek to provide basic mental health services to restore people to social function. Thus, the primary therapeutic goals aim at crisis resolution, diminution of disabling symptoms, short-term therapy oriented to reality coping, and stabilized community maintenance of chronic disorders. Therefore, we do *not* expect the mental health worker with modest training to acquire the skills and abilities for long-term, intensive psychotherapies; however, we expect they can provide modest therapeutic interventions appropriate to functional mental health rehabilitation goals.

2.   What services are to be provided by a community mental health program? In accord with federal and state guidelines, the OCDMH has been organized to provide comprehensive mental health services to all citizens in need. Those who are most disabled receive priority of services to restore them to social function and maintain continuity of care for ongoing function in the community. Thus, the delivery system must be cut of whole cloth, and a functional service program must interweave primary, secondary, and tertiary prevention into it. In this way, *all* staff are involved in a unitary program effort.

To the extent possible, a single staff member assumes overall responsibility for a client to assure that all necessary services are provided over time. This is a generalist approach to service delivery rather than a specialist approach; it is intended as a way to avoid fragmentation and discontinuity of care provision. Thus, the mental health worker becomes a generalist alongside other generalists in a service delivery system constructed to provide a unified program of care.

3.   How are the mental health personnel utilized? Traditional mental health services have been staffed in accord with established mental health professional disciplines. Each discipline was assigned roles and tasks in accord with assumed skills of each discipline. Such a utilization pattern is often dysfunctional because a staffing pattern is built in terms of a "team of disciplines" which ignores actual services to be delivered, skills required, and the role constellation of skills. Further, discipline identity is no assurance of a person's skills or of ability to perform a specific role constellation of skills relevant to a service. Finally, in community mental health we have new skills required, new role constellations, and new patterns of service delivery for which disciplinary team concepts are not functional.

Therefore, in OCDMH we stress construction of staff deployment in relation to the service delivery unit. The *services* to be delivered define the *skills* required. The skills in turn are organized into roles. We then turn to staffing patterns in terms of functional roles. Certain roles require a specific discipline (such as a licensed nurse). On the other hand, many roles can be filled by persons from various disciplines including generic mental health workers. Thus, selection for a role is based primarily on the skills and knowledge of a particular person to fill the role. It should be clear that we are not describing a multidisciplinary or interdisciplinary staffing pattern, but rather a function-oriented staffing pattern. In this way, a mental health worker is selected for a job role on the basis of experience, knowledge, and skill to perform the particular tasks in that functional job role. There is, as a result, no mental health worker role per se.

4.   What are the roles of mental health staff? As mental health worker personnel have been trained to perform many tasks associated with traditional mental health disciplines, there has been inevitable confusion about roles which have overlapping skills. Some traditional professional staff have seen the sharing of skills and tasks as a threat to their roles. Indeed, the literature refers to this as role "boundary-busting" leading to "role diffusion" and "role confusion" (Dinitz & Beren, 1971; Gottesfeld, Rhee, & Parker, 1970; Wagenfeld & Robin, 1976).

In the OCDMH we do not support the notion of "role leveling"; that is, that everyone performs the same tasks, reduced to the lowest common denominator. Rather, we promote the concept of "skilled role differentiation." In this situation, there are certain general skills everyone possesses, and there are degrees of increasing skill and knowledge for more complex tasks. Staff members are assigned to roles that match their skills; those with more skills focus their work on complex tasks. Although there is a rather broad degree of overlap of both skills and tasks, the roles remain separate; thus, we minimize everyone's doing the same thing.

5.   Is the mental health worker role unique? The early rhetoric of the mental health worker movement stressed the uniqueness of such nonprofessional or paraprofessional personnel. In part, that rhetoric stressed the concepts of community advocacy, community representation, and community action on the part of the new coterie of mental health workers.

We believe that such rhetoric can be deceptive and even destructive. It can support the notion that community aspects of a program can be relegated to mental health workers and ignored by traditional professionals. It may be assumed that such community services can be performed by mental health workers in isolation from the rest of the program. It may be hoped that merely by employing mental health workers, a community-based service program would be assured. Basically, such rhetoric may promote a split between mental health workers and other staff. Even more importantly, it may ignore the fact that a community-involved service program must be constructed as a system-wide effort involving the total program (Cowen, 1977). The use of mental health workers is the consequence of a system-wide, community-integrated program, not the cause.

Published data support our analysis, for role and staff conflict is reported when mental health workers are solely responsible for community involvement (Bloom & Parad, 1977); they remain isolated from the rest of the service delivery system and ultimately have no impact (Hardcastle, 1971; Maierle, 1973). However, when there are shared skills and tasks with other staff and a program-wide commitment to community involvement, there is an integration of mental health workers in terms of values, attitudes, working relations, and community effort (Robin & Wagenfeld, 1977; Sarata, 1977). Therefore, although we do not consider the mental health worker role as unique, we do stress that the mental health worker staffing pattern allows us to recruit unique persons.

6.   Who are the professional mental health staff? The current literature exhibits much confusion about new mental health manpower. They are variously called nonprofessionals, paraprofessionals, new professionals, or subprofessionals. We find this issue more than a semantic quibble, because it reflects the confusion about the identity of the individual mental health worker. The various labels attempt to describe levels of education or types of tasks performed. Yet these attempts miss the mark, for the professionalization process involves the development of values, ideals, and ethics of role behavior, not graded education or tasks (Halmos, 1973). Since the full-time mental health service worker is a career person, we identify this worker in terms of the criteria of a professional (Moore, 1970): (a) The practitioner sees his work as a full-time occupation. (b) There is a commitment to a calling. (c) There is identification with peers in a formal organization. (d) There is useful knowledge and skills based on specialized training or education. (e) There is a service orientation. (f) There is autonomy restrained by responsibility.

We have found that in our utilization of mental health workers, it is important to clarify their identity as mental health professionals. They are not primarily identified in terms of their community of origin as is the volunteer (O'Donnell, 1970). Instead, their identity is based on their new function and not on their past life; for instance, they are not just ex-alcoholics or ex-addicts (Pattison, 1973). Their responsibility to clients should not be based on personal inclinations, but rather on professional norms of universal responsibility (Andrade & Burstein, 1973). To underscore and emphasize the norms of professional identity and conduct, we have developed a professional code of ethics for all staff. All new staff must read and sign an agreement to work in accord with the code which is applicable to all service staff as mental health professionals. In a word, the OCDMH defines the mental health worker as a professional.

7.   What is the system base for mental health workers? Many experimental programs have shown that mental health workers can be recruited, trained, and used to provide a wide range of mental health services. Such programs disappear when there are no permanent positions, no career ladders, and inappropriate access or pay. Therefore, in 1970 we developed a mental health worker career ladder personnel series which was officially adopted and has been utilized since. Several aspects are noteworthy: (a) It provides for an entry level training position (MHW I) that allows for 50% time spent in formal education/training. (b) It provides trade-offs between formal education and/or life-work experience for entry qualifications. (c) It provides career mobility into supervisory and administrative positions. (d) It provides four rungs, each containing a range of salaries, making possible incremental compensations for increased competency. (e) It provides appropriate salary levels commensurate with other professional staff. Thus, as shown in Appendix A, there is a career relevant institutional base for the ongoing utilization of mental health worker personnel.

8.   How are mental health workers recruited? Past program experiments have emphasized recruitment of mental health workers to provide jobs for the poor. Usually such jobs have been temporarily funded by federal, state, or local grants. To recruit poor people just to create jobs is not a sound avenue toward the development of new mental health manpower. A poor person, per se, is no more or less appropriate for employment in mental health than a middle-class or rich person! On the other hand, we reject reverse bias which would automatically disqualify a poor person. For example, in 1976 we implemented a WIN-sponsored (work incentive) program in which we successfully identified six trainees from the welfare rolls who became excellent mental health workers.

Similarly, some programs extol the value of recruiting community leaders nominated by their peers. Again, our experience has been negative. Peers may nominate buddies, friends, or relatives on the basis of personal relationships rather than personal qualities relevant to mental health service. Further, we have found that persons who are community leaders do not usually fit well into community mental health services, for the two types of roles reflect very different behavior styles and coping traits. In a sense, the effective political community leader must develop personal insensitivity in order to lead in times of turmoil; the mental health worker, on the other hand, must learn personal sensitivity in order to help others.

For this reason, we have over time developed criteria for recruitment of mental health worker trainees (MHW I) based on personal attributes and experience that we find relevant to successful mental health work.

In contrast to this, when we recruit for journeyman (MHW II), we place additional emphasis on the specific job role. Thus, a MHW II for alcoholism services would have recruitment criteria involving knowledge and experience in alcoholism; recruitment for an inpatient position would emphasize different criteria from that for a community outreach clinic position. Thus, we stress specific recruitment criteria defined for the specific job. This enables us to maximize the unique strengths, background, and experience of an individual that would suit the person for that particular role. As one can see, the decision to hire MHW I trainees or journeymen MHW II staff is related to the immediate program needs for critical staff, the particular unique skills and knowledge required in a specific job, and the availability of personnel funds to enroll a new group of MHW I trainees.

9.   How are mental health workers initially trained? We have found that training is intimately related to recruitment. When illiterate persons are recruited, we have had to spend an inordinate and inappropriate amount of time devoted to basic reading and writing skills. When persons with primarily a political orientation rather than a service orientation have been recruited, we have had major problems in their motivation toward learning mental health skills. In contrast, when we have recruited on the basis of relevance, we have found that training is highly effective.

The strategic value of training MHW I personnel within a service agency rather than hiring mental health workers after graduating from an AA-degree program in a junior college has not yet been resolved. We have found that junior college graduates often have minimal actual supervised work experience in global areas of competence. In contrast to this, when training MHW I personnel within the system, we are able to recruit trainees with relevant prior experience and skill and provide them with intensive didactic and work training that rapidly moves the trainee into a competent and high level of performance relative to the requirements of the job.

In many localities, however, it may be the case that junior colleges are more effective than small community mental health delivery systems, for the latter do not usually possess a sophisticated training organization within their structure. In addition, small mental health delivery systems may prove cost-ineffective since they usually train a relatively small number of mental health workers.

In the basic training of the novice MHW I, we now use the following format. An entire first year is devoted to training. Half of the time is focused on learning specific skills and knowledge pertinent to specific tasks, an approach different from the traditional college curriculum which emphasizes general principles and concepts. (See Appendix B which lists the basic first-year courses taught by OCDMH staff.) The other half of the time is spent on each of four major clinical services of a catchment area. There is careful one-to-one supervision of the trainee's clinical work by skilled clinical supervisors. Rotation to each of four services provides a blend of different clinical experiences. However, the trainee remains in one catchment area with the training supervisor throughout the year to provide an overall coherence of clinical perspective and to assess progress in actual function. (See Appendix C which presents standards for judging competencies of trainees.) It should be noted that if the MHW I wishes to acquire junior college credit toward an AA degree for the training received in OCDMH, such credit can be arranged by the staff.

Subsequent to successful completion of this full year of clinical training and education, the MHW I is eligible for promotion to a permanent journeyman position. In OCDMH we only begin a cycle of training when we have planned and committed permanent positions for eventual placement of the trainees. Thus, there is justification for the program cost of training a group of MHW I personnel, and the trainees have reasonable expectation that they can indeed embark on a career in mental health service once they've completed the program.

We have thus far trained no fewer than four persons in a group. We believe that a group of six is optimally desirable so that a functional peer-support relationship can be developed in the group of trainees. A smaller number considerably reduces the possibilities of mutual learning and support.

10.   What is the ongoing training for mental health workers? We have found that although initial training does indeed prepare the mental health worker to begin full-time employment, it does not provide sufficient training. Therefore, we have developed an extensive in-service training program that is ongoing. The in-service training program consists of *modules,* each of which is a specific unit of skill and knowledge relevant to the conduct of a specific clinical task; for example, family crisis intervention, management of violent clients, and evaluation and triage of alcoholics (see Appendix D). Each module is conducted for 10 weeks in a three-hour session each week. A pretest and posttest are given, with course content based on learning objectives embodied in the tests. Each training module is open to all OCDMH staff and personnel from any other human service agency or any county agency; however, in the latter case, the content of the module must be relevant to the worker's clinical role. If a person wishes college credit, he must personally pay the registration fee but no tuition is charged. An attendance rate of 70% and passing the posttest are required for a formal certificate of completion. College credit

toward an AA, BA, or MA degree can be obtained for the majority of modules. This unique arrangement has been made with local colleges and universities as part of their community outreach activities. One staff person is assigned to negotiate personally with the schools for credit arrangements. This specific job assignment highlights the importance of providing a structured administrative channel for the development of this aspect of the program.

A yearly schedule of modules is constructed on the basis of needs assessments conducted with the OCDMH staff. Approximately 20 modules per quarter are offered. Thus, the mental health worker is afforded a rather broad array of continuing training in job-specific skills and knowledge that will build further competence and prepare for career development. It should be noted that this arrangement also encourages peer learning from other kinds of professionals both within OCDMH and other human service agencies and that it reinforces the development of professional collegiality and identity in the mental health worker.

11.   Where is the system locus for mental health worker development? A system-wide utilization of mental health workers truly involves multiple components of the entire mental health delivery system. Each aspect of mental health worker utilization must interdigitate with each other aspect. Thus, there must be a central administrative locus of authority for planning, development, organization, and implementation of mental health workers' utilization. In OCDMH that locus is in the Training, Consultation and Education Division, which serves as the institutional locus for ongoing monitoring of mental health worker development.

In summary, we have raised a number of system-wide issues that needed to be addressed in order to affect system-wide utilization of mental health workers as integral components of the mental health delivery system.

THE OCDMH MODEL FOR UTILIZATION OF MENTAL HEALTH WORKERS

There are 13 key aspects of this model:

1.   The delivery system is based on the concepts of comprehensive community mental health services.
2.   Primary, secondary, and tertiary prevention activities are built into the direct service units for each specific service component.
3.   Community-linked services are built into the fabric of the entire service delivery system.
4.   All staff are involved in both direct and indirect services, including preventive services, outreach services, and linking of clerical services to community resources.

5. All staff are expected to provide generalist services so that clients receive unified care that avoids fragmentation and discontinuity.
6. Staff deployment is based on roles derived from service needs. There is some overlap of skills and tasks; however, functional role differentiation based on personal skill, knowledge, and ability is stressed.
7. The mental health worker role is not defined as unique, but we seek to recruit and utilize unique persons as mental health workers.
8. The mental health worker is defined as a professional who is engaged in a professional career in mental health service.
9. A career personnel series for mental health workers has been developed to provide appropriate careers in mental health service.
10. Recruitment of trainees is initiated when probable permanent career positions will be available; selection criteria focus on suitability of personality and experience to mental health task performance.
11. Recruitment of journeyman mental health workers is based on terms of specific job requirements.
12. Initial training emphasizes basic mental health skills and concurrent supervised clinical experience in a range of mental health services.
13. Ongoing in-service training programs focus on job-relevant skills and knowledge and are provided to enhance job performance and further career development.

SYSTEM-WIDE ASSESSMENT OF UTILIZATION

Extensive data have been reported on the use of the mental health worker, and problems of system-wide assessment have been identified in terms of complex variables (Figa-Talamanca, 1975; Guttentag, Kiresuk, Oglesby, & Cohn, 1975; Kaslow, 1972). However, our intent is more simple: to demonstrate with some basic data how mental health workers provide a core element of the OCDMH delivery system.

First, we can examine the types of clients served by the OCDMH delivery system. About 90% of all patients come from the lower socio-economic classes who cannot afford private mental health care. The percentage figures on the ethnicity of clients seen approximate the county-wide demographic distribution; this fact indicates that minority clients are being proportionately served by OCDMH. Indirect services include consultation, training, education, and liaison activities with the community. It should be noted that over 18,000 community people were provided these indirect mental health services in 1975–1976. In short, we suggest that the OCDMH delivery system provides both direct and indirect services to critical target populations. Further, we find that over 50% of our clients have psychotic diagnoses; yet the average number of client visits is six. Thus, the service delivery system is oriented toward the disabled client; it primarily provides short-term reality-oriented therapy intervention.

Second, if we examine the types of clinical services offered, all 12 community mental health service components are in operation with mental health workers filling positions in all 12 components. For example, journeyman MHW II staff perform the following clinical functions in a representative outpatient service: (a) walk-in intake evaluations; (b) mental status examinations; (c) psychosocial history and evaluation; (d) formulation of working diagnosis; (e) case formulation of initial treatment plan; (f) individual, marital, group, and family therapy; (g) crisis intervention; (h) formal case evaluation for emergency commitment; (i) sexual counseling; (j) community consultation and education; and (k) provision of in-service training materials.

The management of patients on medications merits special comments. At the time of initial evaluation, or thereafter during the course of treatment, the mental health worker may assess the need for a psychiatric evaluation and/or medication evaluation. A collaborative referral is made to the attending psychiatrist. If medication is prescribed, the mental health worker is responsible for monitoring the effect of the medication on the clinical course of the patient, as well as monitoring possible drug side effects. The patient is regularly seen by the mental health worker who is responsible for primary clinical care; in addition, the patient is also evaluated on a regular basis by a psychiatrist. Thus, there is shared professional collaboration.

Third, the impact of this pattern of manpower utilization and deployment has been beneficial. There has been an opportunity to develop flexible role groupings in which personnel can shift assignments in accord with clinical service needs. New roles can be developed as innovative services are organized.

This pattern promotes personal growth, skill acquisition, and professional development for the mental health worker; as a result, he or she can move into new assignments on the basis of acquired skill, knowledge, and experience. In addition, the mental health worker can provide an increased opportunity for the traditional professional to learn new skills, attitudes and functions relevant to community-oriented services. We find that traditional professionals do not give up or give over their clinical skills to the mental health worker, but rather carve new role configurations in accord with their professional abilities. We also find that this pattern tends to decrease the need for the middle-level professional trained at the Master's degree level. Although fewer PhD or MD professionals are required, doctoral-level staff members assume more important functions as consultants, supervisors, and administrators. In summary, our data show that fewer total professionals are utilized, and, thus, we must conclude that fewer professionals are required.

Fourth, if we examine the employment of mental health workers in relation to other staff, we find that they are a major manpower component. In 1976, with approximately 600 full-time employees of OCDMH, there were 6 MHW Is, 184 MHW IIs, 7 MHW IIIs, and 13 MHW IVs; there were 210 mental health workers in all. Thus, over 35% of the OCDMH staff were in mental health worker (MHW) categories. An examination of the distribution of MHW IIs by service modes dramatically illustrates how the mental health

Table 11–1   Outpatient Manpower Costs by Discipline
(FY 1974–75)

	Staff member month of effort	*Cost to OCDMH*
Psychiatrist	122	$366,000
Psychologist	98	172,000
Social Worker	192	250,000
Nurse	108	135,000
MHW IV	2	3,000
MHW III	18	19,000
MHW II	345	311,000
TOTAL	910	$1,256,000

worker provides the core staffing for major clinical components. These workers comprise a sizable majority of the work force in alcoholism, inpatient, and methadone maintenance programs. Furthermore, they comprise one-half of the drug abuse work force and slightly more than one-third of the outpatient service delivery staff.

When we examine the outpatient service component where the mental health worker group is the lowest, we still find that they provide a proportionate share of the clinical case load; more specifically, the outpatient mental health workers comprise 37% of the work force and provide 42% of direct service. When we break down the actual clinical components, we see that the mental health worker provides a broad range of direct clinical services in the outpatient component. In fact, they provide half the evaluative services and a substantial majority of the group therapy services. Furthermore, they provide almost one-third of individual and family therapy services and more than one-fourth of the therapy services to collateral others.

Finally, in terms of cost effectiveness we can examine Table 11-1, which shows that in the outpatient services the mental health worker provided 40% of service hours, yet salary costs were only 25% of manpower costs.

The data in Table 11-1 indicate that in the OCDMH delivery system the mental health worker provides a broad range of direct clinical services, is a major manpower component, is deployed in all the service delivery elements, and is a cost-effective source of manpower.

CONCLUSION: ADVANTAGES AND LIMITATIONS TO THE UTILIZATION OF MENTAL HEALTH WORKERS

We believe that we have developed and demonstrated a successful model for the institutionalized system-wide utilization of mental health workers. We believe that several factors account for our relative success in institutionalization:

1. The OCDMH administration has provided consistent support.
2. There has been an explicit administrative locus in the Training, Consultation, and Education Division for the ongoing development of the mental health worker program.
3. The service delivery system was originally organized and implemented in accord with community mental health principles that integrate new manpower concepts.
4. The overall deployment of mental health manpower in the system has been consonant with the full and appropriate utilization of mental health workers.
5. Attention has been given from inception to system-wide manpower issues so that explicit steps were taken to define and resolve system issues in the development of mental health worker personnel.
6. The Training, Consultation, and Education Division has had sufficient staff to provide system-wide consultation on program development, to monitor manpower utilization, to provide assistance in recruitment, and to provide both initial and ongoing training/education within the system boundaries.

We have found advantages of the mental health worker program to be as follows:

1. We can recruit unique persons on the basis of skill and experience.
2. We can deploy personnel on the basis of function.
3. We can enhance innovative community mental health service delivery.
4. We can achieve cost effective manpower distribution.

We have found the limits encountered to be as follows:

1. The current surplus of traditionally and highly trained and experienced persons has produced disadvantageous formal competition for available jobs with those with less formal education.
2. Mental health workers are not the complete answer to program innovation and cannot be expected to produce such programs.
3. Mental health workers with limited education and experience can be as shortsighted and chauvinistic as traditional professionals.
4. Mental health workers neither aspire nor work toward highly complex roles that would require extensive further education and experience.
5. Mental health workers need ongoing training to enhance their skills and abilities. We have found marked limitations to the repertoire of the person with very limited training, and we find that intensive initial training does not suffice over long-term career employment.

Finally, we wish to emphasize strongly the importance of a central Training, Consultation, and Education Division that is committed to *overall* manpower development for the system. The development of mental health worker personnel is *not* isolated from the system, but is an integral part of a coordinated manpower program. Thus, the strength of the system-wide manpower program gives strength and success to the mental health worker component.

In conclusion, we find that the utilization of mental health workers is a valuable and central aspect of the OCDMH service delivery system. We do not find the mental health worker concept a threat to established mental health professions, nor do we find it a panacea. We believe it is now the appropriate time to move beyond the rhetoric that attacks or glorifies the mental health worker concept; it is instead the time to accept this concept as a vital part of the larger fabric of community mental health services.

NOTE

[1] This work has been supported by Grant #5 T41 MH 12939 from the Paraprofessional Training Branch, National Institute of Mental Health.

REFERENCES

Albee, G. W. *Mental health manpower trends.* New York: Basic Books, 1959.

Alley, S., & Blanton, J. A study of paraprofessionals in mental health. *Community Mental Health Journal,* 1976, *12,* 151–160.

Andrade, S. J., & Burnstein, A. G. Social congruence and empathy in paraprofessional and professional mental health workers. *Community Mental Health Journal,* 1973, *9,* 388–397.

Arnhoff, F. N., Rubenstein, E. A., & Speisman, J. C. (Eds.). *Manpower for mental health.* Chicago: Aldine, 1969.

Baker, E. J. The mental health associate: One year later. *Community Mental Health Journal,* 1973, *9,* 203–214.

Bloom, B. L., & Parad, H. J. Values of community mental health center staff. *Professional Psychology,* 1977, *8,* 33–47.

Cowen, E. L. Primary prevention misunderstood. *Social Policy,* 1977, *7,* 20–27.

Cowne, L. J. Approaches to the mental health manpower problem: A review of the literature. *Mental Hygiene,* 1969, *55,* 176–187.

Dinitz, S., & Beren, N. Community mental health as a boundaryless and boundary-busting system. *Journal of Health and Social Behavior,* 1971, *12,* 99–108.

Egan, G. *The skilled helper.* Monterey, California: Brooks/Cole, 1975.

Figa-Talamanca, I. Problems in the evaluation of training of health personnel. *Health Education Monographs,* 1975, *3,* 232–250.

Fisher, W., Mehr, J., & Truckenbrod, P. *Human services: The third revolution in mental health.* New York: Alfred Publishing Co., 1974.

Gartner, A. *Paraprofessionals and their performance.* New York: Praeger, 1971.

Gottesfeld, H., Rhee, C., & Parker, G. A study of the role of paraprofessionals in community mental health. *Community Mental Health Journal,* 1970, *6,* 285–291.

Grosser, C., Henry, W. E., & Kelly, J. G. (Eds.). *Nonprofessionals in the human services.* San Francisco: Jossey-Bass, 1969.

Guerney, B. G. (Ed.). *Psychotherapeutic agents: New roles for non-professionals, parents, and teachers.* New York: Holt, 1969.

Guttentag, M., Kiresuk, T., Oglesby, M., & Cohn, J. *The evaluation of training in mental health.* New York: Behavioral Publications, 1975.

Halmos, P. (Ed.). Professionalization and social change. *Sociological Review Monographs.* 1973, *20.*

Hardcastle, D. A. The indigenous nonprofessional in the social service bureaucracy: A critical examination. *Social Work,* 1971, *16,* 56–63.

Hesse, K. The paraprofessional as a referral link in the mental health delivery system. *Community Mental Health Journal,* 1976, *12,* 252–258.

Jones, E. Social class and psychotherapy: A critical review of research. *Psychiatry,* 1974, *37,* 307–320.

Kalafant, J., & Borato, D. R. The paraprofessional movement as a paradigm community psychology endeavor. *Journal of Community Psychology,* 1977, *5,* 3–12.

Kaslow, F. W. (Ed.). *Issues in human services.* San Francisco: Jossey-Bass, 1972.

Lorian, R. P. Socioeconomic status and traditional treatment approaches reconsidered. *Psychology Bulletin,* 1973, *4,* 263–270.

Maierle, J. P. The politics of supporting paraprofessionals. *Professional Psychology,* 1973, *4,* 313–320.

Matarazzo, J. D. Some national developments in the utilization of nontraditional mental health manpower. *American Psychologist,* 1971, *26,* 363–371.

Moore, W. E. *The professions: Roles and rules.* New York: Russel Sage Foundation, 1970.

O'Donnell, E. J. The professional volunteer versus the volunteer professional. *Community Mental Health Journal,* 1970, *6,* 236–245.

Pattison, E. M. A differential view of manpower resources. In G. E. Staub & L. M. Kent (Eds.), *The paraprofessional in the treatment of alcoholism.* Springfield, Ill.: Charles C Thomas, 1973.

Pattison, E. M., & Elpers, J. R. A developmental view of mental health manpower trends. *Hospital and Community Psychiatry,* 1972, *23,* 325–328.

Pearl, A., & Riessman, F. (Eds.). *New careers for the poor.* New York: Free Press, 1965.

Reiff, R., & Riessman, F. The indigenous nonprofessional: A strategy for change in community action and community mental health programs. *Community Mental Health Journal Monograph,* 1965, No. 1.

Robin, S. S., & Wagenfeld, M. O. The community mental health worker: Organizational and personal sources of role discrepancy. *Journal of Health and Social Behavior,* 1977, *18,* 16–26.

Sarata, B. P. V. Job characteristics, work satisfactions, and task involvement as correlates of service delivery strategies. *American Journal of Community Psychology,* 1977, *5,* 99–109.

Sobey, F. *The nonprofessional revolution in mental health.* New York: Columbia University Press, 1970.

Wagenfeld, M. O., & Robin, S. S. Boundary busting in the role of the community mental health worker. *Journal of Health and Social Behavior,* 1976, *17,* 112–122.

Young, C. E., True, J. E., & Packard, M. E. A national study of associate degree mental health and human service workers. *Journal of Community Psychology,* 1976, *4,* 89–95.

Appendix A   Mental Health Worker Personnel Series

Level	Entry requirements	Salary per month
MHW I	Ability to read, write, and understand English. Ability to speak Spanish is required of some assignments. Appointments may be restricted to residents of specific areas or a member of a particular socioeconomic or cultural group.	$693–903
MHW II	Two years as a Mental Health Worker I for Orange County.	$881–1,177

Or

Education
Completion of an Associate of Arts degree in community resources, human services, behavioral sciences or other related field which has included field work experience.

Or

Experience
Two years of experience which would have provided one with a high degree of insight into individual or group problems such as delinquency, alcoholism, drug abuse, old age, or domestic relations and their effect on mental health. (College study may be substituted for the required experience on the basis of one year of college for six months of experience.)
Special Requirement: Ability to speak Spanish is required of some assignments. Appointment may be restricted to residents of a specific area or members of a particular socioeconomic or cultural group.

MHW III	Two years experience as a Mental Health Worker II for Orange County.	$981–1,312

Or

Education
Completion of an Associate of Arts degree in community resources, human services, behavioral sciences or other related field which has included field work experience. (Additional qualifying experience may be substituted for the required education on a year-for-year basis.)

Or

Experience
Two years of experience which would have provided one with a high degree of insight into individual or group problems such as

Level	Entry requirements	Salary per month
	delinquency, alcoholism, drug abuse, old age, or domestic relations and their effect on mental health. (Upper division college study in community resources, human services, behavioral sciences or other related field may be substituted for the required experience on a year-for-year basis.) *Special Requirement:* Ability to speak Spanish may be required for some assignments. Appointment may be restricted to residents of a specific area or members of a particular socio-economic or cultural group.	
MHW IV	Three years of experience as a Mental Health Worker III for Orange County. *Or* *Education*[a] Completion of a Bachelor of Arts degree in community resources, human services, behavioral sciences or other related field which has included field work experience. (Additional qualifying experience may be substituted for the required education on a year-for-year basis.) *Or* *Experience* Three years of experience which would have provided one with a high degree of insight into individual or group problems such as delinquency, alcoholism, drug abuse, old age, or domestic relations and their effect on mental health. (Graduate study in community resources, human services, behavioral sciences or other related field may be substituted for the required experience on a year-for-year basis.)	$1,277–1,719

[a] Some employees on the MHW IV level have MA degrees.

Appendix B Didactic Training Curriculum for Mental Health Worker I Trainees (One Year)

1. Clinical Interviewing
2. Humanizing Death and Dying
3. Responding to the Hostile Client
4. Helping Skills
5. How to Use the Psychosocial History and Treatment Plan in Counseling
6. Multiple Approaches to Psychotherapy
7. Differential Diagnosis
8. Group Process and Personal Development[a]
9. Psychiatric Medications for Nonphysicians
10. Introduction to Group Psychotherapy
11. Brief Family Intervention
12. Behavior Modification Techniques
13. Assertion Training
14. Rational Emotive Psychotherapy
15. Crisis Intervention
16. Working with the Aging
17. Life Styles of the Heroin Addict and Poly Drug Abuser
18. Treating Relationships

[a] All modules are for 10 weeks, 3 hours per week, except #8, which is ongoing throughout the program period.

Appendix C Mental Health Worker I—Training Program
Assessment of Demonstrated Competencies

Employees are rated by their supervisors on a 5-point dimension. When the supervisor is not able to rate the employee's performance, the note, "not applicable," is made. The five points on the dimension are: (a) unsatisfactory; (b) needs improvement; (c) average; (d) above average; and (e) outstanding. The competencies on which ratings are made are listed below.

1. Knowledge of abnormal behavior.
2. Knowledge of mental health vocabulary.
3. Knowledge of human growth and development.
4. Knowledge of mental health problems.
5. Familiarity with major issues in psychotherapy.
6. Knowledge of various techniques in psychotherapy.
7. Knowledge of sociocultural differences and crosscultural similarities in terms of individual and group functioning.
8. Knowledge of different methods for assessing sociocultural milieu.
9. Understanding of the structure and function of OCDMH.
10. Knowledge of community resources.
11. Ability to identify conflicts between individuals and within a larger association.
12. Ability to identify disordered behavior.
13. Ability to write case reports.
14. Ability to analyze case studies.
15. Ability to use various techniques in psychotherapy.
16. Ability for selective use of proper treatment modalities.
17. Ability to incorporate new skills.
18. Ability to critique and propose reforms about programs within OCDMH.
19. Ability to use both OCDMH and community resources effectively.
20. Demonstrated skills in indirect services.
21. Ability to use supervision as a teaching opportunity.
22. Ability to use supervision as administrative management.
23. Ability to function as a member of a team.
24. Awareness of own personal lifestyle.
25. Greater awareness of self.
26. Sensitivity with others.
27. Ability to evaluate self experiences to further own development.
28. Ability to evaluate own preferences for different treatment modalities.
29. Ability to evaluate self in comparison to past experiences.
30. Awareness of own involvement in group activities.

100s   GENERIC MENTAL HEALTH KNOWLEDGE (requires decision making)

01s   *Theoretical Knowledge*
101   Theories of Human Behavior
102   Psychodynamics
103   Psychopathology and Psychodynamics
104   Psychopathology: A Behavioral Perspective
105   Clinical Depression
106   Dreams: Function and Interpretation
107   Group Dynamics
108   Psychotic Reactions—An Overview
10s   *Technical Knowledge*
110   Medical Terminology
111   Psychiatric Medications for Nonphysicians

200s   GENERIC MULTIPHASIC TREATMENT SKILLS

201   Active Listening
202   Clinical Interviewing
203   The Function and Use of Role Playing in Counseling
204   Differential Diagnosis
205   How to Use the Psychosocial History and Treatment
206   Introduction to Group Psychotherapy
207   Short-Term Group Psychotherapy

300s   SPECIFIC THEORETICAL TREATMENT SKILLS

301   Brief Family Intervention
302   Advanced Brief Family Intervention Seminar
303   Behavior Modification Techniques
304   The Application of Behavior Modification to Case Work Practice
305   Assertion Training
306   Advanced Assertion Training
307   Rational Emotive Psychotherapy
308   Advanced Rational Emotive Therapy Seminar
309   Gestalt Therapy Techniques
310   The Use of Transactional Analysis (TA)
311   Helping Skills
312   Anxiety Reduction in Clinical Practice
313   Basic Patient Communication
314   Family Systems Therapy
315   Art Therapy

400s   POPULATION SPECIFIC TREATMENT SKILLS

01s   *Crisis Situation*
401   Crisis Intervention
402   Rape Crisis Intervention Counseling
403   Suicide
404   Handling the Hostile Client
405   Professional Treatment Skills in Alcoholism
406   Alcoholism Today—A New Look at an Old Problem
407   Identifying Addictions
408   Major Issues in Addictive Behaviors
409   Life-Styles of the Heroin Addict and Poly Drug Abuser

400s   POPULATION SPECIFIC TREATMENT SKILLS (continued)

   10s   *Deviant Populations*
   410   Serving Patients Released from Prison Systems
   411   Treatment of Child Abuse
   412   Introduction to the Treatment of Sexual Dysfunction
   413   Adolescent Drug Experience

   20s   *Developmental Disabilities*
   420   Introduction to Sign Language of the Deaf
   421   Advanced Sign Language of the Deaf
   422   Working with the Aging
   423   Humanizing Death and Dying
   424   Psychosocial and Vocational Implications of Hearing Impairments
   425   Introduction to Interpreting for Hearing Impaired Client

   30s   *Nonpsychiatric Populations*
   430   Introduction to Group Counseling for Women
   431   Advanced Group Counseling for Women
   432   Marital Therapy
   433   Cardiopulmonary Resuscitation

500s   ADJUNCTIVE NONCLINICAL SKILLS

   01s   *Planning and Evaluation*
   501   Systems Approach to Mental Health Planning
   502   Fiscal Program Management and Budgeting
   503   Effective Residential Care Management
   504   Introduction to Program Evaluation
   505   Introduction to Social Research Design and Statistical Measures
   506   Program Development and Education

   10s   *Process Functions*
   510   Clinical Supervision
   511   The Art of Consultation
   512   Consultation Procedures for School Counselors

   20s   *Forensic*
   520   Drug Abuse Laws and Resources

   30s   *Support Services for Nonclinical Staff*
   530   Productive Communication
   531   Creative Communication
   532   Practical Assertion Training

600s   PREVENTION-DIRECTED SKILLS

   01s   *School Involvement*
   601   Rational Emotive Education
   602   Advanced Rational Emotive Education Seminar
   603   Rational Self-Counseling with Children
   604   Promoting Mental Health in the Classroom

   10s   *Parenting Knowledge and Skills*
   610   Parenting: Emotional Growth and Behavioral Management
   611   How To Get Your Child To Do What You Want
   612   Step Parenting/Foster Child

   20s   *Community Organization*
   620   The Process of Change in the Community

THE ROLE OF A CONSULTATION AND EDUCATION PROGRAM IN PROMOTING COLLABORATION BETWEEN PROFESSIONALS AND PARAPROFESSIONALS AND BETWEEN AN URBAN COMMUNITY AND ITS MENTAL HEALTH CENTER

Bernard Bandler, MD*
Ruth M. Batson, EdM†
Lyda S. Peters, EdM‡

This chapter describes an unusual consultation and education program that serves as a vehicle for creating a collaborative relationship between a mental health center and the community that it serves. In this program, paraprofessionals function as full-time representatives of the community and play a vital role in making the collaborative outcome possible.

The chapter presents the history of the program and the theoretical assumptions on which the program is based. Major sections discuss the background and selection of the first director (an indigenous paraprofessional) and the details of how professionals and paraprofessionals have worked together both in providing services and in implementing in-service training programs. Other sections describe problems encountered by the

*Professor Emeritus of Psychiatry, Boston University School of Medicine, Boston, Massachusetts 02118

†Associate Professor of Psychiatry, Boston University School of Medicine; Principal Investigator, New Careers Training Program, Boston University Division of Psychiatry and Dr. Solomon Carter Fuller Mental Health Center, Boston, Massachusetts 02118

‡Assistant Professor of Psychiatry, Boston University School of Medicine; Project Director, New Careers Training Program, Boston University Division of Psychiatry and Dr. Solomon Carter Fuller Mental Health Center, Boston, Massachusetts 02118

new program and the factors that have contributed to its success. The chapter concludes with recommendations for similar programs in other settings. (The current operations of the program are described in more detail in chapter 5 of a companion volume, *Case Studies of Mental Health Paraprofessionals: Twelve Effective Programs.*)

The Consultation and Education (C & E) Program described in this article provides a viable and effective model for creating a collaborative relationship between the mental health center and the community that it serves. The community members and mental health center staff, personnel, and planners collaborated in the design and the delivery of services and as a result, the services are simultaneously relevant to the needs of the community and are well designed and delivered. As full-time representatives of the community, the paraprofessionals employed in the C & E Program have always been crucial in making this collaborative outcome possible.

The Consultation and Education Program began in 1970 as part of the Division of Psychiatry of the Boston University School of Medicine (Bandler, 1966). This program was under the auspices of the Commonwealth of Massachusetts Training, Treatment, and Research (Community Mental Health) Center. It is presently a program of the Dr. Solomon Carter Fuller Mental Health Center. The Fuller Mental Health Center serves an inner city catchment area in the South End, Back Bay, Roxbury, and Dorchester parts of Boston, Massachusetts. It maintains its affiliation with the Division of Psychiatry of the Boston University School of Medicine, although as a state-funded program, it is under the auspices of the Commonwealth of Massachusetts' Department of Mental Health. Many of the residents of the catchment area are members of black, Hispanic, and other minority groups, and many of the residents receive low incomes. Thus, the mental health center's professionals, for the most part, differ in cultural background from the residents of the catchment area. The C & E Program staff members have taught mental health skills to staff members of community organizations and have provided community education services. In addition, the C & E staff members have educated the Mental Health Center and Division of Psychiatry staff about the community and have provided direct services when these services have not been provided by other agencies in the catchment area.

This chapter describes the innovative C & E Program, focusing on its historical origins, the period when it began, the struggle to make it viable and a recognized service component of the Boston University Division of Psychiatry as one of the first mental health center programs, and its attempts to cement its recognition both within the community structure and mental health system. The chapter also outlines the contributions made and programs developed by the C & E staff of professionals and paraprofessionals, thereby illustrating that true collaboration between a community and its mental health center was achieved. The time period covered is primarily from January, 1970 (the date of the employment of the first C & E director) through 1975 (when the first director resigned). The initial section on history and function, however, includes a description of earlier planning processes.

It is important to include a word about definitions. For the purposes of this source book, paraprofessionals are defined as BA and sub-BA level service delivery personnel, excluding nurses. The C & E Program seldom uses the term "paraprofessional"; instead it refers to job classifications and titles such as community mental health worker (sub-BA level), community coordinators (sub-BA level and BA level), and social workers (BA level and above). For the purposes of this article, the concept of paraprofessional can be interchanged with descriptive phrases such as community mental health worker, new professional, new careerist.

The clearest distinction that can be made involves a degreed versus a non-degreed status; paraprofessional belongs in the latter group. This definition enables secretaries to be classified as paraprofessionals and makes them eligible for training programs and other activities to upgrade their responsibilities. A good deal of work was carried out within C & E to help each staff person recognize his/her contribution and importance as a member of the unit or team and subsequently, as a participating member of the total C & E staff. The inclusion of secretaries (who had their own unit within C & E) within the staff integration process, equalized the opportunity structure for all staff members. The secretaries, accordingly, participated in: in-service training; development of training seminars; tutoring; bilingual interpreter assignments; courses in psychology and social work; activities of the New Professionals of Massachusetts, Inc., special C & E projects. Some secretaries even became interns in some Boston University training programs and students in the Boston University New Careers Program. Because of this inclusive staff integration, some were upgraded to community mental health workers and classified as paraprofessional staff while still occupying secretarial positions.

THE HISTORY AND FUNCTIONS OF THE C & E PROGRAM

The Consultation and Education (C & E) Program was the first for which a federal grant application was submitted by the Boston University Commonwealth of Massachusetts Community Mental Health and Retardation Center (now the Dr. Solomon Carter Fuller Community Mental Health Center) in 1969. Planning for the center began in 1956 under the leadership of Bernard Bandler, MD, then professor and chairman of the Division of Psychiatry at the Boston University School of Medicine, in collaboration with the community, the state, the university, and the Division of Psychiatry. Federal and state funds had already been provided for a building in which some services would be located and which would be the major locus of training and research. The funding of the federal grant by the National Institute of Mental Health

(NIMH) enabled the staffing of the C & E Program to be carried out. A significant part of the C & E Program included the provision for the training and employment of neighborhood community mental health workers.

This Community Mental Health Center was envisaged as a coordinated series of programs designed to offer mental health services to the total community, which included both the inner city black community and a large Hispanic population. The center would provide services directly to individuals and to families, and indirectly to specific agencies (such as the Roxbury Multi-Service Center) and to broader institutions such as the school system, the health system, and the judicial penal system. The programs at the center would intersect with all agencies, organizations, and institutions which touched people's lives. Most people, it was hoped, would be helped through consultation and referral to those agencies and institutions by the provision of limited direct services within the framework of these organizations. Thus, most people would be helped without the need for referral to such mental health center programs as outpatient and inpatient services.

The Consultation and Education Program was thus seen as central to the Community Mental Health Center; the liaison network with and within the formal and informal structures for the community. Personnel from C & E would consult with people and organizations comprising the community structures, educate them about mental health, and in turn, be educated by them about their needs, problems and priorities. C & E would provide limited direct services within the framework of these structures, and would also serve as a major vehicle for communication and as a formal system of linkage between these community structures and the administration, the programs, and the services of the Mental Health Center. The program would function as a vital interface between the community and the center, as well as an information resource about the community to the rest of the center. Lastly, it was anticipated that C & E would play an important role in program development for and policy formation in the center because of its experience with and knowledge of the community. In light of their varied functions, the personnel of C & E would include: the traditional mental health professionals—psychiatrists, social workers, psychologists and nurses—as well as educators, epidemiologists, and community mental health workers.

The models of mental health made explicit in the application were conceived of as a complementary series. The first one was the traditional "medical model" of mental illness as illustrated by schizophrenia, manic depressive psychosis, and the organic psychoses. But within this model the focus of attention was directed to the individual as the person/in family/in social context. The person does not exist in isolation but rather is understood only within the confluence of the biological, psychological, and the societal perspectives. Even the so-called "medical model," as conceived by Dr. Bandler, took full account of the social structures and the societal processes.

The second model was the "developmental model." It views the individual from the perspective of the life span from birth unto death. Health is defined as an ideal, namely optimal growth, development and functioning. Illness is defined as failures in and disturbances of growth, development, and functioning. The individual does not develop in isolation according to this model. Individual development evolves within the processes and dynamics of family development, and family development resonates to the development and disturbances in the community. By disturbances of development in the community we have in mind the relative powerlessness of minority communities and the oppressive nature of the societal institutions which impinge upon and envelop the community. The "developmental model" is more comprehensive than the "medical model," but the two are complementary. The most inclusive model as stated in the application was the "ecological model." That model considers individuals, families and social context as a totality in their dynamic and mutual adaptations. It evaluates the total ecology in terms of human values, human living, and human satisfactions. The intramural services tend to fall under the medical-diagnostic treatment and the developmental model. The extramural activities and programs fall under the ecological model. The ecological model considers the major locus for mental health activities to be in the community and mental health to be inevitably linked with these overall factors: health, education, employment, the legal-penal system, recreation, religion, social and psychological welfare, community organization, planning and politics, housing, job training, and the problems of poverty and of urban and rural life. Therefore, all activities in some way are seen as impinging upon mental health.

The role of community mental health workers and their importance in the program originates from these conceptualizations and from the realities of minority communities. The Community Mental Health Centers Act of 1963, which provided for community mental health centers, sought to replace the geographically isolated and remote mental hospitals by community mental health centers which were geographically accessible to those people they hoped to serve. But availability, accessibility, and utilization are much more than a matter of geography. Geographical availability does not solve the problems caused by cultural and psychological availability and distance. Physical distance can be reduced by location. The psychological and cultural distances are untouched by location. Consequently, a mental health center located in a community may continue to be isolated and remote, an alien and colonial enclave in the midst of the community. It is crucial that the personnel of the center win the confidence and trust of the people in the community and that they appreciate their cultures, their languages, their history, their traditions, their life styles, and their customs. A well-trained professional does not automatically possess this knowledge; he must humbly acquire it and serve as apprentice to the community. Recognition of one's limitations and ignorance does not come easily to any of us, particularly in one's area of genuine competence, nor does it come easily to professionals. Since one of the functions of the community mental health workers was conceived of as that of educators of the professionals about the community, it may well be that an almost impossible task was assigned to them.

The community mental health workers had many roles. They were advocates of patients within the morass of systems such as welfare, housing, schools, legal-penal, health and employment in which people lived and through which they attempted to move. They educated people about the complexities of these systems including the mental health system, and facilitated their clients' passage through these systems. They helped people establish linkages to each other and to agencies and to institutions. And lastly, through their training, they were to provide some direct mental health services to individuals and to families.

It was important to remain aware of certain reality-based dangers for the community mental health workers. A danger was that they were embarking on dead-end careers. There is an excess of rhetoric about career ladders and about vertical and horizontal mobility. But the realities of effecting changes in university procedures on recognition and certification and of state and civil service job classification and salaries are formidable. The certificates given by some human service training programs are counterfeit currency which cannot be cashed when applying for a job. The C & E administrators discussed with different schools at Boston University the possibility of their collaboration in the programs so this assistance would increase the probability that the mental health workers upon graduation would have a valid degree. They discussed with the state the possibility of changing job classifications in mental health. But institutional change, even from within and when one has status is a slow and laborious task.[1]

In order for the community mental health workers effectively to teach the professionals with whom they work about the community, two conditions are necessary. First, mutual trust and respect must be established between paraprofessionals and professionals. And, secondly, the members of both groups must recognize that they have much to teach and to learn from each other. The professional must be aware of the limitations of his/her knowledge about the community and the handicaps of some of his/her attitudes. The community mental health worker, in many ways, is a professional about the community. But both arrogance and false elitism may well inhibit the professional's capacity to learn. Likewise, the community mental health worker must be aware of the genuine knowledge and skills of the professional in mental health. A failure to recognize this valid source of knowledge may well stand in the way of the community mental health worker and the professional mental health worker's potential collaborative efforts.

There is another barrier blocking the development of mutual trust and respect among the community mental health workers; here, the fault lies with the professional. That barrier is racism, existing both in the professional's personality and in society. In an ideal center both the selection of personnel relatively free of racism and education about racism are crucial responsibilities of top administrators and directors of programs. These outcomes do not always occur. Thus, racism and the reactions that it evokes are often recognized by members of the community, minority professionals, and community mental health workers. The community frequently deals with racism by confrontation. Potential clients of the center deal with racism by refusing to use it. But paraprofessional community mental health workers are confronted with a very different task. The members of the community are remarkably intuitive in their perception of the fact and behavior of racism. The recognition of the unconscious nature of some peoples' racism may help in the educational process of bringing it to awareness and of effecting change. To give this responsibility to community mental health workers in a setting in which they are in intimate contact with racism, and yet simultaneously are low people on the totem pole, is virtually an impossible task. One must develop mutuality of respect and of learning/teaching; these are necessary if worker and professional intend to learn from and collaborate with each other. If these conditions are not met, there is a great danger that all may go their separate ways.

The application for C & E was developed in collaboration with the advisory board of the center and with nine community organizations, including the South End Neighborhood Action Program, the Roxbury Multi-Service Center, and Model Cities (Bandler, 1969). Their staff and directors participated in all stages of its evolution, and their formal letters of approval accompanied the application. Throughout the application process there existed a genuine sharing of power.

Once the application was approved by the National Institute of Mental Health and funded, the crucial process of selecting personnel began. A selection committee was formed: half appointed by Dr. Bandler as chairman of the Division of Psychiatry, and half by the community. After deliberating, it was decided that each group would have an absolute veto. It takes half a minute to write this sentence; the process took almost half a year. The committee decided that excellence rather than academic degrees would be a requisite in choosing the director of the program. Thus the joint committee selected Mrs. Ruth Batson (later Professor Batson) as the director of C & E, and interviewed and approved all personnel of the program, including Ms. Lyda Peters as director of training (later director of New Careers), until Dr. Bandler reached the age of retirement at Boston University.

One final word about the Division of Psychiatry—although the division was in favor of many features at the center, it was sharply divided about community psychiatry. Many equated community psychiatry with social action which they felt was beyond the knowledge and skills of the psychiatrist. A carefully planned conference failed to resolve the differences (Foley, 1972). The issue of racism was not confronted nor was the false arrogance of professionalism, and the snobbery of elitism (Alvarez, Batson, Carr, Parks, Peck, Shervington, Tyler, & Zwerling, 1976). The issue of racism had been taken up on one occasion by the community board when it discussed the Kerner Report on Civil Disorders.[2] The discussion became heated and almost tore the board apart. The board continued to function effectively after that but the topic of racism was avoided for quite some time. For many of the medical school, the process of winning the trust of the black and Hispanic communities, of understanding them, and of working together with them remained a problem for the future. The psychological and cultural barriers remained largely intact.

Some Background on the First Director of the C & E Program

Mrs. Ruth Batson formally entered the mental health field via the C & E Program and the Division of Psychiatry as the first black woman without an undergraduate or graduate degree to administer a major federally funded grant under the auspices of Boston University Division of Psychiatry. An additional feature was that she was the first such person to enter this type of system as a tenured associate professor of psychiatry. Dr. Bernard Bandler requested approval by the school of medicine for Mrs. Batson to be in this position so that Mrs. Batson, and the C & E Program, would not exist in isolation within the medical school or the Division of Psychiatry. Dr. Bandler felt that it was essential that the status and power that accompany a high academic appointment be given to her to assure the credibility of C & E and insure Mrs. Batson's leadership position within Boston University. Dr. Bandler was eager to avoid the possibility that C & E would be isolated within the division and shoved off in one corner. He felt that it was necessary to provide optimal conditions for her effective functioning as the director of C & E through the associate professor appointment.

Mrs. Batson became active in community life because of her concern for her children's education. She made a complaint to the Boston branch of the National Association for the Advancement of Colored People (NAACP) and began her career as an activist in behalf of quality education for black children. This educational struggle quickly broadened to include other issues that impinged on the lack of educational opportunity (housing, employment, and adequate income), and she became vocal in the political life of the Commonwealth of Massachusetts and the city of Boston. These activities resulted in her appointment as a commissioner on the Massachusetts Commission Against Discrimination (MCAD), a board which received complaints of discrimination and attempted to resolve them. In 1966 a voluntary urban-suburban busing program was established and called METCO, the Metropolitan Council for Educational Opportunity. She left the MCAD to take the position of associate director of METCO and within a year she became the METCO director. Her educational background included elementary school, high school, and two years of post high school work in preschool education and several courses toward a BA degree. She served on numerous committees, lectured widely, and taught many seminars.

Mrs. Batson had had very little contact with practitioners in the mental health field. As a child, her mother used to refer to Mattapan, the location of the state hospital, in ominous tones. Therefore, she was not only ignorant of what this resource could offer, but also fearful of it, as most persons were. Her work with inner city children forced her to take a closer look at mental health services.

Mrs. Batson had many experiences that led her to conclude that persons such as she needed to be instrumental in teaching professionals about the viewpoints and concerns of the community. For instance, if a black child had any difficulty within the METCO program, no matter how slight, he/she was sent to the school psychologist. In too many cases, the psychologist displayed stereotypic thinking and as the director of METCO, she found herself in a major teaching role. The following dialogue demonstrates the tendency of the psychologist to ascribe school problems to personal and family factors rather than to social conditions.

Psychologist: This child is having difficulty with math.
Batson: This is one of the reasons parents are busing their children —they feel their children have not received a good education.
Psychologist: His disability is most severe. Is his father living at home?
Batson: If I tell you he is or he is not, how will that influence your treatment?
Psychologist: (Silence.)

Also, she came up against the waiting list syndrome. There were children and parents who needed immediate help, and yet the waiting list was a constant and impenetrable barrier. And, in cases where there were sensitive, knowledgeable, and open-minded mental health professionals, one could find no evidence that this knowledge was being transferred to the people with whom they worked —teachers, principals, counselors. For example, there was a question on the METCO questionnaire concerning the child's medical condition and use of medication. This information was included in folders sent to the schools. One student was epileptic and this was stated along with medical instructions. Her condition was under control. The student did not have seizures. The principal of her school called Mrs. Batson to say that he had just read the girl's folder and he could not keep her in the program because of her *mental* condition, referring to the fact that she was epileptic. Mrs. Batson was shocked to discover that a man could go through the educational process long enough to acquire two degrees, be appointed administrator of a school and display this kind of ignorance.

After four years with METCO, Mrs. Batson applied for the position as director of the Consultation and Education Program. She was interviewed by four experienced community people, all of whom lived in the area serviced by the Community Mental Health Center and all of whom were black. Since she was well-known, she sensed that the community screening committee felt it necessary to subject her to strict scrutiny so that if she became the candidate for the director's position, the decision would be based on talent and suitability for the job rather than reputation. While she sensed a clear determination to show no partiality, she felt no hostility and was quite at ease during the interview. Shortly afterwards, she was notified that the community screening committee recommended her to the professional section of the search committee.

She was much more apprehensive about her appearance before the professional screening committee because she had no academic credentials and would be facing an all-white professional group of psychologists and psychiatrists. Her expectations about how the interview would be conducted were the same as with the community screening committee—a group of interviewers would assess her qualifications and discuss with her ideas about the new program position. Instead, she was subjected to a relay type of questioning. One or two individuals were present; when these individuals would leave, others would take their places. She became very ill at ease.

She was drained when she left the interview and felt that the professional committee did not find her qualified. No questions had been raised about her lack of a degree, but one man did question the wisdom of a woman handling this job. So it was with surprise that she received the news that she was being recommended by the combined screening committees for an interview with Dr. Bandler who would make the final decision. After meeting with him, she felt that she would be offered the position; however, she still remembered the professional screening committee's interview and the hostility that she sensed during it. The guts of this job involved the ability to bring together degreed and non-degreed people in a constructive and productive working arrangement. In order to accomplish this objective some of those very people on the professional screening committee would have to be involved and she would need their help and cooperation. They had many things to learn and unlearn about the catchment area population and she needed to learn about treatment resources and methods. They also spoke a strange technical language with which she was unfamiliar. Mrs. Batson did not feel equal to this position and decided not to accept.

She called Dr. Bandler and told him of her decision, and they agreed to meet again. It was at this meeting that he informed her of his plans to undergird her position with a faculty appointment and an appointment to the Division of Psychiatry policy committee. Because she felt sure of his support, she decided to accept the position as director of C & E.

In accepting the position she hoped to accomplish the following goals. (a) To develop a group of workers who, with new skills, could not only answer a manpower service need but would also be sensitive to the issues and problems of the community. These workers would engage in mutual sharing of information and teaching with their degreed co-workers for the greater good of the client. (b) To work with the professionals who were already well-established in the system toward the objective of seriously reexamining their treatment methods, their attitudes, and the effect of their biases and stereotypes on the community they were being paid to serve. (c) To educate the community members about their rights under the mental health system, to assist them through the mental health service maze, and to help them evaluate the services they were receiving. (d) To eliminate the fears and stereotypes that surround mental health treatment and mental illness in the community. It is important to raise the consciousness and improve the awareness of the community concerning those individuals who are emotionally ill and retarded. Too often, these persons are viewed as strange and odd. (e) To eliminate isolated, individual treatment as the only kind of therapy. This kind of treatment ignores the many issues which influence daily living—poor housing, unemployment, inferior education, racism, sexism, and ageism.

THE SELECTION PROCESS FOR STAFF MEMBERS AFTER THE APPOINTMENT OF THE FIRST DIRECTOR

The community screening committee and professional screening committee eventually merged and continued to screen candidates. Mrs. Batson and Dr. Bandler were given veto power over a selection. This arrangement meant that she could not hire a candidate the committee did not recommend; simultaneously she was not forced to accept a recommendation that she did not support.

Because of the recruiting process and state bureaucracy, it was one full year before C & E had a complete staff; this group consisted of about 45 people from a variety of disciplines and backgrounds. The problems inherent in recruiting, screening, selecting, and hiring were serious. The interviewing/screening/selecting process could take as long as three weeks. Once a candidate was approved by the community, the professional screening committees, and by the director, he/she had to be approved by the State Department of Mental Health (DMH). Papers had to be formally submitted to DMH where they went through a series of reviews and were returned to us approved, disapproved, or for further information. This process could take as long as six weeks. There appeared to be more difficulty having professional staff approved and classified than paraprofessional staff. This we can probably attribute to the fact that there was only one job classification—Special Service Assistant—available at that time for paraprofessional community mental health center staff members. Thus, all our paraprofessional staff started in the same job classification and same beginning pay step regardless of past experience. It would take from six weeks to two months to have a professional employee approved and classified in a pay slot agreeable to both the employee and the Department of Mental Health. And then it took an additional six weeks before he/she received the first paycheck. As a result of this cumbersome, time-consuming process, the C & E Program lost some good potential staff members. However, those persons that were hired gained a firsthand understanding of the problems inherent in the state bureaucracy and a solid feeling for consumers of the service area, who themselves must look to this same system for fulfillment of basic survival needs.

About half of the staff was black and most of these individuals worked as paraprofessional community mental health workers and secretaries. The program started with one black psychiatrist and a black nurse who left after a year to take a position in another department and a position in another city respectively. The director was conscious of the growing Hispanic population and attempted to attract Hispanic workers. Two Hispanic secretaries, two Hispanic psychologists, two Puerto Rican community mental health workers, and one Puerto Rican psychiatrist (who had interned with the program for a year) were recruited. The majority of the paraprofessional community mental health workers had had no formal experience in the mental health field, but most had volunteered or worked in the human services area. Most of the psychiatrists were white, had worked previously for Boston University Division of Psychiatry, and were recruited because of their specialties. For example, one psychiatrist was a child psychiatrist who had a joint appointment with the Division of Psychiatry and the School of Education and who was already consulting within the Boston schools. It was hoped that he would facilitate collaboration with the School of Education. Another psychiatrist was recruited because he was an expert on epidemiology and evaluation who had previously been the recipient of a five-year NIMH award for career research. Two of the social workers had worked for the State Department of Public Welfare and two other professionals had recently received their graduate degrees. The ages of the staff ranged from 21 to 50. While the staff members lived throughout the entire catchment area, the majority of the professional staff members lived outside the catchment area.

With the staff beginning to grow, the director now had to turn her attention towards the determination of goals and implementation of program development efforts. She assessed the varied talents, skills, and educational backgrounds of the staff members, knowing that they had to become *advocates* for the community.

SOME UNIQUE STRATEGIES USED BY C & E STAFF

The staff, which consisted of community mental health workers, psychiatrists, psychologists, and social workers, began its exploratory work with the community by visiting community agencies, introducing themselves and describing the new program, and meeting with neighborhood street committees, parent groups, and nonstructured groups in the catchment area. Simultaneously, these types of meetings were taking place within the Division of Psychiatry in an attempt to assess available resources, and to develop strategies that would break down barriers within the departments which appeared to be most resistant. These initial explorations emphasized to the staff the necessity for immediately responding to the needs raised by the community. As a result, the community mental health workers, whose knowledge of their own community was an undisputed valuable asset, and the professionals, with their diagnostic and treatment expertise, could develop a partnership of service that became not only innovative but effective as well.

Unit and Team Structure

Members of the C & E Program staff were assigned to one or more of four center-based units or to one of four community-based teams. Core staff, research and evaluation, education, and children's services units functioned in administrative and coordination capacities. The catchment area was divided into four subareas, and interdisciplinary staff consisting of community mental health workers, educators, psychiatrists, psychologists, social workers, and graduate students were located in team offices within these four areas. These staff groupings consisted of professionals and community mental health workers from the C & E staff. These teams were located in the South End of Boston, Lower Roxbury, and Roxbury-North Dorchester. A back-up team served as a liaison between the area teams and (a) the Division of Psychiatry and (b) Mental Health Center facilities, where direct services were provided. The back-up team was also responsible for C & E activities for the Back Bay area of Boston.

The teams were organized on a geographic basis; community mental health workers who resided in a particular area were assigned to the team located in their area on the theory that their knowledge of the area was an important and needed skill. Hispanic staff members were assigned to the teams for geographic areas with large Hispanic populations. An attempt was made to provide each team with a diversity of staff skills, depending upon the needs of the area. For example, staff interested in programs for children were assigned to an area needing special services for children. When the problems of the elderly became visible in the South End of Boston, the team serving that area was assigned a worker who had demonstrated a special interest and expertise in the problems of the elderly. All teams had a social worker, a psychiatrist, community mental health workers, and, in some cases, a psychologist, depending on the program needs of the team.

Once staff assignments had been made, a team leader was elected. This position carried extra responsibility with no additional pay. No one wanted the job; however, no members escaped serving as team leader, for leadership rotated on a monthly basis. This arrangement was another example of the sharing of power and responsibility by professionals and paraprofessionals. In the beginning, the MD's especially resented their stint as team leaders because they considered it a waste of their time. Even though there were administrative difficulties with team leadership, the process provided good learning experiences. It proved that the program provided equal assignments to staff members, regardless of job titles. Also, it gave the professionals an opportunity to work and learn under the direction of community mental health workers. And, it provided the paraprofessionals with opportunities for the development of new skills.

The Provision of Direct Services by C & E Teams

Even though the mandate of the program was consultation and education, staff members realized that without direct service delivery C & E would be ineffective. The first project developed within the C & E Program demonstrates how an interdisciplinary team can respond as a group with integrity to a specific community need for both direct and indirect services. A C & E team, which was placed in the Model Cities Family Life Center in the Roxbury section of the catchment area, was composed of two paraprofessional mental health workers, one social worker and a social work student, one full-time adult psychiatrist, and one half-time child psychiatrist. There was some initial resistance to the team by the director of the center because he wanted assurance that the professional members of the team (the psychiatrists and social worker) would be available at all times to the Model Cities Family Life Center staff for referrals. In meeting with Family Life Center staff they discovered that many of the referrals were inappropriate and that training was needed so that staff could use their time more productively.

In a meeting with the community board of the Family Life Center, they found great concern over the number of children who were excluded from school either through suspension, expulsion, or a variety of other reasons. These children were reported to be five to six years old. Further discussion with the Family Life Center board, staff, and the C & E team resulted in the decision that a morning group be established for these children. This effort was one of the first collaborative efforts between the C & E Program and the community.

The program was called the Excluded Child Project. The community mental health workers began looking for these children and found that contrary to the opinion of the community board, the greatest need for such a group was demonstrated by boys and girls between the ages of 12 to 14. A meeting of all parties involved led to the decision that C & E would respond to the need expressed by the greater number of people. The first group consisted of seven boys and three girls who met three mornings a week from 10:00 a.m. to 12:00 noon. A community worker acted as a liaison with the parents and soon a parents' group was organized. This group met with the community worker and the psychiatrist. The child psychiatrist served as a consultant to the project. A special education teacher was hired by C & E to work with the students. As a result, many of the parents who had problems with their children within the Boston school system requested support in an effort to keep their children in school and in sensitizing teachers, school adjustment counselors, and principals to the needs of the children. The team responded to these requests, and, as a result, other programs developed which made use of the interdisciplinary resources of the C & E Program.

Thus, what was demonstrated by this team was their capacity to identify a need and then address the problem with a strategy that combined direct services with the consultation and education process. In addition to consulting and developing training seminars for Family Life Center staff, the team provided time-limited therapy for children and families, tutored students, and provided individual and group counseling services to families of the excluded child.

Problems Confronting the New C & E Program

One of the first problems to be faced by the new C & E Program involved dealing with the biased and cumbersome set of state civil service rules and regulations. The C & E Program was federally funded with matching funds from the state. Because of her previous experience as a state employee, Mrs. Batson asked to be paid by Boston University, because she knew that her lack of academic credentials would not qualify her by civil service standards to be the director of C & E. All other staff members were paid, fully or in part, by the State Department of Mental Health. This arrangement led to a protest by the Department of Mental Health stating that a non-state employee could not direct a program staffed by state employees. In the absence of any clear rule concerning this question the issue was not pursued. State job slots had to be matched by unrealistic and unnecessary academic requirements. Thus, good candidates were lost in the process.

The procedure for payment of salaries was so slow that new employees found themselves waiting for as long as eight weeks for their first check. All C & E workers were classified as "temporary" workers. (This arrangement is not unusual in Massachusetts, since many state workers remain on a temporary list for a number of years before becoming "permanent.") As a result, insurance and sick benefits were never clearly defined, and workers were in a constant state of confusion about the amount of the paycheck each week. These problems nearly killed the program before it got off the ground. Mrs. Batson approached Dr. Bandler and requested that a fund be established from which no-interest loans could be made to the employees until they were paid. This very practical recognition of a serious need allowed the program to employ good people whose financial situation might have prevented them from working for C & E. At no point was this fund ever misused or violated.

Resentment toward the program from other components of the Mental Health Center became our next serious problem. Other program directors felt that the first proposal request for funding for Mental Health Center programming should have been for direct services to relieve the seriously overtaxed staff and facility needs. Furthermore, they feared that the C & E Program would, by its community activities, create more work and frustration at a time when the Mental Health Center could not meet the resulting demand for services. Soon the C & E Program became referred to as "Pandora's Box." Some of this resentment was directed toward the director. She was resented partially because of her appointment to the executive committee of the Division of Psychiatry and her associate professorship appointment without "proper credentials." These two appointments stated clearly to the faculty and the community that the C & E Program should be recognized equally with other psychiatry divisional programs.

Dr. Bandler's retirement posed another problem. The program officially opened the first week in January, 1970, and Dr. Bandler was to retire in June. He was viewed as the C & E Program's main support, and the prospect of his leaving was disturbing. The "young" C & E staff felt very alone and insecure. Dr. Bandler was succeeded by Dr. Sanford Cohen as chairman of the Division of Psychiatry and superintendent of the Mental Health Center, and the C & E Program found that the support was maintained. New leadership for the Division of Psychiatry did not dilute the support for C & E. However, it had to be recognized that a new chairman had many things to occupy his time including the need to strengthen his own base of operation. C & E was forced by circumstances to come of age and assume the major responsibility for resolving the internal problems which existed between C & E and other programs within the Mental Health Center and the Division of Psychiatry.

The C & E Program began by making its presence felt in every phase of the planning by the Mental Health Center, as well as in all aspects of the operation of the Division of Psychiatry. All Division of Psychiatry meetings relating to mental health service delivery were attended by representatives from C & E, professionals as well as paraprofessionals; and staff members were assigned to every planning or operational group, depending on their interest and expertise. If C & E staff were not invited, they called and asked for an opportunity to participate; although this procedure caught people offguard, the C & E staff members were never refused. It was a very difficult period because people who had gone so long unchallenged in a very traditional institution seemed to receive even the most innocent question as a serious rebuke.

In spite of many problems it was decided by the C & E staff members that working in concert with the other components of the Mental Health Center and the Division of Psychiatry on common problems was the best way to proceed. They also recognized that the division was another community with needs to be assessed and with concerns regarding how their community structure would function during these changes. While making these overtures, C

& E had to be certain that its own internal structure was functioning in good order. The professionals who worked in C & E had been trained in a very traditional structure. It was naive to believe that similar conflicts would not have to be faced within C & E. These issues were addressed both through the C & E training unit and the team concept.

TRAINING OF STAFF MEMBERS AS COMMUNITY EDUCATORS

The C & E education unit, one of the four original C & E administrative units, played a significant role in assisting professionals and paraprofessionals to work together in a complementary fashion, and this unit is perhaps one of the best examples of collaboration. Training and education for the Consultation and Education Program were conceived and planned for in the original C & E grant. The original approach to training was to include all levels of staff— from the community mental health worker to the professional postgraduate worker. C & E was viewed as a unitary concept but consultation was not seen as identical to education. Consultation consisted of providing suggestions on alternative courses of action. Education, in contrast, was viewed more as a process in which the staff members participated in both introducing and initiating innovative and relevant programs with agencies already receiving consultation services from C & E. The education unit helped to prepare paraprofessional and professional staff members for educational functions.

The limitations in the original grant application involved the conceptualization of the community mental health worker's educational role. For example, it was proposed that C & E educate its own cadre of paraprofessionals who would, in turn, become teachers and trainers of larger groups of paraprofessionals outside of C & E. The question then may be posed as to why they were limited only to the training of other paraprofessionals when, in actuality, they were to become valuable teachers and trainers to educators, psychiatrists, psychologists, social workers, graduate and undergraduate students, medical students, community agency staff, and nurses. These conceptual limitations were overcome mainly because the C & E director, as well as the director of the C & E educational unit, were not entrenched in psychiatric views about mental health training and education; thereby freeing them to develop community mental health worker roles equally to that of professional roles within C & E.

The director of the education unit held an EdM degree with no psychiatric training and developed the training program by asking: What does one need to know when beginning in the mental health field? From this frame of reference, seminars, site visits, and presentations by invited guests were established for all new workers, both professional and paraprofessional. Both groups needed to learn about the other's systems; more of an emphasis was placed on the institutional network of services for the paraprofessional community mental health workers while the professionals' needs were more in the area of community programs and community resources. The training priorities and content of the C & E Program were developed within the education unit. Trainers were recruited from the C & E staff depending on the skills that were needed as the programs were developed. Professionals and paraprofessionals all participated in training, both as teachers and learners. Both the Division of Psychiatry and the catchment area itself were used as training laboratories. For example, orientation of new staff members included visits to the outpatient department's intake and teaching seminars, tours of state hospitals, visits to community agencies, and meetings with community representatives.

As the education unit evolved within C & E, the goals became clear and distinct. They were three-fold: (1) in-service—to educate and sensitize the staff members, both professional and paraprofessional, about the mental health needs of the catchment area residents, and to give the staff sufficient knowledge and skills to meet these needs; (2) community—to educate the catchment area residents about the entire mental health system, its resources, strengths, and weaknesses, and to aid appropriate agency personnel in developing training programs within their agencies to meet with agencies' particular needs; (3) Boston University Medical Center and university—to involve the Boston University Medical Center staff members and university students who work with community residents in an educational program about community culture and mental health.

Some Examples of Collaboration in Training and Education Between Professional and Paraprofessional Mental Health Workers

Training and education are important vehicles through which opposing groups can engage in meaningful dialogue. In doing so, these four generic mental health skills might be developed: establishing relationships, establishing trust, communicating, and understanding. These are four processes that professionals cannot carry on in most urban communities unless they are working in middle-class environments. The people who can establish trust and meaningful relationships are those who live in the community being served and who know the community, its history, and problems. Professionals have a certain body of knowledge and skills relating to mental health service delivery but it is ineffective without the four generic mental health skills. A vital part of C & E is to deliver quality, innovative services to the community, and to instruct professionals about community needs, problems, and issues. We will give examples of how this goal can be accomplished effectively and collaboratively.

1.   The in-service training seminars for the C & E staff members gave everyone an opportunity to share their skills, knowledge, and expertise. Most

of the training seminars were created by staff for staff. Seminars on human growth and development and on mental health consultation techniques were taught by psychiatrists, and these seminars were attended by community mental health workers, secretaries, social workers, and other professional staff. Social workers were given the opportunity to share their unique skills through seminars on community organization, interviewing skills, and casework, which were attended by psychiatrists, community mental health workers, and other staff members. The paraprofessional community mental health workers taught seminars on agencies and community organizations, drug education, and the history of the catchment area; these seminars were attended by the professional staff. Other members of the staff, both BA level and master's level (educators, research assistants, etc.), taught seminars in their particular areas of interest including urban crisis, community crisis intervention, non-verbal communication, religion and mental health, the exceptional child and his parents.

2.   Soon the seminars were opened to community agencies, so another dimension was added to the learning and teaching milieu. We began to experience education taking place among paraprofessional mental health workers, community agency staff, and professional mental health workers. C & E sponsored two seminars, entitled respectively Black and Puerto Rican Culture Series for the C & E staff, the Division of Psychiatry, and community agencies. The six individuals who organized this series included: a psychiatrist, educators, community mental health workers, and a psychologist. Faculty and staff of the Boston University Division of Psychiatry and staff members from community agencies attended; the C & E staff functioned as an interface between these two groups and facilitated for the first time in a formal setting an educational interchange between them.

3.   Collaboration in training between the C & E Program and other departments within the Division of Psychiatry added still another dimension to the relationship between the professional and the paraprofessional. Collaboration between the Department of Child Psychiatry and the C & E Program was demonstrated through the psycho-education unit and the infant development unit, with their respective internship programs. Through the use of observation, practicum experience, and supervision, the interns, who were paraprofessionals from C & E, were trained to become more sensitive observers of children's behavior and more competent at implementing basic psychological test procedures and treatment techniques uniquely suited to assist the learning disabled child and the infant at risk. Interns, furthermore, received more general training in classroom teaching, tutoring, cognitive strategies, interviewing techniques, counseling techniques, and early detection of developmental difficulties. Paraprofessionals from C & E participated as the first interns to these two programs and they were soon followed by graduate students from other departments within the university. This effort marked the beginning of inclusion of paraprofessionals in interdisciplinary training within the Division of Psychiatry and the Mental Health Center.

4.   Further collaboration was demonstrated by a federally funded project for paraprofessional training within the Division of Psychiatry and the Mental Health Center. Entitled New Careers in Mental Health, this program was one of the 11 originally federally funded projects within the Mental Health Center. The program existed for five years; its accomplishments included:

1.   The recruitment and training of over 57 community mental health workers, mainly from minority groups; these workers received associate of arts degrees from Boston University. One half of this group continued their education and have since received either undergraduate (BA level) degrees, or graduate degrees in law, education, social work, and counseling.
2.   The employment of 87% of these community mental health workers in positions within the Division of Psychiatry, the Mental Health Center, or community human service agencies as social workers, education coordinators, counselors, intake coordinators, associate directors of community mental health center programs, community coordinators, community health workers, therapists, and group workers.
3.   The provision of new skills and new services for the mental health center catchment area with a particular emphasis on involving community residents in the training itself, in the design of services, and in the evaluation of the training and services.
4.   The initiating of innovative training programs, focusing on community service and interdisciplinary methods. These programs include a special training and service component in community crisis intervention (Batson & Peters, 1976).

CONCLUSION

In many ways, the Consultation and Education Program is a distinctive community mental health enterprise. It values and facilitates initiative on the part of its staff members in the conception, formalization, and actualization of its various programs. There is sufficient space within its structure for all staff members to function cohesively and collaboratively. It encourages learning and teaching across disciplines, highlighting the unique contributions of the community mental health worker/paraprofessional staff. Because of the extraordinary depth and seriousness of the staff as a whole, its commitment to the community and its impressive support structure, C & E encourages a continual process of individual as well as group self-evaluation.

Because of the serious problems between professionals and paraprofessionals in community mental health programs and comparable organizations, the goal of mutual education espoused by the C & E Program and the procedures undertaken to meet this goal are particularly significant. C & E attempted to eliminate the restrictive nature of a hierarchically labeled and conceptualized staff through cooperative program planning for the community. The results were a considerable disregard for the limitations often imposed on individual strength and creativity by traditional labeling and an unusual support structure evident in the organization.

The C & E model of staff development and collaboration between the community and the Mental Health Center, between the professional and paraprofessional staff members, and between C & E and other programs within Boston University Division of Psychiatry and the Mental Health Center may be easily transferable to a mental health center that is not associated with an academic setting. The basic strategies and central ideas are: (a) a genuine sharing of power between the community being served and the professional community; (b) a genuine acknowledgement of factors that impede quality service delivery such as racism and elitism and a conscious effort to ameliorate these problems; and (c) the implementation of staffing patterns that reflect the service needs and the populations of the particular community through a strong representation of both indigenous and paraprofessional community mental health workers and knowledgeable and sensitive professional staff. The major difference between the two settings, a community mental health center in an academic setting and one that is not associated with an academic setting, is that there would probably be less teaching and research in the latter. If staff members want to move up a career ladder, however, the program must be affiliated, directly or indirectly, with an educational institution that provides academic credit for work-related learning experiences.

Staff cohesiveness and collaboration were most clearly illustrated during the occurrence of outside conflict having a negative impact on issues involving the community or the sensitive and politically aware C & E staff. Such confrontations brought the C & E staff closer together in developing strategies and planning alternatives. It was not unusual to see one or two staff psychiatrists arguing some point in strategy or negotiation with a community mental health worker and then accepting the method suggested after being convinced it was the better alternative. When the staff went public before a university official or administrator at the higher levels of the university or the hospital, it always presented a united front. A psychiatrist might be the spokesperson, when appropriate, or the community mental health worker might assume the leadership role. This staff averaged about 45 people, and it was not unusual to see all 45 sitting in at the vice-president's office, circulating position papers with signatures of the entire staff and others within the division who chose to join forces with them, sending telegrams to political representatives at the local and national level, and confronting the state bureaucracies in welfare, mental health, and human services. The primary issue confronted at all times was that of white racism, which permeated the systems with which the staff members came in contact. Both white and minority staff, whether professional or paraprofessional, joined forces in an attempt to eradicate this cancer. Thus, it can be accurately stated that if a sensitive and knowledgeable staff is selected by a program, and educated about the issues of the community, collaboration among professionals, paraprofessionals, and a community can be more effectively accomplished.

Boston University, the medical school, and the Division of Psychiatry were all affected by the C & E Program and its staff. They were exposed to new views and different methods of handling confrontations. This process helped to put community people on their boards of trustees for the first time. C & E attempted to bring about institutional change as the issue of institutional racism was raised loud and strong. Rather than being pacified, C & E facilitated community demands on Boston University and the division, and assisted the community in identifying and becoming aware of services that they deserved within the institutional structure of the medical center.

Recommendations

Collaboration must begin at the outset of the program—from design through the implementation stages. There has to be a real sharing of power between the community and professionals. Our collaboration began early in the planning stages of the C & E grant when the chairman of the Division of Psychiatry approached community agencies for assistance in developing and approving the grant. It continued through the recruitment and selection stages of the program with an actual sharing of power between two screening committees. The community screening committee was a well-paid group, not volunteer. The professional screening committee conducted their screening during working hours and received salaries from the division at the same time. Because of the seriousness of purpose of the two groups, the program reaped the benefits. Politically sensitive and aware professionals were recruited and hired. Although they needed special types of education, they were educable because the community screening committee selected appropriate professionals. The selection process is crucial. Unnecessary requirements should be eliminated and one must recruit personnel based on competencies, skills, and knowledge, not necessarily credentials. That was the successful aspect for this program.

Support for the program in the early days is essential and can be demonstrated by: faculty appointments for key staff, assignments to important policy and program committees, and open and declared support by key professionals for a nontraditional approach to developing innovative programs which respond to community needs. Institutional status as respected faculty members should be given to psychiatrists and other professionals who choose to work in a community mental health program. As service staff members in a C & E Program, they should be viewed by administrators within medical schools as equal in status to those faculty members who work in research and teaching capacities. Often, if a psychiatrist was hired for this program, he was viewed with some skepticism by his colleagues in other departments because of his "community" psychiatry status. Some psychiatrists would consequently spend time in divisional activities in order to prove their competencies in areas other than community psychiatry.

Overt administrative support sometimes alienates other programs if it continues too long. At some point, that type of support must gradually be reduced from running interference to a kind of maintenance support. When this outcome is possible, a program has reached its full potential and own level of maturity.

One must recognize the Mental Health Center as a culture with fears, resistances, ignorances, strengths, and weaknesses. C & E should view itself as a consultant and educator to this institutional community also. Active participation by C & E staff in all phases of Mental Health Center operations should take place, and if not invited the program should volunteer to participate. This should take place simultaneously with community and agency C & E activities.

Administrators and staff must face all problems openly, uncomfortable, political, or otherwise, that arise from within and from without the program. It should be recognized that both the degreed as well as non-degreed workers bring certain biases and stereotypes with them. This fact must be confronted directly through working together, sharing resources and information, and in mutual learning and teaching situations.

The team concept is a very important factor because it gives smaller groups of interdisciplinary staff an opportunity to get to know each other on a more personal basis, establishes trusting relationships, and allows for the sharing of authority and responsibility. It allows for both a formal and informal learning and teaching setting. Administratively one must not shy away from delegating equal responsibilities to the professional staff, especially the psychiatrists, in making the team concept viable in practice.

In summary, the recognition that developing and maturing as a program and staff through working together is the most important way for people to discover what they each can do. The process of building a viable, community-oriented program creates both self and community respect.

Notes

[1] The full accreditation of community mental health workers did not occur as originally conceived until 1972, with the establishment of the federally funded New Careers program. It was at this point that paraprofessionals finally gained access to the new job classifications which had been established within the state system as well as within Boston University Division of Psychiatry and University Hospital. They also, by this time, received recognition for academic work through the attainment of an associate of arts degree from Boston University. Some staff members continued to progress, while working for the Mental Health Center, to master's level degrees.

[2]U.S. National Advisory Commission on Civil Disorders. *Report.* New York: Dutton Publishers, 1968.

REFERENCES

Alvarez, R., Batson, R. M., Carr, A. K., Parks, P., Peck, H. B., Shervington, W., Tyler, F. B., & Zwerling, I. *Racism, elitism, professionalism.* New York: Jason Aronson, Inc., 1976.

Bandler, B. Evolution of a community mental health center. In B. Bandler, MD (Ed.), *Psychiatry in the general hospital.* Boston: Little, Brown and Company, 1966.

Bandler, B. The reciprocal roles of the university and the community in the development of community mental health centers. In R. W. Atkins (Ed.), *How the university can aid community mental health.* Rochester, N.Y.: University of Rochester, 1969.

Batson, R. M., & Peters, L. S. *Community crisis intervention: Case study of a training program.* Boston, Mass.: Boston University, 1976.

Foley, A. F. (Ed.). *Challenge to community psychiatry: A dialogue between two faculties.* New York: Behavioral Publications, 1972.

VOLUNTEERS AND SELF-HELP

Chapter 13

THE NEW VOLUNTEER

Karen A. Signell†

Unlike paraprofessionals, who are regular paid staff members, volunteers give time "free" or for token reimbursement and are often affiliated for shorter-term periods with mental health agencies. The author of this chapter has worked with volunteers for a number of years, particularly in innovative outreach and preventive programs, and illustrates her generalizations about volunteers with illuminating examples drawn from personal experience.

The "New Volunteer" differs from the traditional volunteer in characteristics that include socioeconomic background, reasons for volunteering, career aspirations, and the expectations regarding payment. The central purpose of this chapter is to guide paraprofessionals and professionals in selecting, training, supervising, working with, learning from, and interacting in ethical fashion with the diverse set of persons who are now performing volunteer work in mental health. The chapter includes discussions of the ethical and political issues in volunteerism, as well as guidelines for working with volunteers who are members of advisory boards or consumer committees. It concludes with a set of recommendations for the use of volunteers.

*This paper is based on the author's experience as a clinical psychologist, North County Mental Health Center, San Mateo County Mental Health Services, San Mateo, California. The author wishes to acknowledge contributions by Antoinette K. Palladino, M.P.H., and Dorothy A. Staff, M.P.H.

†Currently the author is in private practice in San Francisco and a contract faculty member at The Wright Institute, Berkeley, California.

I recall the turning point in our mental health center's professional-volunteer relationship. It illustrates the dilemma inherent in the use of volunteers in a community mental health center and hints at the problems to be encountered in the creation of the position of paid volunteer.

> After working with volunteers in the community, I approached my two colleagues at the clinic and announced, "I think volunteers should be paid. We're working side by side doing the same thing, yet I'm paid and they're not. It's a gut reaction. It just doesn't feel fair to me." They countered by reminding me of the long tradition of volunteerism. Some people, they pointed out to me, *prefer* to volunteer, and take special pride in their status. In return for their labors, volunteers receive much respect and appreciation. Far from changing my mind, that argument only brought home to me the bias in our view of volunteers. "You're thinking of women's time as 'free,'" I told them, "and you're assuming that women are happy to work for the reward of a pat on the head."
>
> "If you pay volunteers," said my colleagues, "you'll run into problems. As it is, they can come and go as they please; they can say what they really think. And we professionals have to be nice to them. But if we begin to pay them, they'll lose their independence." "But these people can't afford to work for free," I argued. "Each time they work it's costing them two or three dollars for babysitting and gas." "All right," they finally agreed, "let's try to get money, at least to cover expenses. But we may all lose something in the long run."

We did get small stipends for volunteers, and our experience in the following years proved both myself and my colleagues to have been accurate in our predictions. Some volunteers were at first afraid to be paid. They did not feel they were worth it and thought too much would be expected of them. But we insisted upon paying, and this concrete evidence of value we placed on their work strongly bolstered their self-images and encouraged them to make plans to seek good jobs or schooling afterward. Not only did the money help to ease their financial situation, but as it was for most the first money they had earned on their own, it gave them a strong sense of independence. Yet, in the process, volunteers did lose some autonomy vis-a-vis the agency and its professionals (See also Kanter, 1967).

The term "volunteers" as used in the following discussion denotes people who give time "free" or for token reimbursement. The chapter will cover a number of kinds of volunteer, omitting from discussion the fund raiser, and adding another, the citizen board member.

The range of volunteers generally available has broadened due to recent trends in society: the participation explosion, the shorter work week, the women's movement, unemployment, increase in the elderly population, the advent of student work-study programs, and new federal programs. The current value placed on personal and social development in our society has drawn the new volunteers to their local mental health centers. The mental health professionals, for their part, appear more visible and accessible now with their emphasis on the community, collaboration, self-help, and advocacy. Within this context, volunteering itself is changing. It is becoming institutionalized with pay, training, and specialization; in the process, dilemmas of professional attitudes and ethics arise and must be dealt with.

This paper will address the questions "What's in it for us?" and "What's in it for them?" As both the engaging of volunteers and volunteer work itself are seen as peripheral or "extra," consideration of motivation and morale, on both sides, becomes crucial. Following, in this chapter, attention will turn to practical issues: how to find volunteers, examples of the kinds of work they can do, selection and training, and a special section on volunteers as board members. After a discussion of ethical and political issues, general recommendations are given.

My main experience has been to work collaboratively with volunteers to establish innovative programs, especially primary prevention; however, this chapter will also cover volunteer work with the full array of mental health services, including children, outpatient therapy, day hospital, etc. Examples will illustrate the use of mental health processes that have emerged in working successfully with volunteers: working with strengths, forming group cohesion among volunteers, establishing mutuality between professionals and volunteers, and role modeling. The recommendations drawn from these examples are for: (1) time-limited volunteer experience; (2) mutuality of purpose; (3) an emphasis on innovative, collaborative projects; and (4) a reaching out to obtain a balance of volunteers.

Examples come mainly from one community mental health center near San Francisco which serves an isolated, lower-to-middle-income suburban community with substantial minorities; an occasional example is taken from other mental health centers in the same general area.

VOLUNTEERS VS. PARAPROFESSIONALS

It is important that volunteers be distinguished from paraprofessionals, for the two groups of service personnel play *different* roles in community mental health. When appropriately selected, trained, and supervised, members of both groups are essential to the delivery of the full array of services needed by consumers. Volunteer services should not replace or partially supplant paraprofessional ones, nor should paraprofessional services replace or partially supplant volunteer services.

While also raising attitudinal and ethical dilemmas for professionals, paraprofessionals differ from volunteers in terms of several central characteristics. Volunteers work free of charge or for token reimbursement, while paraprofessionals are salaried as regular staff members; without proper safeguards, volunteers thus are in danger of being exploited, while paraprofessionals are potentially susceptible to cooptation. Volunteers work (or should work) for time-limited periods, while paraprofessionals often pursue a career or else work for longer periods of time with mental health centers. Within an appropriate organizational framework, volunteers can contribute to shorter-term service innovations, while paraprofessionals can assist both in the initiation and the implementation of longer-term structural changes in a mental health center.[1] Finally, volunteers receive shorter-term training, while paraprofessionals ideally receive a combination of longer-term training and extensive supervised on-the-job experience.

Paraprofessionals and volunteers also share central characteristics. Persons in both categories can provide valuable "indigenous" skills and resources. These strengths include: knowledge of the community; an array of local personal contacts; the trust of catchment area residents and organizations; the ability to communicate with members of local subcultures; and an "aprofessional," intuitive style of service delivery.[2]

WHAT'S IN IT FOR US?

The first time I was asked to take on volunteers, I flatly refused. The chief of our community mental health center would have to find someone else, I insisted, as I was already overburdened as a therapist. I did not need the extra burden of training and supervising lay people. Now I feel very differently about that "burden." The change came about when the use of volunteers grew out of my own needs in the natural course of my work, where it made immediate sense.

The satisfaction of working with volunteers, I find, is similar to that of working with students. The problems, too, are similar, in that one must find extra time to meet with them, must find space in which they can work, and there is a high initial investment of energy and time in orientation. Yet, like students, volunteers are eventually capable of substantial output, and their enthusiasm brings freshness to my work day. Whereas field placement students, in their pursuit of learning, draw out our highest ideals and skills as teachers, volunteers, on the other hand, with their freedom and personal relationships to their work, remind us of our personal relationship to our own work. Volunteers can lead us again to commitment, caring, sense of community, and the satisfaction which sometimes get lost in our pressured, routine and rolebound relation to colleagues and clients. There is, of course, a "burden" involved in working with volunteers, as their selection and training require a heavy output of energy. Added to this, very often, is a lack of encouragement from colleagues and little or no incentive from the bureaucracy.

In the long run, however, a volunteer work force can stretch our time as professionals. Volunteers can cut a clinic waiting list. They can embark on innovative community outreach programs, prove the efficacy of these programs, and at the end of their period of service, leave a new program or justify a new position as a legacy for the agency and the community. So, volunteers' very practical contribution of work accomplished cannot be denied. But there are also wider reaching implications to this collaboration. Time spent with volunteers from the community is a direct investment in educating citizens about mental health and encouraging knowledgeable citizen participation. Perhaps the strongest educational program any mental health center can have in the community, with the greatest spinoff, is the education of community volunteers.

WHAT'S IN IT FOR THEM?

Two pictures from history come to mind when I think of "volunteer." One image is the society lady with time on her hands, who wants to "do good." She represents a long tradition of women's charity work in this country, which was sometimes tokenism but in other instances constituted impressive social reform (Jane Addams and Margaret Sanger). A second image is the mother who volunteers at school or other community organizations to do routine office work or routine caring for others. Neither of these stereotypes is useful in identifying the contemporary volunteer emerging with the participation explosion. The new volunteers are decidedly more various, including men and women, young and old, from lower and upper income levels. Rejecting the prospect of dead-end, "put in time" work, they demand specific experience. Most are in transition, so that volunteer work serves as a brief but important stepping stone to what they really want.

New volunteers fall into four groups, each group receiving different benefits from being volunteers.

One group is expatients or other recipients of outpatient or inpatient services. They know how it feels "to have been there," and they want to help others. These may be teenagers who had drug problems and then volunteered to manage a teen hotline, or day-hospital patients who co-lead patient groups. Their crucial need is to consolidate their position of identifying with their healthy side, and shift from the patient role to the helping role. They need close personal contact with the professional, either consultation or apprenticeship, in order to identify with the professional and his or her work. The personal quality of this contact, in turn, allows the expatient to maintain a personal quality of empathy with patients.

Another type are volunteers who approach the mental health center saying they "want experience." They are typically (but not only) middle class and are interested in mental health as a career. They want experience as a transition step to a job or school. Often there are specific motivations: The high school or college student wants to look over mental health as a career field. The ex-social worker with grown children wants to try out her skills again and get recommendations for jobs or further training. A newly graduated, unemployed mental health worker hopes to be on the spot if a job opening occurs. For these people it is important to identify false hopes and clarify mutual expectations. Since they are usually oriented toward a traditional career, for example, therapist, they need firsthand experience working with patients to find out their suitability for the field or to update their skills, and they need to observe and work closely with the professional as a role model. The most important thing for the less experienced is training and supervision; for the more experienced, participation, respect, and power commensurate with their ability and contribution to the agency take precedence.

The third group are those who say they "want to be useful." We need to recognize their situation as they define it: they do not have a useful place in society. Sometimes their predicament is caused by a current crisis situation such as temporary unemployment or recent divorce. Sometimes it is the result of a normal developmental stage such as adolescence or old age in which the people find themselves with time on their hands, young adulthood in which often it is difficult to find jobs, or the period of self-questioning when students temporarily drop out of school. In some cases the feeling of alienation may arise from a more chronic situation created by personal inability or social disadvantages; the isolated unemployed single parent is a prime example of this condition. In any case, the people seek work to give meaning to their lives and perhaps also to stave off depression and social isolation. They need to feel important and know that their contribution is worthwhile to others in the mental health center. And they need to belong to a social network. Whether their duties are gathering statistics, doing clerical work, or being a member of a citizen's board, they need to belong to a group effort and have some kind of regular contact with others.

The last group are those with heretofore untapped potential in the community whom we professionals usually find in the course of community outreach and preventive programs. They are very able people, but we need to search them out and entice them into mental health work. Women, new arrivals in the community, ethnic minorities—these are groups whose members, because of their ascribed status or position in society, have not yet become active in the community or work world. We often find them when they take their first step toward participation by attending a mental health education course, a parent-teen rap group, a women's consciousness-raising group, a minority group meeting, or a welfare rights group. Many of these people are lower-income women whose children are almost grown and who, never having had an opportunity to do interesting paid work, lack confidence in their abilities. Without formal education, experience, or even clerical skills, they might have considered seeking work as dime-store clerks or bank tellers, low-expectation jobs that may not be commensurate with their potential. They need to have their life experience recognized as valuable whether it be child raising or participation in a particular culture or community network. They need their special interests heard, and they need intensive training as a group in a way that promotes social cohesion, high standards, and a strong sense of common purpose.

RECRUITMENT AND NON-EXPLOITIVE FUNCTIONING OF VOLUNTEERS

This section describes the routes by which volunteers become involved in community mental health work and provides examples of the kinds of work volunteers can do. (See also NIMH, 1970; Siegel, 1973.) Examples illustrate how the needs and strengths of volunteers can be matched with programs.

Mental health workers, in the natural course of work, have immediate access to volunteers among recipients of services; and they can try using untrained, "on-the-spot" volunteers on a small scale:

> A day-hospital wanted aftercare groups for expatients in their transition from hospital to community and social groups for more chronic patients in need of social experience and group support. Former day-hospital patients were asked to lead the groups. Staff, as advisors, met regularly with the volunteers. However, when the groups met there were no professional staff present, which truly handed responsibility over to the volunteer leaders. Over the course of many years, volunteers co-led the groups in teams of two, three, or four. They planned outings and accompanied the groups on various activities. While providing a useful service they also derived other satisfactions for themselves: an opportunity to learn leadership from the advisors, and to form close working relationships with other volunteers as co-leaders.

In the following example we see not only how people receiving services can be introduced into volunteer work but the kinds of contributions they are uniquely equipped to make.

> As a community psychologist leading discussion groups with kindergarten parents about their children entering kindergarten, I often paused in the course of discussions, sometimes because I did not know an answer, sometimes to see if other kindergarten parents would answer. I noticed who contributed ideas and opinions, and when the next year came I invited those parents who had participated most actively in the previous groups to co-lead the newly formed discussion groups. Sometimes it was those who had been the most anxious—kindergarten parents themselves who were the most helpful to others, because they were eager to share their strong feelings and could be role models for others. I found that parents

could really hear something when it came from another kindergarten parent as co-leader. The idea had credibility and it was put in a directly usable way. For example, a mother of eight told with great conviction what other parents could anticipate from various kinds of children. Other parent volunteers could translate general principles into practical techniques: "When my child is angry I give him a hammer and a bunch of nails and he goes and pounds them into the back porch." "If I really want to listen to my child's feelings, I squat on my heels and look into her eyes and she knows I'm listening." The kindergarten parents also knew effective community organization. They volunteered to go up and down the kindergarten registration lines in Spring to tell other kindergarten parents about the discussion groups, and they telephoned other parents before meetings (Signell, 1972).

These times of increased unemployment among professionals have made available the services of mental health workers and other professionals who call mental health centers to volunteer. There is an overabundance of such applicants, which is a problem in itself, and their being accepted as volunteers raises touchy questions of status and political ramifications.

A mental health agency had so many calls from mental health professionals wanting to volunteer at the center that they named a head of volunteers to sort out requests. Highly experienced professionals sought part-time work, newly graduated professionals wanted to accumulate supervised hours for their license, some wanted advanced training, others wanted a job and couldn't find it. At first they all volunteered time free and the volunteer staff grew. The clinic waiting list disappeared. After a year or two the volunteers wanted pay and received an agreement for token payment of about $2.50 an hour. They were mollified but resentful. It was a corrosive situation with a large group of volunteers covertly wishing each staff person would leave and vacate a position. When they chafed at feelings of low status and powerlessness, they were named "associate staff" with a representative on the administrative committee and the power to review potential volunteers. However, each supposed step forward actually heightened the basic inequity of the system. Later, when potential volunteers called and offered free services the paid volunteers, dissatisfied as they were, protected their positions by staving off those requests—a lifeboat ethic to which they themselves were subject.

This example illustrates the tremendous output that professional volunteers can have, and yet it also shows the dilemmas. This kind of problem may call for radical monetary or political solutions such as sharing salaries or forming half-time positions, but these are at most problematic and stopgap. A practical solution in the foreseeable future for agencies with professional volunteers is to put time limits on volunteering. Then, whether volunteers received token monetary benefit or not, one would have a large number of volunteers and high turnover. One would ensure a high ratio of personal, social, and educational benefits to service given, and thus alleviate the exploitation factor.

If one recruits volunteers for *time-limited* positions, then volunteers are perceived as *trainees* and direct recipients themselves, rather than professionals. The agency has responsibility to provide experiences to prepare them for the "real world." Then, like a good parent, the agency must insist they leave the nest, and in the process, make room for others. The volunteers cannot hold false expectation of the agency or prolong their "internship" beyond its usefulness to become instead an exploitive situation, corrosive for haves and have-nots alike.

The third way to find volunteers is for the professional to take initiative in recruiting community members for special projects to fill gaps in programs. Volunteers in this situation can be immensely productive, for while the bureaucracy exerts pressure on staff to continue the "safe" course of traditional services, volunteers with their freedom and new ideas are in a position to risk and spearhead innovative or extra programs.

> The Children's Service wanted activity clubs for latency age children. The clubs would supplement therapy and provide social experiences for children to improve peer relationships, helping them, for instance, learn to talk instead of hit. The Children's Service asked professors at a nearby college to send them students from the departments of psychology, recreation, education, and music. At first students came as volunteers, just for the experience. In later years students received incentives in the form of course credit, small stipends from the college or from work-study programs. It was hard work and it made a difference to students to receive something tangible for their efforts.

> Another factor contributing to the success of the program through the years is our recruitment of a mix of students to ensure a strong support system. Student volunteers worked in groups of two or three, always a graduate student among junior college students (who find it hard to set limits alone).

> In recruiting we did not pass by students who were in a stage of adolescent rebellion themselves, since most are to some extent. Rather, the therapists offered consultation and emotional support so they could learn to handle their anger when children were difficult and destructive and thus assume the adult role. Nor in recruiting did we pass by volunteers from various cultural backgrounds that expected too little or too much from children, but instead therapists offered intensive consultation to convey expectations of normal behavior for certain ages and appropriate discipline. With strong backup most students recruited stayed the entire year. Only on rare occasions was a student unsuited because of time limitations or sociopathic tendencies, an example being the kind who tries to protect children from

"those bad authorities" but finds the children themselves turn on their "champion"!

The special needs of youth once again provided the impetus as described in the following example, for a successful involvement of volunteers in establishing a service.

> The mental health center, reacting to community pressure and our own concern about teenage drug abuse, brought together all the energetic people we could find: personnel from church and court, concerned parents, and teenagers. We pledged a room, telephone, training, and consultation for a drop-in center and hot-line if they would volunteer to run it. Through the years this service took a great investment of staff time, but staff were willing to give time to the venture and the tremendous output was highly gratifying. Thousands of calls a month were handled.

A final example illustrates a volunteer program structured to avoid exploitation of volunteers and provide them with maximum benefits while making productive use of their abilities.

> The preventive service wanted to give community courses on parent-child communications skills. To have large-scale impact we recruited a corps of volunteer instructors through various means: word of mouth, an ad in the newspaper, referrals from ministers, nursery school directors, school counselors. We gathered 18 parents. Two were interested in community organization aspects of arranging classes; the other 16 took the course on parenting skills, then intensive training on how to teach courses (Signell, 1975).

> When this first group taught parents, they generated new volunteers. From each class they recommended one or two parents as new instructors, and thus the system could perpetuate itself despite high turnover in instructors. In this way, volunteer instructors were able to reach over 2,000 parents in the community.

> An important aspect of the program was the expectation that volunteer's involvement was time limited. During training and teaching the first courses, instructors were still learning and gaining a great deal for themselves. After this, their continued teaching of courses could have become mere exploitation of them as unpaid workers. Most volunteers were eager to move on, at this point, using the experience as a stepping stone to paid jobs, returning to school, or community organizing. In retrospect, I believe, we should have made career counseling an intrinsic part of the program as volunteers left. A few volunteer instructors remained because we offered horizontal or vertical volunteer mobility. We recruited them to collaborate on more advanced activities: training courses for new instruc-

tors, developing a parent-teen course, making a film, consulting other centers on starting programs.

A survey of 36 instructors showed that the program met volunteer needs for changes in self-image, acquisition of skills that are useful in the community, self-confidence in a group situation, feelings of belonging, and friendships (Signell, 1976).

Toward a Balanced Variety of Volunteers

The traditional approach of self-selection needs to be supplemented by reaching out to bring a variety of new community people into relationship to the mental health center. Formal recruitment of the general public can be accomplished through news articles, the local or federal volunteer agencies,[3] church groups, PTAs, nursery school parents, the local or state Mental Health Associations. We seek out people with special skills in the arts or interpersonal relations. Informal contacts occur during the course of community work. For example, I noticed a young woman at a women's consciousness workshop who spoke openly about her former alcoholism and her constructive work with AA and co-alcoholics. I jotted down her name and later asked her to become a VISTA volunteer specialist on alcoholism.

One must seek out male volunteers. Young students and retired men are more available, but the middle-aged blue and white collar working man can sometimes be persuaded to offer his services. Our first contact with some men comes through their wives. For example, a volunteer mentioned her husband's interest in creative writing although he worked nine to five as a salesman. The head of volunteers was alert to the need for male volunteers and did not assume that because of his full-time job he would be unavailable. She interviewed him, and he led evening group meetings in writing therapy for day-hospital patients.

Selecting and Interviewing Volunteers

Whether volunteers are self-selected or selected by professionals, interviewing the volunteers to determine their interests and skills calls for common sense and imagination rather than grim-faced methodical selection procedures. Mental health professionals are sometimes very concerned about selection as a difficult or problematical process, but in our experience we have had only rare difficulties (e.g., someone too angry or narcissistically talkative to be a group leader). We find it more worthwhile in the long run to emphasize and to put effort into training and consultation backup. The most important aspect of selection is a very practical one: to determine whether a volunteer can realistically make a time commitment.

A head of volunteers needs to orient staff members who will be interviewing volunteers. Otherwise they may fall back upon professional roles and patterns of diagnosis, therapy, or selection that are more appropriate for use with patients, students, or professional job applicants. For example, a therapist may probe, as with a patient, into a volunteer's deeper motives, when all that is necessary is to take the volunteer's word at face value.

TRAINING

We consider orientation, training, and supervisory backup for volunteers to be as serious a commitment as the training and supervision of students. Our senior mental health educator, from her many years' experience working with volunteers in mental health agencies, developed the following viewpoint.

> No community mental health center has a right to take on untrained paraprofessionals—including volunteers—without providing organized training that can lead to career development. This means that someone must be delegated the specific responsibility of planning and implementing training and follow-up consultation, including career counseling (Palladino, Note 1).

TRAINING BY INDIVIDUAL SUPERVISION OR APPRENTICESHIP

When a volunteer is working alone with individual cases it is important to provide equally intensive one-to-one supervision, training, or apprenticeship. The supervisor can provide emotional support as well as modulate the emotional involvement and responsibility of a volunteer (See also Reding, 1967).

> Volunteer "big brothers" met with individual, disturbed children ages 4, 5, and 6, while the mother was in therapy. So that the volunteer would not be overwhelmed with responsibility he was exposed only to brief orientation and progressive learning confined to a simple behavioral level. For example, volunteers were encouraged to use common sense: "Be firm, keep contact, tell the child to hold your hand. If the child has a tantrum in a grocery store, how can you stop it? Sure, pick the child up and take it out!"

Although we need to share our skills and knowledge with volunteers, it is a mistake to prolong orientation or give them too much initial training. Professionals seeking to educate volunteers are sometimes tempted to emphasize pathology or give lectures on symptomatology, diagnostic categories, the effects of prescription drugs, etc. It is not only unnecessary but may make the volunteer feel overwhelmed, inadequate, afraid of mental illness, and distant from patients. It is more useful for the professional to be a "reachable model" for the volunteer. To assuage qualms on the part of professionals and volunteers it is better for volunteers to have some immediate brief work experience and use these examples as a springboard for relevant learning, rather than be subjected to lectures or theory initially. These can be apprenticeship experiences, where the volunteer can observe the professional; collaborative work side by side; role-playing practice of typical situations; or on-the-job training.

TRAINING IN A GROUP

Educating volunteers in a group is efficient for the professional. The following example shows how a group can provide volunteers with a group identity, social network, and a strong enough position to give feedback to the agency or take advocacy positions in the community. We started with a clearly defined problem, role for volunteers, and purpose, followed by intensive and relevant training.

THE VISTA VOLUNTEERS PROJECT

The Problem

When the state hospitals closed there was an influx of severely disturbed people into the community. Research showed high rehospitalization rates and inadequate use of community resources, especially patients' primary social unit, the family. We sought to reduce rehospitalization through home visits and linking patients with community resources.

Initial Steps

I first asked the day-hospital head nurse to experiment with the use of volunteers on a small scale. She selected a few former day-hospital patients who soon proved their worth, allowing us to obtain a VISTA grant for 10 volunteers.

Selecting "Reachable Models"

Instead of requesting professionals from the general pool of VISTA volunteers, we selected local people who had firsthand experience as patients or members of self-help groups in our community. Thus they could be reachable models for patients. We purposely searched for a wide range of reachable models, both young and old, from various backgrounds and races.

Role and Purpose

The role of volunteers was to be "advocate friends" for patients, providing a bridge between patients and their families, agencies, and self-help resources. The volunteers' purpose was not only to help individuals but also to leave the following legacies when they finished the project: (a) provide proof that links between patients and resources are useful enough to justify permanent positions in the county budget for community workers, (b) establish new self-operating groups in the community, (c) have an impact on health professionals to be more receptive to using community resources in the course of their professional work.

The First Six Weeks

It was crucial to have a strong training program consistent with the purposes. The first six weeks of training are particularly important, and during this time four areas were emphasized.

Orientation.   Volunteers had personal, individual introductions to all staff, including clerical staff. We placed an equal emphasis on contacts with community self-help groups, so that the mental health center was not seen as the only source of treatment but one among many resources.

Identity.   Each volunteer was given a specific identity as a specialist for a community resource (alcoholism and AA, suicide prevention center, housing, jobs, etc.). This contributed to clarity about roles and a way for volunteers to introduce themselves to professionals and patients.

Role-play practice.   A six-week training course provided volunteers with role-play practice of skills—listening to feelings, setting limits, using their own experience as a basis for empathy and advocacy—and also further role definition and practice explaining who they were to patients, therapists, and community resources.

Group cohesion.   Volunteers learned to work with a partner and as a group. Work assignments were made in pairs, threes, or fours, with time on the job for mutual support, collaboration, and consultation. We also insisted that they meet weekly as a group without us supervisors. This fostered independence, group solidarity, honest feedback to us, and a firsthand experience for them in a self-help group without professionals. Different volunteer pairs rotated as group leaders which provided experiences for them in leadership and peer supervision—which we as outsiders could not give.

Research and Results

Volunteers collected research on their interventions. They listed each link attempted and its success (e.g., referral for medication, job placement). These hard data were used to justify positions in the future and also for the volunteers' own use as an index of their productivity. At the end of the project they left a report on their legacy, describing liaison structures developed between agencies and noting the establishment of self-help groups in the community (e.g., a center for alcoholics and co-alcoholics, a childcare center, a new emergency hot-line).

Impact on Staff

Volunteers also educated professional staff in a profound way. Illustrative are three instances in my personal experience:

1. One volunteer was working with patients in the emergency room. A former inpatient herself, she protested with eloquence the heavy medication of patients and made other astute observations about the hospital system and alternatives of which I had been unaware. She, other volunteers, and staff became strong advocates for establishing the new inpatient hospital on a more humane basis.

2. On another occasion, I was conducting an initial interview with an outpatient couple. They had a severe alcohol problem but equally strong denial. As an outpatient therapist I was frustrated and stymied until I asked our volunteer specialist on alcoholism to join us. Having had firsthand experience with alcoholism, she immediately sensed the situation, and the patients knew that she was aware of the problem. We collaboratively conducted outpatient treatment, and she took the couple to AA. In the process, she taught me a great deal about how to work with alcoholic families.

3. Another instance took place on emergency duty. A woman rushed into the center after having broken windows and doors and having made threats. Two police officers came close behind, bringing an ambulance in which to strap her down for the 20-mile trip to the hospital. The volunteers intervened and insisted on finding alternatives. While I kept the police waiting, one volunteer telephoned the woman's relatives and convinced them to drive to the hospital. Another volunteer, seeing how terrified the patient was, went over and put an arm around her, letting her know her feelings were understood. The nurse came over and did likewise. Finally the woman relaxed a little and said she would go to the hospital without restraints if they would accompany her. The important impact this incident left on our staff was the strength of conviction we got from the volunteers that we must forego the safe and easy traditional bureaucratic solution and search for alternatives, that we must risk ourselves, as our volunteers did, and be patient advocates too.

TRAINING STAFF TO WORK WITH VOLUNTEERS

In educating staff regarding volunteers it helps to have a clear statement from a high administrative level that the education of volunteers and collaborative work is, in itself, an important part of the community mental health services and outreach to the community.

It is also important to orient and train staff about specific groups of volunteers and their work.

> In the case of the VISTA volunteers, we explained to staff that they were selected for their ability to have rapport with clients, their firsthand experience with therapy or self-help groups, and their knowledge of community resources. We described their background and the intensive training program in which they had participated. We gave staff written lists of the volunteers' specialties and typical functions such as home visits or taking a patient to AA for the first time. We also listed inappropriate tasks for volunteers (e.g., they should not be asked simply to transport a patient; they should not have to take sole responsibility for a patient; they should not do more flunky work than others in the center). We discussed with professional staff and also put in writing what the volunteers needed from them. This helped staff go their halfway in establishing collaborative working relationships with the volunteers (e.g., VISTA volunteers need before-after exchange of ideas, mutual respect for each other's specialties).

Staff who train volunteers for community work or join with them in a common cause need to be reminded to use good group process. The best incubation for high moral and collaborative work is a warm, mutually responsible and supportive atmosphere. At the same time, staff should guard against being patronizing; the volunteers need their work to be taken seriously, and realistically high standards should be set for them. Our old roles and professionalism should give way to a more informal directness in our relating. Joining in a common cause, with similar dedication, means doing whatever one does best without preconceptions, and it means sharing the "dirty work." Collaboration essentially calls for principles of democratic participation. Because volunteers' main identity is with their group cause (not with a profession or the agency), processes that promote group identity and independence are important. These include small group process, meeting without the professional, working in pairs.

BOARD VOLUNTEERS

Another kind of volunteer often overlooked by professionals is the community representative who gives his/her time free (or for token payment) on citizen advisory boards or consumer committees involved in the administrative tasks of planning, reviewing budgets, and hiring. The following are recommendations for a well-functioning volunteer board:

1. Structure the board to consist of a majority of nonprofessionals so that professionals do not overrun the others. However, a board should have the option of inviting experts when necessary, or else it will be unable to reach decisions and will become dysfunctional. To make policy, board members need the experience, and the liaison function, of also being members of working committees composed of a combination of nonprofessionals and professionals.

2. To avoid eventual infighting, recruit on the basis of mental health goals, not race or other criteria. The message, then, is that goals, not power issues, are important. Recruit from widely differing sources, including consumers and volunteers who have close working knowledge of the system and a commitment to general mental health goals.

3. Assure "new blood" and regular turnover of members by inserting a written policy in the bylaws specifying an explicit length of service, for example, three years, and get rid of loopholes which would allow the reelection of members.

4. Have provisions to fire board members who do not fulfill minimal functions such as attending meetings. Without these requirements one is subtly communicating that members' role or representation of the community is not important.

5. Make sure the administrator orients new board members and also provides for input and exchange with various staff.

6. Delegate responsibility to a community mental health center staff member to train the board and be liaison. Training should include orientation to the history and function of the center and the board, processes of running a board, and the best access to needed information.

7. Give board members access to information as complete as that available to the administrator. Otherwise the board is a sham.

8. To avoid divisiveness or the domination of one person, which is common to boards, have a staff member initiate goal-oriented process, such as the group process method of writing down individual needs, then meeting in small groups to arrive at consensual ranking of needs and goals.

9. As a motivational factor and a way to help board volunteers get to know each other personally, precede board meetings by the social event of eating together.

10. Be alert to absenteeism and other signs of demoralization as an indication that board members may feel they are not having sufficient impact. If board members perceive that they are having impact commensurate with their efforts, they will keep coming.

ETHICAL AND POLITICAL ISSUES IN VOLUNTEERISM

It may be that the institution of volunteerism itself has the effect of diverting energy and lulling us into an unrealistic view of societal problems and processes for change.

If we look at the areas in our society in which volunteerism is common, we see that it is much used and encouraged in the social services. In space programs, on the other hand, or national defense, the concept would be summarily rejected and probably has never even been considered. We might ask, then, whether the federal government's strong support of the volunteer movement (through the ACTION agency, which encompasses VISTA, Foster Grandparents, etc.) is not an indication of the low value placed upon social services in general. And the crucial question is whether this financial support encourages short-term hit-or-miss efforts by the powerless in areas such as innovation in the social services, community organization and aging, where we actually need long-term substantial organized efforts on the part of established power.

In other words, by using volunteers are we settling for tokenism and obscuring the need for major governmental commitment?

One way to turn the situation to our advantage might be to use volunteers to spearhead pilot projects that will later become established programs. Actually that is the intent of ACTION programs and often the political outcome of letting loose volunteer spirit in a community. For example, in our community when the board of supervisors tried to cut the mental health budget it was our volunteers who spoke up in the political arena. For the individual practitioner, then, or a particular clinic, the orientation might be toward the use of volunteers' services as a way to engender substantial change.

A second element we should examine is: *who* volunteers? And the answer is: mostly women. This confronts us with the exploitation that stems from the sexist nature of our society. The National Organization for Women (NOW) has examined (1975) some of the forms this exploitation takes. For example, volunteering may represent an extension of the woman's traditional role as unpaid helper and nurturer at home to unpaid helper and nurturer in the community at large! It may serve to keep women in a state of arrested development and protect them from moving into the adult world, the "real world" with its expectations and responsibilities as well as rewards and power (Adams, 1971; Gold, 1971). NOW points out that full-time volunteering keeps a woman from earning her living, thus perpetuating her economic dependence and her second-class-citizen status. Considering recent developments—the cutting of funds and increased unemployment among public service personnel—are we substituting volunteers for laid-off workers in social services? NOW asks, are the volunteers who take the place of laid-off workers saints or scabs? NOW recommends that women be paid, or if they do volunteer that it be for change-oriented actions or causes that shift political priorities in the direction of women's individual or collective needs.

Some of the benefits to the individual of volunteer work, mentioned earlier in this paper would counteract, to a certain degree, NOW's bleak picture of exploitation. And there still are some general dangers in paying volunteers, as pointed out by the Department of Labor: "The need for reimbursing volunteers in lower income brackets for expenses incurred for transportation, meals, or babysitting seems obvious. But when more than expenses, yet less than the prevailing wage is paid, volunteers are in reality underpaid employed workers" (NOW, 1975, p. 14).

However, the question of the exploitation of women should not be ignored. Perhaps the most encouraging prospect for correcting this situation is the interest in volunteering in the social services that is beginning to come from many more sectors of the population, so that women will not, eventually, form the bulk of volunteer workers. As this gradual change takes place, however, we should remain alert to the possibility that we might substitute for the sexist exploitation of women a similar unprincipled use of other segments of the society, such as young people, the elderly, and ethnic minorities.

The distribution of work among volunteers should also be examined, for the mental health system may be merely replicating society's prejudices if it keeps women and uneducated or disadvantaged people in the most menial positions and gives the decision-making power and interesting work to men and the educated or the advantaged.

One final, and usually unacknowledged, factor which may affect one's selection and use of volunteers is projection, the attributing to others of the characteristics one does not claim in oneself. What personal or social characteristics (temperament, ethnic origin, behavior) distinguish the volunteers from the staff? The answers to this question, in helping us become aware of how we characterize volunteers, can give us information about what deficiencies the staff may perceive in themselves. These projections on volunteers are often positive, and may represent staff's unacknowledged wishes for themselves.

ATTITUDES AND VALUES

I wish to touch briefly upon certain attitudes and values held by staff and volunteers which affect their relationship and work. The first is professionals' fear of volunteers. Some fear is justified, as volunteers do indeed comprise a threat to staff and the status quo in many ways, challenging staff values and their accustomed ways of viewing patients or community. Some uneasiness is inevitable, then, and it may be manifested in various ways: procrastination about using volunteers, denial of volunteers' presence, the use of jargon, relegating volunteers to compartmentalized areas of the clinic's functioning. The most common response of us professionals is to be patronizing. We may attribute a mystique of special knowledge and freedom of option to the volunteer and not assert our own knowledge, freedom or power; we may do all the "dirty work" or administrative work.

Another problem is devaluing volunteers' time and, by implication, devaluing volunteers as persons. Since it is a fact that a professional's time is expensive and the professional has a high status, in contrast to the volunteer's time which is free and whose status may be lower, there can be a natural tendency to waste the volunteer's time and consider the professional's time, opinions, and person as more important. This treatment, while it may be tolerated by volunteers, clearly conveys disrespect for them. Conversely, a professional needs to let volunteers know if he or she feels disrespected around issues of time, expertise, and division of labor.

O'Donnell's (1970) study of professionals and lay volunteers shows striking differences in culture, values, and perceptions of each other which can interfere with working relationships. Briefly, professionals saw laymen as "uninformed hearts" while laymen viewed professionals as "unfeeling heads." Professionals saw laymen as limited in their understanding; laymen viewed professionals as hesitant or unwilling to act or get their hands dirty. Professionals and laymen may fall into the roles of therapist and patient in relating to each other and the work situation. The assumptions about therapist-patient roles may hamper working together in community organizing. The major difference between the two groups is that professionals tend to place value on knowledge and striving for harmony while volunteers prefer action and confrontation. To the extent that either group dominates, the other will be discontented. The best chance for mutual influence is for both professionals and lay volunteers to collaborate in new situations or projects outside the professional's usual territory (Feldman, in press), thus putting the professional on a more equal footing with the volunteer.

RECOMMENDATIONS

1. That volunteering in one position be *time limited* to safeguard against exploitation and insure that volunteering is a transition and not a dead-end, underpaid job. A volunteer made this telling observation: "Volunteering lulls people. I outgrew it years ago, but I lack the courage to get out."

2. That there be a written agreement between the mental health center and the volunteer on purpose and mutual obligations. This promotes self-respect, dignity, and clarity. It is an antidote to illusions of charity on either side and legitimizes the self-interest of each party. It forces the mental health system to clarify what it wants from volunteers, to specify

work to be done and indicate the desired side effects of volunteers' close contact with the system (e.g., volunteers' becoming resources in the community or mental health advocates). The volunteer too needs to define expectations, such as gaining experience, feeling useful, becoming part of a social network, serving as advocate for a constituency.

3. That volunteer work be mainly reserved for innovative work done in the spirit of collaboration rather than traditional basic services which require the kind of long-term coordination, planning, and concentrated effort that only paid workers can give in well-funded programs. The volunteer is in a unique position to see unmet needs in the community and new ways to meet them. When volunteers work in innovative programs which they personally care about and helped design, then the relationship between worker and work is shifted from "doing for" to "doing with." When the mental health professional also has an interest in a similar program, then they can work side by side and learn from each other in collaboration on a mutual cause. This collaboration forges strong personal links between mental health and community people, and keeps each abreast of recent developments in the other's sphere.

4. That the mental health system observe *who* its volunteers are, and soul-search any imbalances in kinds of people they are, the work they do, and the way we perceive them. There are various hazards. The easiest to spot is possible exploitation in an overrepresentation of women or men, young or old, uneducated or educated, poor or rich, lay or professional people, Anglo or minority. Selective recruitment can be used to correct the imbalance. Another hazard is reliance on cultural stereotypes, manifested in work assignments according to prejudice, for example, assigning work on the basis of sex or level of education rather than ability. A third hazard is unconscious attitudes in the staff, who may, without recognizing it, view volunteers as patients, may overprotect the volunteers or otherwise patronize them, and may attribute various qualities to volunteers that are missing in themselves, rather than seeking to develop these qualities.

NOTES

[1] Chapter 12 in this sourcebook, by Bandler, Batson, and Peters, describes the use of paraprofessionals to induce and perpetuate structural changes in a community mental health center.

[2] Chapter 14 in this sourcebook, by Frank Riessman, describes in some detail the features of this "aprofessional" style.

[3] National Student Volunteer Program, ACTION, 806 Connecticut Ave., Washington, D.C. 20525, (800) 424–8580, for information/consultation on the use of students as volunteers in local mental health centers; United Way of America, 801 No. Fairfax St., Alexandria, Va. 22314, (703) 836-7100, for information/materials on use of local volunteer agencies.

REFERENCE NOTE

1. A. K. Palladino, Personal communication, May 1977.

REFERENCES

Adams, M. The compassion trap. In V. Gornick, & B. K. Moran (Eds.), *Woman in sexist society.* New York: Basic Books, 1971.

Feldman, R. E. Collaborative consultation: A process for joint professional-consumer construction of primary prevention programs. *Journal of Community Psychology,* in press. (Available from R. E. Feldman, Social Action Research Center, 18 Professional Center Parkway, San Rafael, California 94903.)

Gold, D. B. Women and volunteerism. In V. Gornick, & B. K. Moran (Ed.), *Woman in sexist society.* New York: Basic Books, 1971.

Kanter, D. Volunteerism and problems of domain in the American mental health movement. In P. L. Ewalt (Ed.), *Mental health volunteers.* Springfield, Ill.: Charles C Thomas, 1967.

National Institute of Mental Health. *Volunteers in community mental health* (PHS Publication No. 2071). Washington, D.C.: U.S. Government Printing Office, 1970.

National Organization for Women. *Volunteerism.* Washington, D.C.: National NOW Action Center (425 13th Street, N.W., Suite 1001). Also in *Ms.,* February 1975, p. 73. (Summary)

O'Donnell, E. J. The professional volunteer versus the volunteer professional. *Community Mental Health Journal,* 1970, *6,* 236–245.

Reding, G. R., & Goldsmith, E. F. The nonprofessional hospital volunteer as a member of the psychiatric consultation team. *Community Mental Health Journal,* 1967, *3,* 267–272.

Siegel, J. M. Mental health volunteers as change agents. *American Journal of Community Psychology,* 1973, *1*(2), 138–158.

Signell, K. A. Kindergarten entry. *Community Mental Health Journal,* 1972, *8,* 60–70. Also in R. H. Moos (Ed.), *Human adaptation.* Lexington, Mass.: D. C. Heath, 1976.

Signell, K. A. Training nonprofessionals as community instructors. *Journal of Community Psychology,* 1975, *3*(4), 365–373.

Signell, K. A. On a shoestring: A consumer-based source of manpower for mental health. *Community Mental Health Journal,* 1976, *12,* 342–354.

Chapter 14

SELF-HELP[1]

Frank Riessman*

Self-help groups provide an alternative to services delivered by agencies. Based in the community and controlled by community members, these groups employ "aprofessional" strategies in helping members to retain or regain states of positive mental health. The self-help movement is rapidly proliferating in response to the needs of people for group support in dealing with concerns ranging from the daily problems of living to the process of community reintegration following discharge from a mental hospital.

The author of this chapter is the co-director of the National Self-Help Clearinghouse, and is in an excellent position to present a broad overview of the self-help movement. Perhaps the central theme of the chapter is that the services offered by self-help groups complement those provided by agencies, and that members of self-help groups and employees of agencies can assist and learn from one another. Two sections of the chapter focus, respectively, on models for professionals and for paraprofessionals who wish to work with self-help groups. The chapter concludes with a directory of self-help groups relevant to mental health; this directory should prove useful to agency employees who wish to locate area self-help resources relevant to clients' needs.

The self-help mode is particularly relevant at the present time because it is economical, nonprofessional, and apparently effective. Currently, there are over a half million different self-help groups. There are self-help groups for

*Professor, Queens College, City University of New York.

parents who abuse their children, isolated older people, drug abusers, young people in search of identity and jobs, patients who have had heart attacks or mastectomies, parents of handicapped children, suicide-prone people, smokers, drinkers, over-eaters, patients discharged from mental institutions, underachieving children who need tutoring, and more. Self-help groups are defined by Katz and Bender (1976) as:

> Self-help groups are voluntary, small group structures for mutual aid and the accomplishment of a special purpose. They are usually formed by peers who have come together for mutual assistance in satisfying a common need, overcoming a common handicap or life-disrupting problem, and bringing about desired social and/or personal change. The initiators and members of such groups perceive that their needs are not, or cannot be, met by or through existing social institutions (p. 9).

The rapid proliferation of self-help groups not only reflects the decline of traditional institutions such as the family, the church, and the neighborhood, which perform integrating functions, but it also reflects the inadequacy of the formal caregiving institutions in meeting the needs that arise in the absence of these bonding structures. Because the major problems in mental health currently relate to feelings of alienation, isolation and lack of identity due in part to the breakdown of traditional small groups like the family, community, and neighborhood, the small self-help units may play an important role in filling the resulting vacuum. In addition, since the specific mental health problems of the period relate to various forms of addiction such as drugs and gambling, self-help groups are important and have frequently been recommended by the traditional agencies as the treatment of choice. Other more specific mental health related issues such as the loneliness of parents without partners, widows, suicide-prone individuals, and the special needs of women and men who have formed consciousness-raising groups are other areas for which the small group mutual aid orientation appears beneficial.

Many of the mental health problems have a chronic character, and so the usual episodic forms of mental health intervention may be less appropriate than the continuous, all-embracing interventions of the mutual aid form. In addition, mutual aid is also indicated for the general problems of living. Modern problems do not necessarily take the form of a specific disorder such as alcoholism, but in many cases are more diffuse problems of living, experienced by many women and men in consciousness-raising groups, by the large number of people who use the coping books, and by members of the various encounter groups. Furthermore, there are the unique problems of specific groups, such as parents of retarded children, parents without partners, people who are dying, young people with identity problems, older people facing death, midgets, and ex-offenders. In fact, the failure of the correctional system and the difficulties of postprison existence has led to organizations such as The

Fortune Society for ex-offenders, and various types of self-help groups have been developed for delinquents.

The trend toward deinstitutionalization in the mental health field has important implications for the mutual aid modality. Former mental patients need organizations such as Recovery Incorporated and other types of small units to aid them in their adjustment and transition to everyday life. The recent concern for dealing with the emotional problems of the dying has led to self-help units usually attached to hospitals. Special problems related to sexism, racism, and ageism have led to a great variety of self-help activities ranging from the Gray Panthers and women's groups to youth hotlines and various kinds of co-ops. Concerns with parenting, aggression, and sex behavior have brought forth a great number of self-help books in these spheres.

Mutual aid groups appear to integrate a great variety of approaches to behavior change, derived from multiple levels of experience. Some utilize traditional principles based on will, inspiration, and the demand for action and motion. They all use the principles of group reinforcement and group support; they all demand reciprocity and mutual helping; they seem to be rooted in role theory and behavioristic models; they are strength-based and call upon the coping abilities and the strengths of the individual to overcome the pathology, the crisis, or the problem; they use simple principles or persuasion ideologies, such as the AA's Twelve Steps, that tend to demystify complicated mechanisms; they provide corrective emotional experiences through the group and through cooperation, mutuality, and helping; they are not episodic but rather continuous. They fill time and structure the day; they emphasize socialization and commitment rather than formal training; they provide models (the old-timer, the helper); they fight relapse or regression; they diffuse and share leadership; they use their own resources of skills, the resources of the consumer; and they attempt to build a new way of life, a subculture, a community, a movement.

SELF-HELP AND THE PROFESSIONAL

Implicit in the self-help thrust is a profound critique of professionalism. Traditional professional models, whether in psychotherapy, education, or other services, are seen as outmoded for modern needs, and the traditional relationship between professionals and consumers is not only inconsistent with the participatory ethos emerging out of the sixties, but also seems to correlate with inefficient and ineffective service delivery. Self-help mutual aid groups have developed, in large measure, because of the unwillingness and inability of professional organizations to deal with these and other problems, their limited reach with regard to various populations, their overly intellectualized orientation, and their excessive credentialism. Although the entire ethos of the professional orientation is very different from the more open, inexpensive, activistic, self-help orientation, both have valuable attributes in an integrated practice—each is needed; however, most service practice has been largely professionally based. The self-help orientation provides a needed paraprofessional dimension as a dialectic balance in a practice which has become overly professionalized. This is not to reject the value of professional knowledge, system, organization, evaluation, each of which is limited in the self-help perspective; the two together could make a significant dialectic unity and a far better practice.

Mutual aid groups use much more subjective, peer, informal, gut-level approaches; disclosures are shared, and the participants are judgmental with each other. In essence, the self-help approach reflects a series of dimensions which might be termed "aprofessional." Table 14-1 demonstrates this by presenting a schematic, ideal type contrast of the professional and the aprofessional.

The aprofessional dimension is not only a powerful counterbalance to the *intrinsic* limitations of professional interventions, but it also serves to reduce some of the difficulties in professional approaches which are not intrinsic, but which are related to the way the professional functions in our society. In this case, we are referring to the elitism, the tendency to mystify, to maintain a monopoly and high cost for professional service; to be removed, particularly from low-income and rural populations; not to be sufficiently accountable and relevant to the consumer, frequently applying outmoded practices because these are the ones in which they, the professionals, have been trained. Any aprofessional approach is likely to be much more consumer-centered, immedi-

Table 14–1 Professional and Aprofessional Characteristics

Professional	*Aprofessional*
1. Emphasis on knowledge and insight, underlying principles, theory, structure	1. Emphasis on feeling
2. Systematic	2. Experimental: based on common sense, intuition and folk knowledge
3. Use of distance and perspective, self-awareness, control of "transference": objective	3. Closeness and self-involvement: subjective
4. Empathy, controlled warmth	4. Identification
5. Standardized performance	5. Extemporaneous, spontaneous performance (expressions of own personality)
6. "Outsider" orientation	6. "Insider" orientation; indigenous
7. Praxis	7. Practice
8. Careful, limited use of time, systematic evaluation, curing	8. Slow, time no issue, informal, direct accountability, caring

ately relevant, demystified, not held in an imperialistic manner, non-elite, more directly accountable to the consumer, at least in terms of direct satisfaction, and, of course, far less expensive.

Much of the professionals' training and socialization move them away from the dimensions of identification, deep concern, full involvement and caring which often derive from nearness to the client, feeling like the client in a highly direct, indigenous fashion. Actually, indigeneity, a characteristic emphasized a great deal in the sixties with the development of the paraprofessional movement, is a very important component of the aprofessional dimension. And while this indigeneity or nearness may result at times in over-identification and an impairment of perspective, it also contains a valuable component in human service practice.

One of the major dangers that the self-help movement will face in the coming decade is the fact that it may be much more closely allied with the professional and institutional structures. We have noted the positive potential in this alliance, particularly if it is to work in its best form with the unity of the aprofessional and professional modalities. But while this is a worthy ideal and worth striving toward, there is no question that there will be all manner of deviations from it, and that in many cases agencies which are led by professionals will attempt to dominate and socialize self-help groups to the existing professional norms. The self-help approach may then become an appendage of the professional structure, losing much of its spontaneity, vitality, innovativeness, small group character, and flexibility.

Not all professionals wish to do this however. It is noteworthy that Gerald Caplan's Harvard group, which has quite successfully fostered the development of the Widow Program (Silverman, 1970), has set a tone whereby the self-help groups are to be independent and are not to be controlled and modeled by the professional.

MODELS FOR THE PROFESSIONAL

There are a great variety of potential models where the professional is instrumental in self-help activity:

1. In the assertiveness training model, a professional psychologist usually trains a group of lay people to become assertive themselves, and then to train others to be equally assertive. Frequently, the women—and they are usually women—who are trained in this manner help various members of women's groups, such as consciousness-raising and support groups, to develop assertive skills. The lay trainers may return from time to time to the professionally-led group for added training. The multiplier effect of this model is fairly obvious: a small number of professionals have an effect which radiates out to many groups.

2. In the peer group rap session model there is usually one professional who trains a large number of youngsters to help each other through mutual or reciprocal counseling, which is sometimes called co-counseling. The professional adviser functions in a backup role in the rap group meetings as well as in other community and school meetings in which the youngsters help other members of the community. This model is well developed in the Woodland High School in Hartsdale (Petrillo, 1976).

3. In the youth-tutoring-youth and children-teaching-children model in education, the professional trainer or teacher plays an important role in setting up the program, training the participants, and providing general backup services and support. Nevertheless, the participants have enormous freedom to develop their own curriculum for tutoring other children, meet in their own groups, discuss their problems, and develop techniques for dealing with them (Gartner, Kohler, & Riessman, 1973).

4. In Recovery, Inc., an organization for mental patients funded in 1937 by Abraham Lowe, a medical doctor, it is stipulated that the professionals should not hold office or become leaders of Recovery, Inc. (They may and sometimes do become members.) In the course of its history, the organization has moved from what was a highly professionally supervised association during its formative years to a much more independent one without professional supervision. At first the groups were located in hospitals, but the fact that the doctors asked members to report back to them on other members' behavior during the sessions forced the groups to be moved away from the hospitals and into the community. Nevertheless, in 1970 some 33% of its members came from professional referrals, a figure which has now gone up to about 50%.

5. In Parents Anonymous (for child abusers), a professional is typically involved as backup support and is available for consultation, who is called a "sponsor."

6. In various types of social action groups, such as tenants' organizations and welfare rights groups, professional organizers have frequently played a major role in forming the groups, catalyzing them, assisting them with advice, organizational training, and skill development. Thus, it is clear that professionals, and for that matter, paraprofessionals, can play a number of roles in relation to self-help groups.

SELF-HELP AND LOW-INCOME GROUPS

Much of human service practice in the self-help area has been directed toward a middle class clientele, and it may very well be that a careful systematic analysis of the way self-help groups function might lead to suggestions for modification that would enlist and hold low-income clients. It is widely believed that the self-help mutual aid movement typically fails to attract low-income members, and that it is largely a middle class movement. Certainly, this appears to be true for many of the traditional mental health-oriented groups such as Recovery, Inc.; and historically it is probably true of Alcoholics Anonymous and most of the other "anonymous" groups. But, perhaps, a more careful analysis is needed.

Low-income groups in the United States have expressed their interest in self-help in a great variety of ways: in the Home-Town clubs of Puerto Ricans living on the mainland; in black associations and tenants' groups; in anti-crime groups and safety patrols; in groups such as the Sisterhood of Black Single Mothers and Debtors Anonymous; in organizations such as Fightback, which includes unemployed persons who rehabilitate housing for themselves and members of their community. Other mutual aid groups include the Welfare Rights groups; the veterans groups; the youth groups and gangs such as Chicago's Blackstone Rangers; the ex-offender groups such as the Fortune Society; the storefront churches; the informal, shared child care groupings; and the "rap groups." Moreover, children in low-income communities learn extremely well by teaching other children; in fact, the successful youth-tutoring-youth designs were originally developed among the poor during the 1960's anti-poverty program. Not all these examples match the more classical definitions of mutual aid, but in many cases they have much in common.

The point, of course, can be made that low-income populations seem to be drawn more to social actions in neighborhood and ethnic support groups rather than to the traditional mental health groups led by professionals. But is it true that the low-income populations do not have these other problems? Does alcoholism, for example, not prevail in low-income communities? Is drug addiction not a concern among the poor? Is hypertension and diabetes not a problem among the black community? Is mental illness a middle class phenomenon? Are there no battered wives in the ghetto? Are the families of alcoholics in low-income communities comfortable? Are there no lonely parents without partners in working class and low-income communities?

Perhaps these problems need to be met through the development of new forms and new styles of mutual aid. Thus, groups in the human service areas such as Alcoholics Anonymous might be much more effective in reaching the low-income populations if they added a social dimension and were less narrow in their appeal and function; the self-help movement could be greatly expanded if it could reach severely underserved populations by modifications of its style. The implications are enormous.

MODELS FOR THE PARAPROFESSIONAL

The neighborhood mental health paraprofessionals who have done effective work with low-income populations in outreach activities, group work, counseling, and various therapeutic interventions may be the key ingredient for reaching low-income consumers. The Queens College Mental Health Program is training paraprofessionals to assist in fostering self-help groups in low-income communities. Central to the training model is the development of group skills and knowledge in the following areas:

- Group structure
- Phases of group development
- Leadership patterns and leadership styles
- Development of group norms and sanctions
- Peer help and the helper therapy principle
- Group purpose and function
- Group task behavior and decision making
- Group conflict and agreement (handling of differences)
- Setting of limits
- Group size
- Tools of group interaction (sharing, disclosure, feedback)
- Verbal and non-verbal listening
- Group problem solving
- Instrumental versus expressive functions
- Development of self-reliance and interdependence
- Seating and use of physical space
- Use of program activity
- Role(s) of the group worker

Paraprofessional community workers are being trained to develop relationships to self-help modalities in a variety of ways. At the simplest level they may *refer* their clientele to an existing group; such as Parents Anonymous, Gambler's Anonymous, Recovery, Inc., or the Gray Panthers. If there is need for such a group in the community and none exists, the paraprofessional may (with the cooperation of the national organization) form such a group in the local area.

Paraprofessionals may also be of value in community work by developing new types of groups, such as groups of people on methadone maintenance, youth groups for young people with various problems, sewing clubs for women who are isolated and lonely, and transition groups for mental patients (and their families). These groups would probably be temporary and the paraprofessional would have the task of helping them get started and become autonomous. She/he would then phase out, lest the clients become lifelong patients.

The following are types of self-help groups that the paraprofessionals would work with: transition group for "patients" returning to the community; groups focused on auxiliary parties; groups whose target population comes to a community mental health program with other presenting problems or does not come at all; and groups whose activities are directed toward social and community problems. In the first of these groups there is a variety of transition activities, often likely to be a part of a deinstitutionalization program, and designed to be part of a spectrum of services moving persons toward greater functional autonomy. In the second of these groups, there is a focus on the needs of persons related to the individual with a problem; for example, the children of an alcoholic (Alanon) or the parents of mentally disturbed children. In the third grouping, a program might be developed for a group that shared a common condition (e.g., widowhood). These individuals may be served by a community mental health program for some other matter or may have had no previous contact with the program.

Conclusion

In essence, then, the mutual help groups combine a great variety of sociological and psychological principles involved in changing behavior. In their typical form, they are not concerned with exploring the childhood causes of problems. Their emphasis is on present behavior, in some cases on current symptoms, but most of them are concerned not only with reducing or controlling the symptoms, but also with building positive mental health, integrated human relations, honesty, and the like.

The power of self-help, mutual aid groups is related to the fact that they combine a number of very important properties: the group process, the aprofessional dimension, the use of indigeneity, and the implicit demand that the individual can do something for him or herself. The implication is that people need not be passive; they have power, particularly in groups, to demand the individual do something for him/herself and for other group members. At its best the group permits dependence while it also fosters autonomy and independence; it, furthermore, demands action and work from its members while it also gives support. The focus in this sort of group should not be on one particular leader or professional but rather should be on the peer group itself.

Note

[1]The terms "self-help groups," "mutual aid groups" and "mutual support groups" are used synonymously.

References

Gartner, A., Kohler, M., & Riessman, F. *Children teaching children.* New York: Harper & Row, 1973.

Katz, A. H., & Bender, E. I. *The strength in us: Self-help groups in the modern world.* New York: New Viewpoints, 1976.

Petrillo, R. Rap room: Self-help at school. *Social Policy,* September/October, 1976, 7(2), 54–59.

Silverman, P. R. The widow as a caregiver in a program preventive intervention with other widows. *Mental Hygiene,* October 1970, *54*(4), 542–545.

The following directory has been excerpted from a more inclusive one prepared by the staff members of the National Self-Help Clearinghouse. The directory provides a partial listing of self-help groups whose activities are relevant to the goals of mental health centers. The list has been prepared to assist persons wishing to contact self-help groups. Where possible, the Clearinghouse has provided the address of the organization's national office; most of the national offices will provide a list of their member groups. It has been the experience of the Clearinghouse staff members that people in self-help groups are very generous in sharing information and otherwise assisting others in need.

The co-directors of the Clearinghouse are Frank Riessman (the author of the preceding chapter) and Alan Gartner (the author of Chapter 4 in this source book). The Clearinghouse staff members not only assist individuals interested in self-help groups, but also publish reports, papers, a newsletter, and offer a variety of other relevant services.

The newsletter, the *Self-Help Reporter,* is of special note. Issued bimonthly, it contains original articles, notices of relevant conferences and workshops, portrayals of individual self-help groups, and descriptions of newly available materials and sources of funding.

Materials and information can be obtained by contacting: The National Self-Help Clearinghouse, 184 Fifth Avenue, New York, New York 10010.

Self-Help Groups Relevant to Mental Health

Abused Women's Aid in Crisis
GPO Box 1699
New York, New York 10010

Addicts Anonymous
Box 2000
Lexington, Kentucky 41991

Alanon
P.O. Box 182
Madison Square Station
New York, New York 10010

Alateen
200 Park Avenue South
New York, New York 10003

Alcoholics Anonymous
AA World Services
P.O. Box 459
Grand Central Station
New York, New York 10017

American Schizophrenia Association
Huxley Institute
114 First Avenue
New York, New York 10021

Association for Children with Learning
Disabilities
5225 Grace Street
Pittsburgh, Pennsylvania 15236

Association for Children with Retarded
Mental Development
902 Broadway
New York, New York 10010

The Bridge, Inc.
231 West 83rd Street
New York, New York 10024

Buxom Belles International
20515 Westover
Southfield, Michigan 48075

Center for Independent Living
2539 Telegraph Avenue
Berkeley, California 94704

Checks Anonymous
Box 81248
Lincoln, Nebraska 68501

Congress of People with Disabilities
170 Broadway
New York, New York 10038

Delancey Street
3001 Pacific Street
San Francisco, California

Diet Workshop
28 Merrick Avenue
Merrick, New York 11566

Divorce Anonymous
P.O. Box 5313
Chicago, Illinois 60680

Drop-Outs Anonymous
3876 East Fedora Avenue
Fresno, California 93726

Emotional Health Anonymous
4328 Cumnor Road
Downers Grove, Illinois

Emotions Anonymous
P.O. Box 4245
St. Paul, Minnesota 55104

The Fortune Society
29 East 22nd Street
New York, New York 10010

Gamblers Anonymous
P.O. Box 17173
Los Angeles, California 90017

Gam-Anon
P.O. Box 4549
Downey, California 90241

Gray Panthers
3700 Chestnut Street
Philadelphia, Pennsylvania

Help
2310 Locust Street
Philadelphia, Pennsylvania 19103

Human Growth Foundation
28 Sylvia Lane
Plainview, New York 11803

Institute for Rational Living
710 Magnolia Drive
Clearwater, Florida

International Parents' Organization
c/o Alexander Graham Bell Association
  for the Deaf
1537 35th Street, N.W.
Washington, D.C. 20007

La Leche League
9616 Minneapolis Avenue
Franklin Park, Illinois 60131

Mothers of Young Mongoloids
713 Ramsey Street
Alexandria, Virginia 22301

Nar-Anon Family Group
P.O. Box 2562
Palos Verdes Peninsula, California 90274

Narcotics Anonymous
P.O. Box 622
Sun Valley, California 91352

National Association for Autistic Children
169 Tampa Avenue
Albany, New York 12208

National Association for Down's Syndrome
628 Ashland
River Forest, Illinois 60305

National Association for Gifted Children
8080 Springvalley Drive
Cincinnati, Ohio 45236

National Association for Help of Retarded Children
405 Lexington Avenue
New York, New York 10017

National Association for Retarded Children
2709 Avenue E, East
Arlington, Texas 76011

National Committee for the Prevention of Alcoholism
6830 Laurel Street, N.W.
Washington, D.C. 20012

National Association of Recovered Alcoholics in the Professions (NARAP)
P.O. Box 95
Staten Island, New York 10305

National Association to Aid Fat Americans
P.O. Box 745
Westbury, New York 11590

National Congress of Organizations of the Physically Handicapped
7611 Oakland Avenue
Minneapolis, Minnesota 55423

National Foundation for Sudden Infant Death
1501 Broadway
New York, New York 10036

National Society for Autistic Children
c/o Ruth Dyer
169 Tampa Avenue
Albany, New York 12208

Neurotics Anonymous International Liaison
Room 426
1341 G Street, N.W.
Washington, D.C. 20005

Overeaters Anonymous
2365 Westwood Boulevard
Los Angeles, California 90064

Parents Anonymous
2810 Artesia Boulevard
Redondo Beach, California 90278

Parents of Large Families
54 Miller Street
Fairfield, Connecticut 06430

Parents United
840 Guadelupe Parkway
San Jose, California 95110

Parents Without Partners
7910 Woodmont Avenue
Washington, D.C. 20014

Phobia Self-Help Groups
White Plains Hospital
41 East Post Road
White Plains, New York 10601

Prison Children Anonymous
129 Jackson Street
Hempstead, New York 11550

Prison Families Anonymous
134 Jackson Street, LL4
Hempstead, New York 11550

Project Release
202 Riverside Drive, #4E
New York, New York 10025

Recovery, Inc.
116 South Michigan Avenue
Chicago, Illinois 60603

Retarded Infants Service
386 Park Avenue, South
New York, New York 10016

Schizophrenics Anonymous
1114 First Avenue
New York, New York 10021

Self-Help Social Clubs
American Conference of Therapeutic Self-Help
Windridge Farm
West Genesee Turnpike
Elbridge, New York 13060

SHARE Community Limited
Self-Help and Rehabilitation Employment
170 Kingston Road
Merton Park
Wimbledon, London SW19 3NX, United Kingdom

Self-Help Enterprises
220 South Bridge Street
Visalia, California 93277

Sisterhood of Black Single Mothers
P.O. Box 155
Brooklyn, New York 11203

South County Help Phone, Inc.
P.O. Box 582
Great Barrington, Massachusetts 01230

Sudden Infant Death Syndrome Foundation
310 South Michigan Avenue
Chicago, Illinois 60604

Synanon
P.O. Box 786
Marshall, California

Take Off Pounds Sensibly
4575 South Fifth Street
Milwaukee, Wisconsin 53207

Weight Watchers
175 East Shore Road
Great Neck, New York 11023

Widowed Inc.
1406 Spring Rock
Houston, Texas 77055

Widow-To-Widow
c/o Laboratory of Community Psychiatry
Harvard Medical School
Cambridge, Massachusetts

Index